MODERN RETINAL LASER THERAPY:
PRICIPLES AND APPLICATION

Modern Retinal Laser Therapy: Principles and Application

Jeffrey K. Luttrull, MD

Ventura County Retina Vitreous Medical Group, Ventura, California

Founder of LIGHT: The International Retinal Laser Society

Medical Director, Vision Protection Institutes

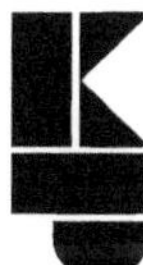

Kugler Publications/Amsterdam/The Netherlands

Jeffrey K. Luttrull's Financial Disclosures:
Ojai Retinal Technologies, LLC: Management, equity
Retinal Protection Sciences. LLC: Management, equity
Vision Protection Institutes, LLC: Management, equity
SDM™ and Vision Protection Therapy™ are registered trademarks of Ojai Retinal Technologies, LLC

ISBN 978-90-6299-942-2

Kugler Publications
P.O. Box 20538
1001 NM Amsterdam, The Netherlands
www.kuglerpublications.com

Kugler Publications is an imprint of SPB Academic Publishing bv, P.O. Box 20538, 1001 NM Amsterdam, The Netherlands

Table of Contents

Common Abbreviations and Definitions

CW
: Continuous wave. Laser applied in a constant and uniform release and application of energy throughout the duration of exposure. CW is the fundamental laser mode used for conventional RPC treatment, although visible wavelength and high-duty cycle microsecond pulsed laser can produce identical effects.

DC
: Duty cycle / pulse frequency. Periodicity of pulses within a train of pulses.

MPL
: Microsecond pulsed laser. Pulsed laser applied in a fixed periodicity using pulse lengths long enough to allow intracellular heat dissipation to preclude melanin vaporization and cavitation, but short enough to preclude heat spread outside the area directly exposed to the laser. While SDM refers to a specific subtype of MPL designed to accomplish the goals of MRT (effective, maximized/optimized, and safe as reliably sublethal to the RPE), MPL is non-specific with respect to effects of treatment, with effects varying widely. MPL effects may range from MRT to suprathreshold retinal photocoagulation depending upon the laser parameters for MPL employed.

MRT
: Modern retinal laser therapy. The concept and execution of applying uniform laser thermal photostimulation reliably sublethal to the RPE to activate a restorative response, then clinically maximizing this response by confluent treatment of large geographic areas of the retina to achieve *en masse* recruitment and transformation of dysfunctional retina.

RPC
: Retinal photocoagulation. Thermal laser damage to the retinal pigment epithelium (RPE), typically intentional, which extends in varying degrees upward into the overlying neurosensory retina (NSR), ranging from clinically inapparent damage to the photoreceptors to clinically visible full-thickness NSR coagulation extending to the internal limiting membrane, depending on the intensity of the laser application. RPC generally also results in similar damage to the choriocapillaris and choroid underlying the RPE, accentuated by significant thermal absorption by choroidal melanin.

SDM
: Low-intensity / high-density subthreshold diode microsecond pulsed laser. The technique of MRT and particular and specific use of microsecond pulsed laser. The archetype of MRT.

Subthreshold
: A retinal laser spot or application that is less visible. Requires qualification with the means of observation to have other than a purely subjective meaning. Ranges from no retinal damage to outer RPC.

Suprathreshold
: A retinal spot or application that is easily visible/prominent. Gray to while full-thickness RPC burn visible by any means, including biomicroscopy.

Threshold
: A retinal laser spot or application that is generally visible. Requires qualification with the means of observation to have other than a purely subjective meaning. Ranges from outer retinal to full-thickness RPC.

VPT
: Vision protection therapy. Regular periodic SDM MRT performed to maintain maximum treatment benefits over time.

For Caesar

All of the clinical applications described below were performed with a laser with an FDA approved IFU (Indications for Use) that includes diabetic retinopathy, diabetic macular edema, retinal vein occlusion, central serous chorioretinopathy, various forms of macular edema, dry (grid) and wet (focal) age-related macular degeneration. Thus, the vast majority of the clinical applications discussed in this text are "on label." "Off label" treatments, identical to those "on label," were offered to patients with different diagnoses in light of well-established treatment safety and a reasonable expectation of treatment benefit. In all cases, where standard of care treatments were available, such as AREDS supplements and anti-VEGF injections, MRT was employed to complement, not replace, the standard of care. In every case, MRT was offered or recommended in the practice of medicine as being in the best interest of the patient according to the treating physician's best clinical judgment.

Testimonials

"This book is a masterpiece compendium of novel ideas on technology that we have been using so long. In it, the pioneer in the field walks us through his experience in opening new applications for modern retina laser therapy. The book demonstrates what we did wrong and what we can do better in the future. A true guide for every forward-thinking retina specialist."

Igor Kozak, MD, PhD
Moorfields Eye Hospital
Abu Dhabi, UAE

I was initially very skeptical of the concept of SDM laser (MRT) for chronic macular diseases. Having now implemented these procedures in my practice for 2 years and seen first-hand the clear benefit they offer to patients, I can confidently recommend this monograph to anyone looking for a way to help their patients with retinal pathology. The concepts presented here are an example of innovative thinking with protection of patients as the highest priority. The scientific arguments made are interesting and compelling. The real-world results of implementing these concepts have demonstrated to me that this is the right thing to do for patients.

Thomas Myers, MD
Riverwood Eye Clinic
Provo, Utah

This book represents the masterpiece of the long-standing Jeff's clinical and research dedication and experience to micropulse laser treatment of different retinal disorders. It's definitely not "an ordinary" scientific text. I am sure that any reader can find it curious and inspiring, even if not always in agreement.
I congratulate Jeff for this extraordinary work!

Stela Vujosevic, MD, PhD, FEBO
University Eye Clinic San Giuseppe Hospital Milan

I have been using SDM laser (MRT) for years and I continue to be positively impressed by it. Currently, I only use continuous wave laser for retinal tears. Diabetic retinopathy used to be managed by photocoagulation and vitrectomy. Now I find that SDM laser and anti-VEGF can control most cases. For age-related macular degeneration, I use SDM to help delay conversion to exudative macular degeneration. Also, it helps to enable longer intervals between anti-VEGF injections for those who convert. This book is a wide-ranging treatise by one of its pioneers. It gives the history, including the author's first experience with it in 2000. It explains how it works and is safe even for use across the fovea. It gives results from published articles detailing years of experience. I would recommend it for anyone involved with conditions of the retina.

Kenneth R. Diddie, MD
Westlake, California

This book may accelerate the sunset of traditional *visible-threshold* laser photocoagulation, and may disprove many mechanisms of action theorized to rationalize indications and outcomes validated by landmark trials such as the Diabetic Retinopathy Study (DRS), the Early Treatment of Diabetic Retinopathy Study (ETDRS), the Macular Photocoagulation Study (MPS) and many other. Modern laser therapy is the evolution from *tissue destroying threshold* laser photocoagulation, which is mostly benefitting patients in clinically significant conditions and should be replaced by *nondamaging subthreshold* laser photostimulation for the therapy of patients at earlier stages of progressive degenerative retinovascular disorders. With his remarkable pioneering work, Jeffrey Luttrull has been the most valuable prophet to prompt the historical paradigm shift from *traditional threshold laser photocoagulation* to modern subthreshold laser photostimulation. Conventional threshold laser photocoagulation should not be used any longer in the treatment of *retinovascular and progressive degenerative disorders* and should be confined to the treatment of structural retinal disorders requiring strong chorioretinal adhesions.

Giorgio Dorin
Cupertino, California

Jeffrey K. Luttrull, MD, has given us *Modern Retinal Laser Therapy: Principles and Applications*. With 108 figures, hundreds of color images, and 13 tables, *Modern Retinal Laser Therapy: Principles and Applications* is a comprehensive book full of concepts that look at laser photocoagulation in a new more modern way that will appeal to the retina specialists. The development of low-intensity/high-density subthreshold diode micropulse photocoagulation has eliminated laser-induced retinal damage (LIRD). Elimination of LIRD as a necessity for effective therapy has basically eliminated adverse events, and has allowed new, more effective/safer treatment techniques, improved outcomes, and the understanding of the therapeutic mechanisms of retinal laser, and new treatment applications.

J. Fernando Arevalo, MD PhD
Professor of Ophthalmology
Wilmer Institute, Johns Hopkins University
Baltimore, MD

The methods for the detection, monitoring, and treatment of retinal diseases, now a major cause of vision loss worldwide, have changed dramatically from the severely destructive laser photocoagulation of the retina inaugurated with the DRS through the advent of repetitive intravitreal injection trials, all aimed at the severe, end-stages of neovascularization and edema. More recently the progressive course of neuronal apoptosis and microvascular injury and occlusion, occurring in multiple retinal layers, has demanded the application of new imaging and functional testing along with less invasive treatment methods that can stop the progressive injury and reverse the vision loss within earlier stages of the disease progression. Since 2000, the healing algorithms of contiguous laser, non-damaging, RPE thermal stimulation have been proven to accomplish this, demonstrating significant prevention of the progression and reversal of the functional loss, agnostic of the cause, whether glaucoma, diabetic retinopathy, vascular occlusion, uveitis, or AMD. Dr. Luttrull has been a leader in the demonstration of the benefits of this laser therapy, and this book represents a compilation of the necessary introduction and application of treatment. It should be read by all ophthalmologists and optometrists as it will become a mainstream of patient ocular care.

Stephen H. Sinclair, MD
Former Chairman of Ophthalmology
Drexel University School of Medicine
CEO Sinclair Technologies, Salt Lake City, Utah

Jeffrey K. Luttrull has written an excellent book covering modern contemporary approach to laser treatment of the retina. *Modern Retinal Laser Therapy* not only provides the knowledge on the principles of action and clinical application of non-damaging laser techniques but also gives us an individual view on the subject—the aspect frequently omitted in scientific publications. One might not agree with all the thesis presented by the author, but cannot ignore the consequence, logic, and scientific background in presenting controversial subjects.

The book is written with literary passion and as such enormously engaging and engrossing, like traveling in a sports car. Take it in your hand, fasten your seatbelt and enjoy the ride.

Maciej Gaweki, MD, PhD
Head of Department
Specialist Hospital in Chojnice,
Dobry Wzrok Ophthalmological Clinic in Gdansk Poland

Dr. Luttrull has succeeded where many others have not by making a complex medical topic both readable and interesting for both practitioner and public alike. If MRT achieves its potential as outlined in this book, it will have most significant impact on the treatment of blinding retinal disease since the advent of anti-VEGF therapy.

Matthew Ward, MD
Riverwoods Eye Clinic
Provo, Utah

Getting to know the author personally in 2011 and following his published papers and congress talks since then, it's with great pleasure that I agreed to write some words about *Modern Retinal Laser Therapy*, a book that summarizes 22 years of history with this fascinating retinal treatment. In this book, written in pleasant language and filled with witty quotes and philosophical analogies, Dr. Luttrull provides the reader with evidence-based data (when available) and interesting logical deductions. It should be an insightful read for even the most skeptical minds. Dr. Luttrull achieves in *Modern Retinal Laser Therapy* an amazing feat. The preface already sets the tone for an unconventional read, one that will challenge the reader's preconceived concepts and background about current retinal physiopathology and treatment. As the author points out, the subthreshold laser treatment, done properly (and here lies its main barrier for a broader acceptance and popularity among retinologists), really works and is harmless. This is why we needed this book to help spread the word even further.

Renato M. Passos, MD, PhD
Departamento de Oftalmologia, Universidade Federal de São Paulo.

Thank you to Dr. Luttrull for this comprehensive overview from one of the most experienced key opinion leaders in retinal laser technology and treatment approaches. This compendium will serve as a great guide for beginners and seasoned retina specialists alike. Most importantly, our patients will benefit from the use of these technologies and techniques in our complex world of pathology.

Veeral S. Sheth, MD, MBA, FASRS, FACS
Clinical Assistant Professor of Ophthalmology
University of Illinois at Chicago

Jeffrey K. Luttrull, MD, is not only a very experienced and excellent ophthalmic surgeon, he is also worldwide recognized as *the* pioneer in modern restorative retinal laser therapy.

In the era of intravitreal anti-vascular endothelial growth factor (VEGF) injections, conventional retinal laser surgery lost ground because of its destructive nature with visible retinal burns inducing permanent scotomas. As a result, new non-damaging laser therapy modalities emerged since 2005 as a safe and tissue-sparing solution for the treatment of retinal diseases and glaucoma. Micropulse laser setting algorithms limitate the transmission of thermal energy, preventing the formation of visible laser burns and scotomas. Its advantages include the ability to apply treatment near the fovea as well as treating the same retinal area multiple times. In many peer-reviewed scientific papers and many presentations during international ophthalmology conferences, Dr. Luttrull demonstrated the clinical efficacy and safety of the micropulse laser modality in the treatment of various retinal vascular diseases.

I strongly recommend ophthalmic surgeons with an interest in restorative retinal laser therapy to read Dr. Luttrull's monograph *Modern Retinal Laser Therapy*.

Jan E. E. Keunen, MD, PhD, EBOD
Em. Professor of Ophthalmology
Radboud University Medical Center, Nijmegen, The Netherlands
Member of the Senate of the Dutch Parliament, The Hague, The Netherlands

As a general ophthalmologist, cornea specialist with an interest in retina, I have been using SDM (MRT) since 2018. I find the procedure effective with an excellent safety profile. A wealth of practical knowledge can be found in *Modern Retinal Laser Therapy*. This book should be on every ophthalmologist's desk for quick reference.

K. Alex Dastgheib, MD
Garden Grove, California

Ophthalmology adopted laser therapy in the second half of the twentieth century and gradually became more sophisticated in terms of wavelength, setting, and clinical application. But generally speaking, conventional laser treatment has not evolved a great deal so far, except for photodynamic therapy and subthreshold laser applications. This is why the laser approaches described by Dr. Luttrull in *Modern Retina Laser Therapy* are absolutely revolutionary. Dr. Luttrull shows that he is a true pioneer in the field of retina laser therapy, thoroughly exploring innovative concepts and demonstrating how laser therapy can be applied in many fields previously considered out of reach in common clinical practice. All ophthalmologists who are fans of laser therapy will enjoy reading this exceptional book.

Maurizio Battaglia-Parodi, MD, PhD
Associate Professor Department of Ophthalmology, Vita-Salute San Raffaele University, Ospedale San Raffaele, Milan, Italy

The book *Modern Retinal Laser Therapy* presents many years of fundamental research on the interaction between laser radiation and ocular tissues. The entire history of thermal exposure to the eye evolves from uncontrolled cryotherapy through light coagulation of tissues to gentle subthreshold infrared exposure. This work … calls for sparing our patients and looks to the future for many years to come. I recommend this book to anyone who is planning to practice ophthalmology.

Dr. Andrii Korol, MD, PhD, DMedSc, Head of Laser Division, The Filatov Institute of Eye Diseases and Tissue Therapy of the NAMS of Ukraine

Dedications

Thanks to God for blessing me with this work; to my wife Christina, the love of my life and the best and most remarkable person I have ever known, my deepest gratitude and appreciation; to my patients, who put their trust in me; to Victor L. Heasley, PhD, Professor of Chemistry, teacher, mentor, and friend of 47 years, who looked at a surly long-haired trumpet-playing surfer with no interest in chemistry standing in the hallway one day in 1975 and inexplicably saw a researcher; and to Harry T. Carneal. If *Modern Retinal Laser Therapy* ever achieves its potential to reduce human suffering in the world, it will be in no small part due to the belief, vision, steadfast commitment, experience, and tireless work of Harry.

For Emily, Miles, and James

Foreword

"*Modern Retinal Laser Therapy: Principles and Applications* represents" the last of scientific series on the most advanced approach to laser treatment of retinal diseases today. Written by the pioneer in the field, it describes the philosophy of the novel treatment from its conception through clinical testing and trails up to the current scientific knowledge. This memorable and triumphal journey has started with the creation of the idea to use nondamaging laser power to launch reparable processes in the human retina. This was in diametric contrast to philosophy of using predominantly destructive laser photocoagulation techniques, which eliminate diseased tissue only in hope to improve natural history of the disease. The novel concept was followed by establishing physical theory by the author and observing a biochemical evidence of retinal repair mechanisms by other groups. Clinical observations on countless number of patients have solidified the theory attesting to the effects of nondestructive and reparative stimulating therapy. The elegance of this approach is that retinal repair is agnostic to initial retinal process leading to damage and is, therefore, applicable for use in various retinal conditions irrespective of their origin.

All of these are presented to the reader in a breathtaking writing style of an ophthalmologist, pioneer, and a philosopher who paved the way to the modern retinal laser therapy. The book also serves to remind physicians how to fight barriers associated with resistance to novelty in science, medicine, and society posed by established authorities. Prior lack of acceptance was also attributable to imperfect assessment of certain qualities of vision following the treatments. With novel technologies to detect subtle vision changes, we are likely to be able to assess more precisely the effects of this therapy on human retina. As such, the author has seen the potential of this new therapy approach that was invisible to others. He is also showing us how impactful ideas are created and nurtured to grow into new therapies to help people.

Apart from the author, the accolades belong also to all the people who helped to investigate various aspects of modern retinal laser therapy such as physical principles, basic laser tissue interaction, imaging outcomes, and clinical data. Their work has supported and corroborated as proof of concept the visionary idea of the author, which has now converted into recognized treatment for retinal diseases. The author has shown us how much we did not know about retinal lasers. For all these reasons, this book deserves utmost attention by ophthalmologists in all fields of our specialty.

Igor Kozak, MD, PhD, MAS
Consultant Ophthalmologist and Clinical Lead
Moorfields Eye Hospital
Abu Dhabi, United Arab Emirates

Foreword

The word "laser" often invokes thoughts of advanced innovative futuristic technology regardless of whether it is used in the context of medical treatments or in fighting space aliens above the stars. In the field of ophthalmology, it has been used now for over 60 years. In fact, one of its first medical uses was in photocoagulation of the retina. Yet, over the last decade and with the advent of intravitreal injection, it has seemingly slowly fallen out of favor in the retinal field. The reasons for this are largely two-fold. First, positive therapeutic effects of intravitreal injectable agents are typically quicker than the effect of a laser treatment. Second, retinal laser has historically been and continues to be damaging to the retinal tissue. That is, until now.

After graduating from medical school, I first entered a residency in diagnostic radiology, with a specific interest in interventional radiology. I was attracted to the minimally invasive and minimally damaging aspect of this field when compared with traditional open surgical approaches to many problems. However, ophthalmology had always been in the back of my mind and I had always admired it as being a delicate field treating a very delicate part of the body. My draw to the field ultimately overcame my interest in radiology, and I was able to transfer to a residency program in ophthalmology after completing a year of a radiology residency.

My first decade of practice in ophthalmology was a traditional ascent of any young physician—a careful and conscientious doctor who executed as best as he could everything that was taught to him in all his prior years of training. I was very much a "by the book" conservative type of practitioner. I was excited and rewarded by the ability to help people while minimizing harm and adverse advents. In my second decade of practice, some of that perspective began to change.

Specifically, I began to question our approach to traditional, damaging, thermal laser photocoagulation. I wondered why such an advanced and innovative part of the medical field still considered a treatment that literally irreversibly burned tissue away acceptable. I cringed as I created large burn marks in the retinal periphery of a patient who need panretinal photocoagulation. But I did it. It was what I was taught and what was deemed to be correct. As intravitreal injection began to dominate my practice more and more, I admired the quick results it would generate in a reasonably safe procedure. However, the displeasure of monthly needle sticking weighed on both my patients' and my own mind. It was when I began to think more about laser. Laser was still less invasive and typically more comfortable to the patient. But why did it always have to be damaging? Why did I have to leave burn marks behind? Surely laser was a more advanced technology than this I thought. Space aliens used it. There had to be a way.

My first introduction to Dr. Jeffrey Luttrull was by way of his article in a 2014 issue of the journal *Retina*, entitled "Safety of Transfoveal Subthreshold Diode Micropulse Laser for Intra-foveal Diabetic Macular Edema in Eyes With Good Visual Acuity." Surely this could not be true. Safe transfoveal laser application in a patient with good visual acuity never crossed my mind. It was not what I was taught. I didn't dare to do it. I was skeptical. But those three words stuck in my mind and stayed with me: *safety, transfoveal*, and *good*—three words that should not go together, like oil and water. I continued to read his work over the years. It was ground breaking. It challenged the field. It should change everything. But why was that not happening? Why did none of my colleagues know about it? Surely it was because it was too good to be true, or some sort of gimmick. I continued to be skeptical. But as I read, and as I followed, and as I learned and educated myself on how it really all worked, that was slowly changing.

It was just at this opportune and somewhat disillusioned crossroads of my now mid-career in vitreoretinal disease that I stumbled upon Dr. Jeffrey Luttrull. I had been practicing in the Los Angeles and San Diego area, and I saw an ad to join his practice. I felt lucky to be both in the vicinity and to be fairly well-versed in the work that he had been doing, so I contacted him. I told myself to remain both objective and open minded. I got the opportunity to talk to him at length and see him at work firsthand with his patients in his office. I was impressed with what I saw. Happy smiling patients that were seeing well. Diabetic patients that were astonishingly stable long term with no visible laser scars and minimal continued intervention. Long-term dry macular degeneration patients that had been seeing him for over 20 years with no visible signs of decay. Wet macular degeneration patients that remained stable despite needing needle sticking at a dramatically decreased frequency that I certainly was accustomed to. Central serous retinopathy patients that were actually being healed and doing well.

I had to be a part of this. I just had to.

On top of all of this, I found Dr. Luttrull to be the quintessential package when it comes to my vision of the ideal doctor. A brilliant mind. A questioning scientist. A calm demeanor. Universally loved and trusted by his patients and his family. An innovator who first and foremost does no harm and is still a traditionalist when it comes to what a doctor should be doing for his patient. An old school with just the right mix of new school. An incarnation of the Hippocratic Oath itself. I trusted him. I trusted myself. I trusted what I was seeing. I was going to be a part of this.

It is here that I present to you the book ***Modern Retinal Laser Therapy.*** I invite you to read it with an inquisitive and open mind as I have. I invite you to trust yourself in your judgment. I invite you to explore a specialty-changing and ground-breaking approach and technology. I invite you to the future.

Sathy V. Bhavan, MD
Vision Protection Institutes
Ventura, CA

Preface

Times are bad. Children no longer obey their parents, and everyone is writing a book.

—Marcus Tullius Cicero

I want to thank you for reading this book. You could be doing almost anything else. If nothing else, this represents a triumph of curiosity over skepticism, a good thing. While we love the affirmation we get from agreement, we learn nothing from it. Thus, it is my hope you will find much in this book disturbing. Progress requires replacing old ideas and practices with new ones. For this to happen, we need to question our ideas and opinions. This is often uncomfortable, at best. As said by more than one ancient Greek and many others since, the more deeply held our ideas, the more important it is to examine them. When you find things in this book upsetting, I hope that your notions have been challenged, and not that I have written drivel. Medical books are usually encyclopedic compendia of consensus. Confirmatory by nature, medical books seldom if ever contain information new to readers. Not this one. Most contemporary readers will find the ideas in this book foreign and controversial. If I am right, later readers will wonder what the fuss was about.

Any reservations and criticisms you may have about the author himself are justified and widely held, as a recent email from a prospective patient attests: "I've spoken to my retina specialist about (SDM), naturally he knew nothing about you. He looked up Dr Luttrull and commented to me that 'if this was real Dr Luttrull would have a professorship at a large university and not be in private practice in a small town like Ventura.'" (Email from CB, August 14, 2022) Thus, you are not alone in your apprehensions. The author's provenance is unimpressive. He has not held or sought any academic position. His experience is mostly unique, and thus his thoughts and conclusions are largely eccentric and mostly unknown to others, let alone tested or shared by them. He belongs to no select clubs. He is in solo private practice in a small town fully engaged in caring for patients. He has no laboratory and no fellows. He has done no randomized clinical trials. The list goes on. However, the author has spent more time thinking about, doing, and exploring clinical retinal laser treatment than anyone in decades, and possibly ever. His bibliography, unique for a solo physician outside academia, documents his journey, and forms the basis for this book.

As noted in the text, you have to do something different to learn anything new. Doing anything different is increasingly rare in our field. The pressure to conform increases daily and the resultant "homogeneity" of practice is hailed as progress rather than the intellectual desertification that it represents, a Faustian assignment of doctors' individual intellects and consciences to institutions, organizations, companies, and for-hire "thought leaders" (Moynihan 2008, Cimberle 2021). This is bad in itself, and a bad thing if medicine is to advance and progress and this progress is to be made via discovery. Homogeneity of thought and practice meets the classic operational definition of insanity, that of (everyone) doing the same things for the same reasons while hoping for a different result—the different thing in this case being learning something new. While solo practice has certain disadvantages, it does facilitate independent thinking. Isolation attenuates the influence of the typically coercive group-think that tends to dominate small groups (the retina specialty is a small group). The author did not choose an affair with retinal laser treatment simply to be different. He had no unusual interest in laser at all. However, at the age of 44 and well into a typical clinical career, retinal laser treatment chose him. A mystery unexpectedly presented itself that piqued his curiosity and demanded an explanation. Understanding this mystery required the persistence of following one thread to the next to the next, and so on, resulting in a clinical career unlike any other. Different things were done. New things were learned. The purpose of this book is to share those lessons with you.

People tend to dismiss observations that do not fit in with their preconceptions. When this happens in science, as it frequently does, belief upstages data and the objectively open mind and science is replaced by religion. The god of this religion against which science contends is the status quo and the perceived wisdom. The struggle between data and dogmatic disbelief and the power of intellectual inertia has characterized the history of the development of Modern Retinal Laser Therapy. Indeed, inertia can be defined as "the inhibition of progress by a dead weight." In science, that dead weight is belief based on convention and authority.

What we have learned from the development of Modern Retinal Laser Therapy has been predicated by the conviction that there are good reasons for the way things are, and thus we have hope of making sense of them. If we do not understand something we observe, we do not simply pass it off as being random incomprehensible nonsense, the pointless product of an accidental and meaningless universe; instead, we realize that all things in nature have a purpose that we simply have yet to appreciate, and that this purpose can be apprehended by reason and investigation. Thus, at times the thinking that leads to our current understanding of the "reset" mechanism of retinal laser action came down to simple anthropomorphic projections such as: "If I was the RPE, what would I do?" Or "If you wanted to design a system to do such-and-such, how would it work?" Such thinking, directed to attempting to understand the underlying wisdom of the processes observed, did not disappoint.

Proof belongs to mathematics and theology. Everything else is probability and uncertainty. Modern Retinal Laser Therapy is neither math nor theology. However, dots can be connected, impressions recorded, observations made, data collected, and within reason, at least tentative conclusions drawn. Modern Retinal Laser Therapy is informed by 22 years of immersion and work in retinal laser therapy. Those 22 years (thus far) represent a professional lifetime, which is not nothing. But compared to the time and number of minds it generally takes to understand even the simplest bit of nature, it is uncomfortably close to nothing. It is hoped that the reader will find the observations based on these years of experience, investigation, and accrued data interesting and useful. *Modern Retinal Laser Therapy* is the report of a journey, not an arrival. The journey is not yet over.

It is important to keep in mind that, fundamental to all that is described in this book, is the fact that SDM, the basis and epitome of MRT is, properly done, harmless—at worst. This is the bedrock for all else, and the main point of separation from everything that went before. Such a level of safety allows consideration and application of MRT wherever existing treatments are nonexistent, poorly effective, or onerous. That is a lot of potential applications. Thus, wherever SDM has been employed it has been safer for the patient than any existing alternative treatment. Where no alternative has existed, failure to act would have allowed the natural history of disease lead to visual loss, while failure of SDM would have resulted in no harm or disadvantage or prohibit any subsequent intervention of any kind. So, why not try? And at every step along the way, Modern Retinal Laser Therapy has exceeded every expectation.

It is my firm belief that Modern Retinal Laser Therapy is the most important development in modern ophthalmology, surpassing even the importance of anti-VEGF medications by virtue of its potential for prevention of all of the most common causes of irreversible visual loss—the chronic progressive retinopathies, as well as the exceptionally wide range of potential treatment indications. Once you stop laughing, consider that nothing described in the Clinical Applications section of this book would have been believed or predicted by anyone not so long ago. So, if you are willing to read on, there is a chance you might conclude my assessment of MRT is not as hyperbolic as it sounds.

Few technologies survive the passage of time. This is good because they are usually displaced by better ones. The anachronism of retinal photocoagulation and current dominance of intravitreal drug injections are presented throughout the following discussion as the main current alternatives to Modern Retinal Laser Therapy. This will change. Eventually, retinal photocoagulation will draw its final breath and be gone. Intravitreal drug injections will also be a thing of the past, sooner than we might think. What does this mean for Modern Retinal Laser Therapy? Almost certainly, a more prominent role. Modern Retinal Laser Therapy will not be defined in relation to its current alternatives. Because Modern Retinal Laser Therapy is harmless, no future treatment will be safer. At the same time, the results of Modern Retinal Laser Therapy are sufficiently robust that the likelihood of another treatment, drug or otherwise, being as effective while also being as safe, are virtually nil. Expect Modern Retinal Laser Therapy to not only survive, but thrive, well into the future.

Jeffrey K. Luttrull, MD
Ventura, California

Modern Retinal Laser Therapy

Overview and summary

1. Modern Retinal Laser Therapy (MRT) is defined by low-intensity direct thermal laser photostimulation of the retinal pigment epithelium (RPE) that is always sublethal to the RPE, exceeds the reset activation of RPE heat shock proteins, is far below the cellular damage threshold; and high-density treatment application over large areas of retina to maximize the clinical effects.
2. The effect of MRT is to improve and normalize retinal function, usually constituting reversal of the disease process. The ability of MRT to improve retinal function is largely independent of the nature of the disease process. MRT is neuroprotective, neuroenhancing, and may be neuroregenerative.
3. Reflecting on these points, there are no adverse treatment effects from MRT.
4. The most important treatment indications for MRT are the chronic progressive retinopathies. These disorders require regular periodic MRT to maintain maximum treatment benefits over time. *Vision protection therapy* has been coined to describe this strategy.
5. MRT is the most useful and widely applicable treatment yet developed in ophthalmology, and the first to be well suited to preventive treatment.

Section I. Principles of Modern Retinal Laser Therapy

The best physician is also a philosopher

—Claudius Galenus

1. Modern Retinal Laser Therapy

The most incomprehensible thing about the world is that it is at all comprehensible.

—Albert Einstein

Modern?

The limits of my language mean the limits of my world.
—Ludwig Wittgenstein

In what sense is "modern" retinal laser therapy "modern"? (Kozak and Luttrull 2015). Like the other one million words in the English language, "modern" has several meanings. Two are most relevant here. Both imply a departure from a less auspicious past in favor of a better, more promising present and future. In the first usage, "modern" refers to what is fashionable, popular; *au courant.* In the second, "modern" implies a past based on tradition, authority, and dogma; supplanted by a new era based on fact, evidence, realism, and reason (Oxford English Dictionary [OED] 1989).

To which "modern" are we referring to when we say, "modern retinal laser"? Despite decades of uniformly positive clinical and laboratory evidence, the precepts and clinical application of modern retinal laser therapy (MRT) remain widely unknown and poorly understood. One needs to look no further than the 21st annual edition of American Society of Retina Specialists *Preferences And Trends* survey, which has never in its history considered anything resembling MRT as a treatment option for any disorder in any clinical setting, despite the fact that retinal laser treatment remains indispensable, and "subthreshold" approaches—the precursor of MRT—now predominate in clinical use (Luttrull and Dorin 2012, Chhablani et al 2018, ASRS 2021). The future has a complicated relationship with the present and the past. While often seen as idyllic and perfect, it is also strange and suspect. Louis Armstrong famously hated bebop. About Dizzy Gillespie he is said to have opined, "I couldn't play that many wrong notes if I tried." And that was before Miles Davis. Despite ample evidence, assertion of MRT principles inflames passions in those still conventionally and traditionally minded (Bataglia Parodi and Iacono 2019, Keunen et al 2020, Van Rijssen et al 2020, Luttrull AJ 2020). Therefore, we cannot mean "modern" in the first sense. Thus, modern retinal laser can only mean that which represents progress based on the transcendence of evidence and new information over tradition. It also implies that we are at a beginning, not an ending, and there is much yet to be done and learned.

But does "modern" retinal laser therapy have a clear and precise meaning representing a real thing; or is it simply another hopeful but fluid and ambiguous adjective attempting to cast favor on one approach over another? Table 1 summarizes the principal attributes, and thus differences, between traditional PC and MRT. Note that the attributes differentiating PC and MRT do not represent extremes of a continuum. Instead, they are distinct and binary (yes/no). Thus, MRT is a noun and not an adjective, representing a specific well-defined entity, a species clearly distinguishable from its predecessor. While future advancements in retinal laser treatment are certain, the divide between PC and MRT is a Rubicon that, once crossed, will not be crossed again. The future of retinal laser therapy, however it may evolve, will always embody the principles of MRT (Caesar 1961, Luttrull and Dorin 2012, Luttrull and Kent 2019, Luttrull et al 2005, 2012, 2015, Luttrull 2016, Luttrull and Margolis 2016, Luttrull 2018, Luttrull, Samples et al 2018, Luttrull, Sinclair et al 2018, Chang and Luttrull 2020, Keunen et al 2020).

As noted, "Modern" does not mean current. There continues to be extensive investigation and scientific publication approaches to retinal laser approaches that do not qualify as "modern" retinal laser therapy, and thus will not be considered here. This is because they are inherently destructive by their nature. This includes nanosecond laser, which is photodisruptive to the RPE (2RT, Ellex, Adelaide, Australia); as is microsecond laser (Selective Retinal Laser Therapy or SRT, Leutronic, Seoul, Republic of Korea). Nor does "modern" apply to short-pulse millisecond CW lasers such as the PASCAL ("Pattern Scanning Laser", Topcon, Tokyo, Japan). This is because each was conceived decades ago during the retinal photocoagulation (RPC) era and designed to cause retinal damage when laser-induced retinal damage (LIRD) was considered necessary for effective therapy. Despite decades of work on these laser modalities by teams of outstanding scientists, progress has rendered these approaches obsolete and

Table 1. Comparison of traditional conventional photocoagulation to Modern Retinal Laser Therapy. Note the absence of shared attributes.

Comparison: Conventional / Traditional vs. Modern Retinal Laser Therapy		
Treatment Attributes	**Conventional[1]**	**Modern**
Retina Damage Hypothesis	Required	Avoid[3]
Mechanism	Unknown[2]	Reset to default / homeotrophy
Intent	Destroy retina	Preserve / revitalize retina
Action	Indirect	Direct
Intensity	High	Low
Density	Low	High
Inflammatory	Pro	Anti
Retinal function	Worsens	Improves
Visual function	Worsens	Improves
Adverse effects	Many	None
Repeatability	Minimal	*Ad infinitum*
Indications	Few	Many

1. Includes traditional photocoagulation, short-pulse and nanosecond continuous wave laser modalities.
2. Invocation of the necessity of laser induced retinal damage prevented an accurate understanding of the mechanism of action. Actual mechanism is same for all retinal laser treatment modalities, "reset to default" homeotrophy.
3. Modern Retinal Laser Therapy defines laser-induced retinal damage as the most serious complication / adverse treatment effect of retinal laser treatment.

clinical application inappropriate by the "modern" definition. LIRD used to be a good thing, the reason laser worked and therefore an absolute prerequisite for treatment. Now LIRD is a complication of treatment, wholly detrimental, and a severe adverse effect (SAE) of treatment to be absolutely avoided. No one saw this coming. Only treatment reliably and predictably safe and thus sublethal to the retinal pigment epithelium (RPE) is eligible for consideration of "modern" retinal laser therapy (MRT). And that is just one aspect of it.

Is it too harsh to say that these damaging laser modes have no clinical future and should be abandoned even now? It is not. This is because there are two insurmountable prohibitions to their use, one practical, the other ethical. Their continued exploration and clinical use bring some urgency to the understanding and importance of these issues.

First, in practical terms, LIRD precludes application of the fundamental principles of MRT, those of low-intensity treatment reliably and predictably sublethal to the RPE, combined with high density treatment confluently applied to wide swaths of the retina to maximize the clinical effects of low-intensity treatment. It is not enough to improve the function of one cell by direct exposure to treatment; the function of the retina as the visual organ must be improved. This is achieved by treating the organ. These

are the foundations that transform retinal laser treatment from a fraught tool for localized destruction with very few potential applications, to a functionally enhancing and restorative treatment with virtually unlimited applications, and the ability to treat early, preventively, and repeatedly, to maintain treatment benefits over as long as the lifetime of the patient. Second, in ethical terms, harm—such as LIRD—can only be justified if the benefits of that harm are more than compensated for by improved outcomes. LIRD uniformly worsens outcomes compared to retina-sparing treatments, as will be shown.

Hippocrates, et al

There is no science, or medicine, without a philosophy (Dennet 1995). Thus, despite continued use, active investigation, and continuing peer reviewed publication, it is also clear that clinical use of damaging retinal laser modes for treatment of CPRs is no longer medically ethical (Edelstein 1943, Varkey 2021). In the following discussion it will be shown that LIRD of any kind or degree has no direct therapeutic effect. It is therapeutically sufficient, but unnecessary. Any and all therapeutic effects of LIRD are indirect, and thus common to laser treatment sublethal to the retina as well and not unique to damaging laser modes. Only the damage is unique. As LIRD is both unnecessary and accounts for all adverse treatment effects, it can only be considered as a complication of retinal laser treatment, and in fact, the most severe adverse effect of retinal laser treatment. In the past and in the extreme, some have argued for the clinical benefit of laser retinal ablation as a direct treatment benefit. The less retina, the less retinopathy, the argument goes. Because our job as ophthalmologists is to improve and preserve visual function, this argument is no longer tenable in the era of retina-sparing alternatives. Just as limb amputation is no longer an acceptable first line of treatment for infection or injury, retinal reduction as a therapeutic strategy is no longer defensible (Edelstein 1943, Varkey 2021).

For retinal damaging laser modes to continue to be justifiable and acceptable, they would have to demonstrate clinical benefits over sublethal therapy that are sufficiently superior to sublethal, retina-sparing treatment, to compensate for the risks and adverse treatment effects inherent from LIRD. Review of the literature demonstrates that the results of damaging laser modes are inferior, not superior, to retina-sparing treatments. Thus, while damaging retinal laser modes may still be effective to some degree in certain settings and for particular indications, in the era of retina-sparing treatments such treatment is no longer ethically or practically justifiable (Edelstein 1943, Sivaprasad and Dorin 2012, Brader 2016, Chen et al 2016, Scholz et al 2017, Guymer et al 2018, Glassman, Wells et al 2020, Varkey 2021).

Key point: Modern retinal laser defines laser-induced retinal damage as unnecessary, impractical, wholly adverse, and thus unethical.

A change of opinions is almost unknown in an elderly military man.

—Lord Kitchener

"Subthreshold"

Note that the term *subthreshold* will find scant use in the following discussion. This is because, although ubiquitous, it is meaningless, archaic, and wholly dependent on convention for its survival. Unlike the "modern" in reference to MRT, "subthreshold" is an adjective that has as many meanings as persons using it, having been applied to everything from conventional PC to photodisruptive nanosecond laser to treatment wholly sublethal to the RPE (Luttrull and Dorin 2012, Chhablani et al 2018). A brief perusal of the author's own work will indicate that he has been as guilty as anyone in this regard. This reflected sage advice early on that the work needed to be presented in anodyne terms familiar to reviewers to gain acceptance, even if inaccurate. "Subthreshold" suggests treatment that is less detectable, but without reference to the method of detection. Absent such a qualifier, it is meaningless. As meaningless, it is prone to abuse. Thus, as a term that confuses and obfuscates rather than clarifies, "subthreshold" will be avoided whenever possible in this text (Luttrull and Dorin 2012).

Key point: Conventional photocoagulation, short-pulse CW, and nanosecond lasers are either inherently or unpredictably damaging to the retina and should be avoided, particularly in the macula.

Also not covered here

In this discussion, we also do not concern ourselves with use of retinal lasers to perform cautery for treatment of such things as retinal tears. Instead, our focus is laser treatment of the retinal disorders that constitute the most important causes of irreversible visual loss worldwide: the neurodegenerations constituting chronic progressive retinopathies (CPRs) (Luttrull et al 2005, 2008, Luttrull and Dorin 2012, Luttrull et al 2012, Luttrull et al 2015, 2016, Luttrull 2018, Luttrull, Samples et al 2018, Luttrull, Sinclair et al 2018, Luttrull and Kent 2019, Chang and Luttrull 2020, Luttrull and Kent 2020, Luttrull et al 2020).

Definition note

In the following text, the acronyms "SDM" (for low-intensity/high-density subthreshold diode microsecond pulsed laser) and "MRT" (for Modern Retinal laser Therapy) will be used both together and separately in various contexts. To aid understanding, SDM can be thought of as the practice currently epitomized, while MRT as the concept and principle.

2. Retinal Photocoagulation

The fact that an opinion has been widely held is no evidence whatever that it is not utterly absurd.

—Bertrand Russell

Why retinal photocoagulation?

The first application of retinal laser treatment for treatment of the most important causes of irreversible visual loss, the chronic progressive retinopathies (CPRs), was in the management of diabetic retinopathy (DR). Prior to the advent of insulin, diabetes, particularly type 1, was an acute, fatal illness. With insulin, diabetes became a chronic progressive disease and the manifestations of long-term diabetes started to present themselves. One of these manifestations was DR, uncommon prior to long-term survival with diabetes (Goldberg and Jampol 1987, Polyzos and Mantzoros 2021). Pituitary ablation could improve some cases of particularly rapidly progressive and/or florid cases of DR but was an extreme measure (Kohner et al 1976, L'Esperance 1978). It is apocryphal that early in the experience of the rapidly growing post-insulin DR epidemic it was noted that eyes with large chorioretinal scars, such as from trauma or congenital toxoplasmosis, appeared to be protected from DR compared to otherwise normal fellow eyes (L'Esperance 1966). This observation gave rise to the idea of creating chorioretinal scarring as a therapeutic measure to treat or prevent DR (L'Esperance 1966, Zweng et al 1971, Townsend et al 1978). It was recognized that laser (or xenon arc) could produce photocoagulation (PC) scars that could mimic the traumatic and infectious lesions that appeared to confer protection. There was no clear understanding as to what it was about chorioretinal scars that conferred a protective benefit against DR other than by possibly simply reducing the amount of available retina for disease. Thus, thermal retinal ablation and reduction appeared to be the obvious goal of retinal photocoagulation (RPC). Early studies of RPC demonstrated benefits from laser photocoagulation compared to no treatment at all, appearing to confirm the therapeutic retinal ablation hypothesis. From this point forward, laser-induced retinal damage (LIRD) was presumed and universally accepted as being both the necessary and sufficient cause of all retinal laser benefits for all indications (Goldberg and Jampol 1987).

One does not need to consult Aristotle to see that the inductively derived connection between retinal destruction and therapeutic efficacy was flawed from inception (Smith 2020). Association was misconstrued as causation. Confusion of association with causation is common in life and has a noble history in science and medicine. Many of these mistaken beliefs arose in what we consider ancient and thus primitive times, persisting for millennia (Brain 1986). Evil or inauspicious maladies had to be released: Dropsy? Bloodletting. Phrenitis? A purge, and so on. What is remarkable about the false premise underlying RPC was that it arose in what we think of as modern times, and further, that it was accepted as self-evident by everyone in the field and unchallenged by anyone of record for nearly 60 years, codifying thinking about retinal laser treatment to the level of a sacrosanct universal doctrine, thinking that survives to this day (Rosenfeld and Feuer 2019, Van Rijssen et al 2019, 2020, AAO 2021, ASRS 2021, Chhablani et al 2022). This is despite the futility of developing a cogent and useful explanation for the mechanism of retinal laser treatment based on LIRD as the precondition. History and Gaus teach that the more widely an opinion is shared, the more likely it is wrong (Lukacs 1942). As noted by Allan Bloom, when we look back in time, the thing we find most shocking and abhorrent about a prior society is the very thing that society took most for granted (Bloom 1987). Thus, the decades universal agreement regarding photocoagulation and the necessity of LIRD should have set off alarm bells for that reason alone.

Because RPC was effective (compared to no treatment) within the narrow confines of expectations and damage-limited early treatment indications, there was little concern regarding the inability to understand the mechanism of action. Rather than raising red flags that the failure of understanding and explanation might indicate a problem or flawed thinking, the failure of LIRD to account for the effects of laser treatment was largely brushed aside, because, after all, it "worked." Thus, this relative lack of curiosity about the mechanism of retinal laser treatment was because there was never any hope or expectation that understanding of the mechanism of RPC would alter its application in any significant way. Laser was cautery, plain and simple. There was only so much you could do and expect from RPC, and the destructive nature of RPC rendered deeper understanding, in practical terms, irrelevant (L'Esperance 1978, Fong et al 2003). In contrast, each of the novel indications for retinal laser treatment spawned by MRT, including treatment for inherited retinal degenerations (IRDs), neuroprotective treatment of the retinopathy of open-angle glaucoma (ROAG), prevention of neovascular conversion in dry age-related macular degeneration (AMD), slowing of age-related geographic atrophy (ARGA), and reversal of anti–vascular endothelial growth factor (VEGF) drug tolerance in neovascular AMD, and possible neuroregeneration, are each the direct result of specific predictions arising only and entirely from understanding the mechanism of action of retinal laser treatment afforded by MRT, and paradigmatic low-intensity/high-density subthreshold diode microsecond pulse laser (SDM) in particular (Luttrull et al 2012, Luttrull 2018, Luttrull, Samples et al 2018, Luttrull et al 2020, Luttrull and Gray 2022). Without understanding the mechanism of retinal laser action, there would be no reason whatsoever to conceive of any of these retinal laser indications. That these novel predictions have each been subsequently validated speaks to the veracity and power of our current theory of retinal laser action and the mechanism of action it describes (Luttrull et al 2015, Luttrull and Margolis 2016). That something works is important. But it really does help when you know what you are doing.

The wonder is not that it does it well. The wonder is that it does it at all.

—Samuel Johnson

You're making the wrong mistakes.

—Thelonious Monk

Photocoagulation: Dr Johnson's bipedal dog

In the late 1960s and early 1970s, retinal photocoagulation for proliferative diabetic retinopathy (PDR)

began in earnest. Initial results were disappointing (L'Esperance 1969, Patz et al 1971). With time and experience, however, conventional RPC damage to the retina was found to be therapeutically superior to no treatment for certain findings, particularly advanced PDR characterized by neovascular proliferation from the optic disk and/or retina (L'Esperance 1978, ETDRS No.1 1985, Bressler 2011).

The presumption of the therapeutic necessity of LIRD for therapeutic retinal laser effects had a stunting effect on clinical application and precluded understanding the therapeutic mechanism of retinal laser treatment (Mainster 1999). The simplest way to understand the deficiencies of PC is to use its clinicopathologic description: severe iatrogenic multifocal chorioretinitis. In what clinical settings, one may reasonably ask, might a diffuse multifocal chorioretinitis be helpful? To paraphrase Dr. Johnson, the surprising thing about RPC was not that it worked well, but that it worked at all (ETDRS No. 1 1985, Boswell 1986, Luttrull et al 2005, Blumenkranz 2014). In the past, the lack of alternatives and poor outcomes absent treatment made the costs of RPC—the many inherent adverse treatment effects and risks—tolerable (Figs. 1-3). However, as retina-sparing alternatives to RPC have become available, these drawbacks relegated RPC to the second or third tier of treatment options behind drug therapies for most indications (DRCRN 2010, Jampol et al 2014, Glassman et al 2020). In the following discussion, it will be shown that MRT, absent the risks, adverse treatment effects,

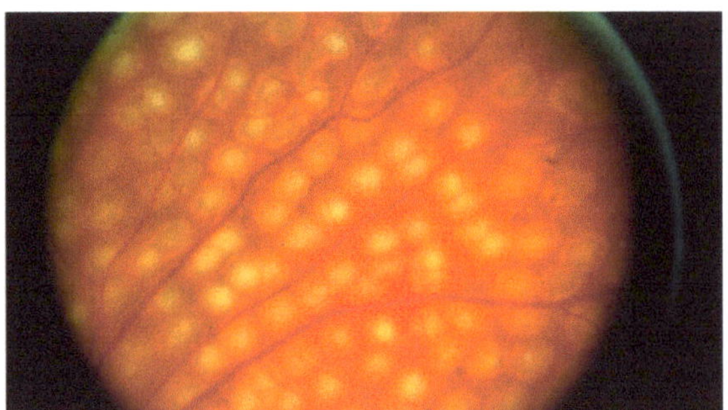

Fig. 1. Acute conventional retinal laser photocoagulation (RPC) for proliferative diabetic retinopathy (PDR). Note grey-white full thickness retinal burns. This photo was taken a few days following treatment. Note the "halo" of photocoagulated retina surrounding the intense central burn. This halo of surrounding photocoagulated retina around each spot would not have been visible at the time of treatment. Thus, the area of destroyed retina from each laser application is larger than the acute burn would indicate.

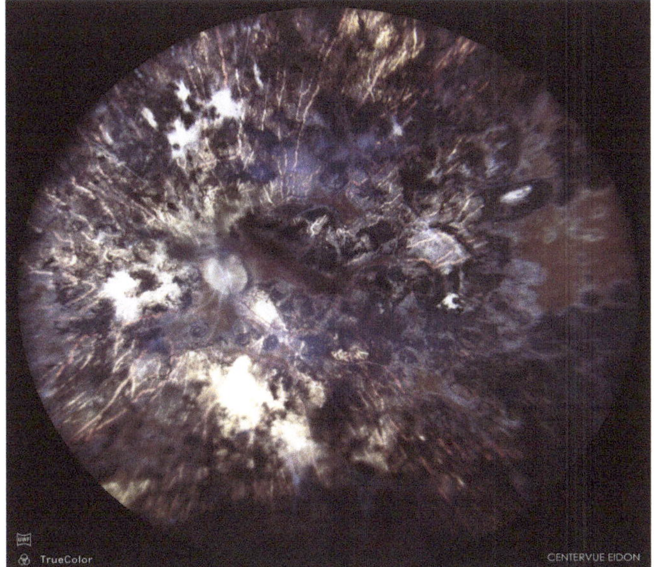

Fig. 2. Left eye of 69 year old woman presenting in 2022 with the complaint of a progressive paracentral scotoma in her left eye. She had undergone conventional PRP for PDR in both eyes in the mid-1970s and lost her right eye to a traction retinal detachment. Visual acuity OD NLP and OS 20/50-. Note nearly complete obliteration of the retina in the left eye. Her recent symptoms were due to progressive expansion of parafoveal RPC scars continuing over 40 years following conventional PRP.

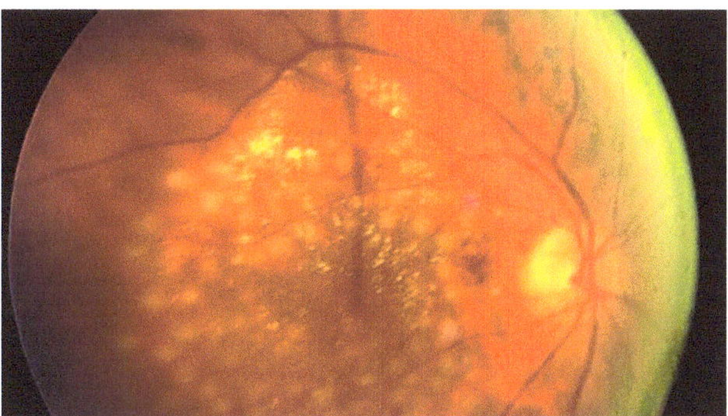

Fig. 3. Acute conventional grid macular RPC for diffuse diabetic macular edema (DME). Note grey-white full-thickness retinal burns constituting an iatrogenic acute multifocal chorioretinits.

and limitations of both RPC and drug therapy, is the most useful and effective therapeutic tool available to us now and in the foreseeable future; for both treatment and particularly for the prevention of visual loss from all the major causes of irreversible visual loss—the CPR neurodegenerations—and many other common clinical disorders besides, by combining the visual benefits of drug therapy with the lasting effects of RPC, but with a far wider breadth of clinical treatment indications than either (Luttrull et al 2005, 2008, Luttrull and Dorin 2012, Luttrull et al 2015, Bressler et al 2016, Luttrull 2016, 2018, Luttrull, Samples et al 2018, Luttrull, Sinclair et al 2018, Luttrull and Kent 2019, Luttrull et al 2020).

Key point: Photocoagulation is an example of confusion of association with causation.

3. The Foundations of Modern Retinal Laser Therapy

Resistance to innovation is clearly demonstrated, not by the ignorant masses, but by professionals with a vested interest in tradition and the monopoly of learning.

—Arthur Koestler

Why isn't everyone doing it (SDM)?

—Daniel Palanker, PhD 2005

Morris and associates reported a 17-year lag from the time a new and superior treatment is first reported, to its general acceptance and implementation by the medical community (Morris et al 2011). The inertia is not technical or informational. It is human. Doctors, like normal mortals, are reluctant to change. Like other humans, they are prone to justification to support such reticence. In medicine, this generally takes the form of "We need more data." Innovators and early adopters are rash and irresponsible. Late adopters, rather than negligent, are given the honorifics of "careful" and "prudent." This inertia has many ramifications. Resistance to progress impairs the ability of new technologies to secure funding and investment to allow them to become established and advance the field. The more marginal the advance—and thus less useful and less important—the more likely it will be accepted and supported (Cao and Langer 2008). Conversely, the more disruptive and important the advance, the more likely it will be rejected (Reza 1961, Christiansen 1997). Gullstrand (an ophthalmologist) denied Einstein (a physicist) the Nobel Prize for physics on several occasions, including for the theory of relativity. Academic publications are rejected because they threaten legacies and offend the status quo (Ravin 1999).

Gaus, a mathematician, had a gift for perspective that can be widely applied. The peak of his normal distribution represents the mean. In culture, this represents the popular and fashionable. In organized medicine, however, the apogee of the bell curve is a consensus called the *standard of care*. Further, it is sacramental, on par with a mother's honor. Any departure is treated as a threat to the status quo (defined as excellence), whether falling to the right or the left of the apogee of the curve (Lukacs 1942, Cover and Thomas 2006, AAO 2021). Because the source of innovation is always an individual, while opposition to innovation in medicine is institutional, the success of even the most important innovation is anything but inevitable (Christiansen 1997). It is not enough to innovate. One must also persevere against active opposition, or even worse—disinterest. Few are willing to pay the price (Hull 1989).

As noted earlier, firm belief in the necessity of LIRD to obtain a therapeutic retinal laser effect was universally held and unquestioned by anyone of record for over 50 years. It continues to be championed by authoritative bodies and accepted by many, if not most clinicians and academics to this day (Van Rijssen et a. 2019, 2020, AAO 2021, ASRS 2021, Chhablani et al 2022). Confusion of association with causation has a long pedigree in medicine and is not confined to modern ophthalmology. For example, a recent study found that the therapeutic benefits of the most commonly used targeted cancer chemotherapies are not actually the result of effective drug targeting, but instead are the result of off-target chemical toxicity (Lin et al 2021). The underpinnings of MRT were presaged in the landmark study of RPC, the Early Treatment of Diabetic Retinopathy Study (ETDRS) (ETDRS 1985). In the ETDRS, nonfocal grid treatment was found to be effective; higher intensity treatment was associated with more frequent and severe SAEs and visual loss; and higher density treatment was more effective than low density treatment. This led to a gradual trend toward less intense RPC and less severe LIRD through the late 1980s and 1990s (Mainster 1999, Jampol et al 2014). However, the goal of treatment remained creation of LIRD. Thus, this evolution was one of style more than substance (Moorman and Hamilton 1999). Other than turning down the temperature, the treatment concepts, techniques, indications, risks, and limitations remained unchanged.

SDM and the discovery of modern retinal laser therapy

If you want something new, you have to stop doing something old.

—Peter Drucker

If at first the idea is not absurd, then there is no hope for it.
—Albert Einstein

Progress is made by lazy men looking for easier ways to do things.

—Robert A. Heinlein

Information theory and MRT

Information theory states that the more unlikely an event, the greater the amount of new information it has to offer (Reza 1961, Jaynes 2003, Cover and Thomas 2006). This is the story of MRT. The new information unlocked by it has barely yet been explored.

Innovation is unlikely. It cannot be anticipated, planned, or systematized. Innovation is rarely the product of experts. The greater the innovation, the more absurd it appears. Innovation always arrives as low-quality data. An epiphany rather than fruition of a well-constructed plan, innovation changes the world in ways incrementalism cannot. Innovation is, by definition, an existential threat to the status quo and vested interests. Thus, innovation is never popular or widely accepted. At first (Christiansen 1997).

Such is the context for the discovery and development of MRT. As a solo private practitioner, the author had no special interest in or knowledge of retinal laser treatment beyond what was common in the field. Like many others, over time, it became clear that minimizing (necessary) laser damage in the macula for treatment of macular edema (ME), due to diabetes or retinal vein occlusion, was just as effective as more intense treatment, and less likely to lead to late visual loss from coalescence of atrophic macular laser lesions leading to geographic atrophy (Mainster 1999). Low-density grid treatment with the continuous-wave (CW) krypton red laser became favored for this purpose. However, despite every effort to minimize and even prevent detectable LIRD, laser uptake and thus damage was highly variable and unpredictable (Fig. 4). One laser spot application might do no apparent damage to retina, either clinically, by fundus autofluorescence photography (FAF), or by fundus autofluorescence photography (FAF), or

intravenous fundus fluorescein angiography (FFA). However, the spot right next to it, only micrometers away and with exactly the same laser parameters, was often obvious by any if not all modes of detection.

The author's long-lived water-cooled gas-tubed argon/krypton laser began to fade due to years of use, progressively losing power. At about this same time there was interest in transpupillary thermotherapy (TTT) for subfoveal neovascular age-related macular degeneration (NAMD). Not wanting to be left behind, the author purchased a new laser for this purpose, a solid-state diode laser 1/100th the size of his argon/krypton laser, featuring a longer near-infrared 810 nm wavelength, a wide-field adaptor for TTT, air-cooling, and a simple 110 V plug rather than a dedicated 220 V power line.

Wednesday, April 19, 2000, the new Iridex SLx 810 laser (Iridex Corp, Mountain View, California) with the large spot aperture was delivered. That same morning, the long-serving argon/krypton laser finally failed completely, unable to muster enough power to make any kind of necessary retinal burn.

Jim Brum, the Iridex sales representative, explained how the machine worked. He noted that, in addition to the large spot capability, it also had a *micropulse mode*. He explained that some people thought it might be useful for treating DME. The author did not know who these people might be. Absent an internet and PubMed, it would be difficult to find out even if he had a mind to—which he did not. Mr Brum explained how by changing the duty cycle (DC), or pulse frequency, the effective power and tissue heating could be modulated beyond the power and duration settings.

The only thing the author knew about 810 nm lasers was that they penetrated tissue more deeply and thus tended to be painful. The author, having just bought a new 810 nm laser, did not want to have to buy yet another laser to replace his dead argon/krypton for indications beyond TTT. So, in hopes of making use of the 810 nm laser for all indications, he decided to try using the micropulse mode to reduce treatment pain and discomfort. As he later learned, he was not the first to do this (Friberg and Vinkatesh 1995). Absent any familiarity with the micropulse (microsecond pulsed) diode laser, a low-intensity treatment strategy, employing a low DC, was chosen.

Lacking information and experience, the laser spot size, duty cycle (DC) and power were chosen by divinely inspired (author's judgement) intuition. Because of the marked

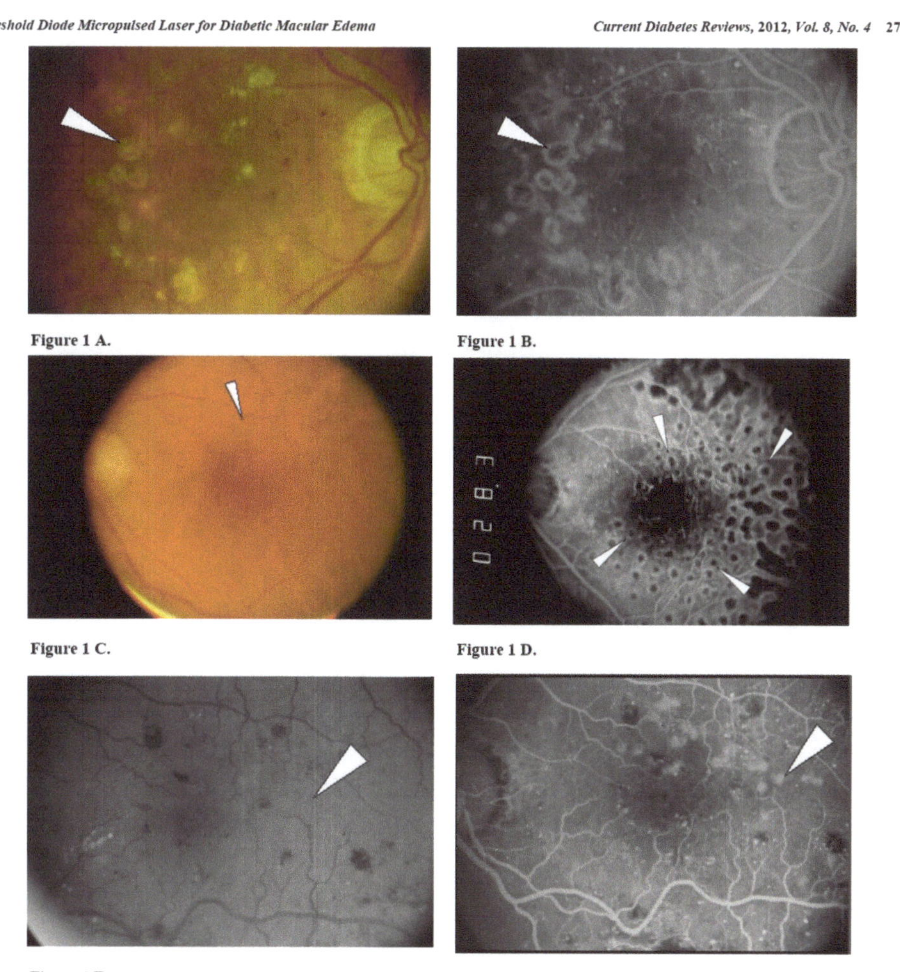

Fig. 4. Examples of "subthreshold" grid photocoagulation for DME performed with continuous wave lasers. Note variability of the laser lesions with regard to uptake and visibility on fundus photographs and intravenous fundus fluorescein angiography (FFA). Courtesy of: *Luttrull JK, Dorin G. Subthreshold diode micropulse photocoagulation as invisible retinal phototherapy for diabetic macular edema. A review. Current Diabetes Reviews, 2012, 8, 274-284.*

reduction in treatment intensity resulting from selection of a 5% pulse frequency (duty cycle) to promote comfort, intuition further suggested use of high-density treatment strategy to maximize the treatment effects. The thought was simply, "If I'm not doing much, I'd better do a lot of it." Rather than focal treatment or a low-density grid of spaced laser spot applications, confluent treatment of all areas of retinal thickening of patients with diabetic macular edema (still avoiding the fovea) was performed. Thus, the conceptual and technical twin pillars of MRT were born simultaneously that first day with the first patients treated for DME. There was no conscious attempt to completely avoid LIRD, or any thought given to the idea that it might be good to avoid retinal damage; or that treatment might still be effective if one could do this. There was no thought that a fundamental change in the conception, understanding,

and use of retinal laser for CPRs had occurred. Changes were simply made in an attempt to make treatment more comfortable, and by so doing, to save money (Luttrull et al 2005, 2008, Luttrull and Dorin 2012).

The laser parameters chosen that first day were wavelength 810 nm, a Mainster macular contact lens (mag. factor 1.05x), 0.78 W power, 125 um spot size, 5% DC, 0.30 second spot duration (Luttrull et al 2005). The terminology for this approach was later adopted on the suggestion of Martin Mainster as "SDM" for "subthreshold diode micropulse laser" (Luttrull et al 2005). Later, the more fully descriptive terminology of "low-intensity/high-density" SDM was adopted, to distinguish SDM from the panoply of other microsecond pulsed laser approaches being used elsewhere (Luttrull and Dorin 2012, Luttrull et al 2012).

Similarly intuitive selection of parameters for panretinal treatment of PDR was also made, that same day. There were patients with PDR that were there that day to be treated. The parameters selected were wavelength 810 nm, Volk 160 contact lens, 500 um spot size (1,000 um retinal spot), 2.0 W power, 0.20 s duration and 15% DC. The higher DC was used to compensate for the upper limit of 2.0 W maximum laser power, so that a larger spot could be used with a reasonable spot duration so as to keep treatment from taking too long. There was concern about a greater likelihood of LIRD (and thus pain) with the 15% DC, but less concern in the periphery that would be in the macula. These parameters for both macular and peripheral SDM treatment remained unchanged for several years (Luttrull et al 2005, 2006, Luttrull and Spink 2006). After that first day upon receiving the micropulsed laser, the author never again performed RPC except for treatment or retinal tears or detachments.

Several patients with DME and PDR were treated that first day. No visible retinal lesions could be seen by contact lens examination, and treatment was—as hoped—comfortable and without pain. A large number of laser spot applications were used in hopes of increasing the clinical effectiveness of the low-intensity treatment, on average 600 spots for DME, placed confluently over the areas of macular thickening seen with the contact lens; and 2000 spots for peripheral treatments (Luttrull et al 2005, 2008). While no laser lesions were clinically visible, the author's concern (he knew little about laser in April 2000) was that these eyes might develop late damage and end up looking and seeing like retinitis pigmentosa. There was also a chance that, absent visible laser lesions, treatment might be ineffectual. But this concern was less, because more SDM, or RPC as rescue could be performed if necessary. Inadvertent laser obliteration of the retina could not be undone.

Most of those first-treated patients returned the following week for treatment of their other eye. Again, there was no clinical evidence of LIRD. However, there was something remarkable. Virtually every patient reported subjectively improved vision almost immediately after SDM treatment. This was described as sharper, clearer vision, and improved color perception. Clinically, only one week after treatment, no clinical change was evident and their Snellen visual acuities (VAs) were also unchanged. So why was this remarkable? Because with many years of experience using RPC in DR, patients never reported early (if ever) visual improvement after RPC. In fact, most patients experienced at least transient visual loss following RPC (macular or peripheral) due to treatment-associated inflammation and loss of functional tissue. Thus, in the absence of visible LIRD, and with novel reports of treatment-associated visual improvement, SDM was continued.

Concerns about late developing damage persisted, and there was a desire to better understand why these patients routinely reported early subjective visual improvement. Thus, in this time before clinical introduction of optical coherence tomography (OCT), various patients agreed to undergo FFA one hour, or one day, or one week, or one month following SDM. In no eye at any point following treatment was there any evidence of LIRD—no early focal or diffuse breakdown of the blood-retinal barrier at the level of the RPE, no pigment clumping by FAF, and no focal atrophy at the sites of laser application. At this early postoperative time after SDM there was no indication by any means available at that time that treatment had been done. This was also no small concern (Luttrull et al 2005, 2006).

At that time in mid-2000, it was the author's custom to see DME patients 6 weeks following macular PC. Continuing this convention, by this time it became clear that this new approach of "low-intensity/high-density" SDM laser treatment for DME and PDR was working. DME was resolving, leakage was decreasing, new vessels and retinopathy were regressing—again despite any evidence (by LIRD) of laser treatment having been performed (Fig. 5).

When Columbus landed in the New World he is said to have thought he had arrived in India as planned. Over subsequent weeks and months came the realization that SDM had achieved something more than patient comfort. Remarkably, the laser settings selected that first day were ultimately found to be in the ideal range for achievement of effective retinal laser therapy without LIRD. Likewise, the high-density treatment strategy, intuitively intended to amplify and maximize the therapeutic effects of low-intensity treatment, appeared to be working, as treatment was clearly effective. How it worked was still a mystery. But, absent LIRD, by exclusion SDM could only work by improving, and thus normalizing, retinal function by selective thermal photostimulation of, and sublethal to, the retinal pigment epithelium (RPE). How it did this was unclear. But there were no other viable explanations for the very clear clinical observations being recorded.

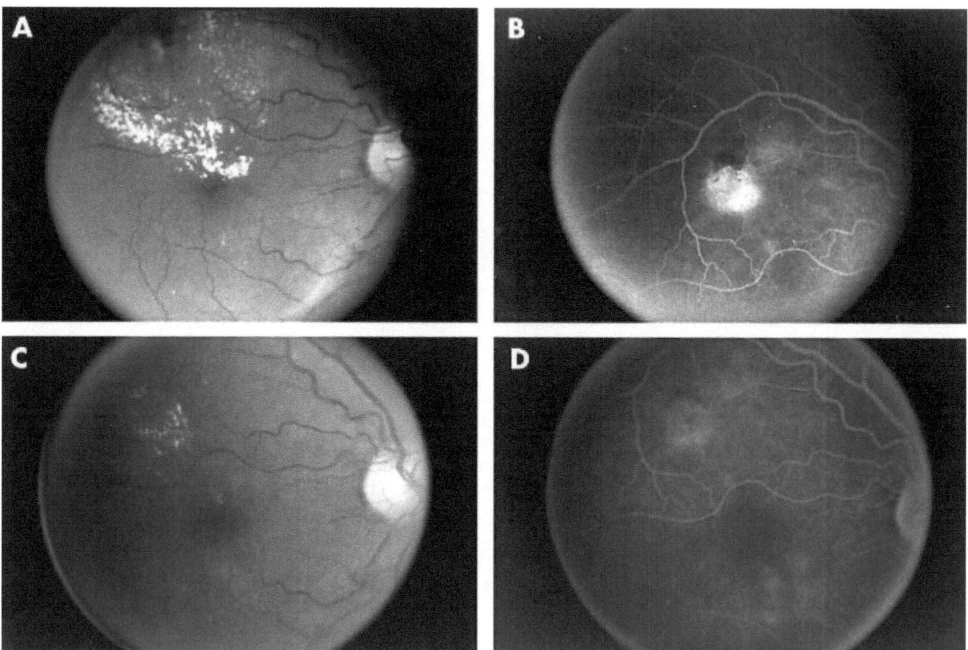

Fig. 5. (A) Preoperative red-free fundus photograph demonstrating clinically significant diabetic macular oedema. (B) Preoperative intravenous fundus fluorescein angiogram. Note prominent focal retinal microvascular leakage. This patient was treated confluently throughout the area of leakage and retinal thickening with 269 applications of SDM photocoagulation. (C) Red-free fundus photograph 10 months following SDM photocoagulation. Note resolution of macular oedema and hard exudates. (D) Intravenous fundus fluorescein angiogram 10 months post-SDM macular photocoagulation. Note persistent but diminished focal microvascular leakage, and absence of angiographically visible pigment disturbance or chorioretinal scarring. From: *Luttrull JK, Musch MC, Mainster MA: Subthreshold diode micropulse photocoagulation for the treatment of clinically significant diabetic macular edema. Br J Ophthalmol 2005 89:1; 74-80.*

In "low-intensity/high-density subthreshold diode micropulse photocoagulation," Modern Retinal Laser Therapy had been born (Luttrull et al 2005, Luttrull and Spink 2006, Luttrull et al 2006, Luttrull and Dorin 2012, Luttrull and Margolis 2016) (Table 1).

Key point: Innovation cannot be planned or "done." Innovation is serendipitous. That is the origin of Modern Retinal Laser Therapy.

Section II. The Mechanisms of Retinal Laser Action

Human subtlety will never devise an invention more beautiful, more simple or more direct than does nature because in her inventions nothing is lacking, and nothing is superfluous.

—Leonardo da Vinci

An invention has to make sense in the world it finishes in, not in the world it started in.

—Tom O'Reilly

4. Pillar I of Modern Retinal Laser Therapy: Low-Intensity Treatment

Clinical observations have informed and established the basis for our current understanding of the mechanism(s) of retinal laser action. First, there has never been a notable difference in clinical outcomes according to laser wavelength, despite the fact that wavelengths below 550 nm are absorbed in the neurosensory retina (NSR) and cause ionizing photochemical cytotoxic damage, while longer wavelengths such as 810 nm are nonionizing and have no neurosensory retinal absorption (Dorin 2003). This suggested that the therapeutic benefits of treatment arise from what they have in common, which is thermal absorption by the RPE. This non-wavelength-dependent photothermal stimulation of the RPE distinguishes MRT from photobiomodulation (PBM), which is nonthermal and wavelength dependent, and thus mechanistically distinct (PBM mediated via photoelectric effects on mitochondrial respiratory chain molecules) (Dorin 2003, Luttrull et al 2005, 2012, Kolomyer and Zarbin 2014, Karu and Kolyakov 2005, Chang and Luttrull 2020). This different mechanism of action in MRT versus PBM is illustrated by the clinical finding that MRT is effective for treatment of diabetic macular edema (DME), while PBM is not (Kim et al 2022) (Table 2).

Second, it has been observed that SDM by thermally affecting the RPE improves retinal and visual function in widely disparate conditions. This indicates that disease-induced but reversible dysfunction of the RPE is a fundamental commonality of most acquired macular disorders and CPRs and retinal neurodegenerations in general (Luttrull et al 2015, Luttrull and Margolis 2016). For example, the phenotypic expression of AMD manifests as primarily as dysfunction of the RPE, DR the neurosensory retina, while open-angle glaucoma (OAG) manifests primarily as an optic neuropathy. Yet all are improved by selective photothermal stimulation of the RPE.

Third, SDM is able to produce robust therapeutic effects absent LIRD in applications traditionally treated by RPC. This indicates that LIRD was unnecessary. As the cause of all adverse treatment effects, RPC thus represents a complication of treatment, and in fact the most serious adverse treatment effect (SAE) of laser treatment, rather than the necessary precondition for effective therapy. Effective therapy absent LIRD eliminated from consideration all prior theories for the mechanism of retinal laser treatment based on prerequisite LIRD (Luttrull and Dorin 2012, Luttrull et al 2012, Chhablani et al 2018).

Fourth, the clinical response of retinal laser photothermal stimulation of the RPE sublethal to the RPE indicates that the effects of retinal laser treatment arise from changes in the function of living RPE cells affected, but not killed, by the laser. Because RPC kills the RPE, the effects of RPC must therefore also be due to cells affected by the laser but not killed. Thus, even if one believed that the laser lesion itself was responsible for the therapeutic effect of treatment—such as improving retinal oxygenation via the choroid by thinning the retina—even this effect (which has not been borne out and cannot explain the effects of retinal laser) would necessarily also have to be mediated by living cells not destroyed by treatment (Luttrull and Dorin 2012, Luttrull et al 2012). Thus, the effects of MRT are direct, elicited by the laser wherever exposed to treatment; while the effects of LIRD are indirect, occurring at the margins of the area of killing by surviving cells either heated but not killed as in RPC, or not heated due to minimal lateral heat transfer from short-pulse CW or nanosecond laser but required to activate to heal and fill the tissue defects created by the laser. In this light,

Table 2. Comparison of attributes of retinal laser treatment with photobiomodulation

	Laser	Photobiomodulation
Wavelength	Any	Visible
Application	Spot	Ganzfield
Wavelength dependent?	No	Yes
Session time/ frequency	Short/low	Long/high
Duration of effect	Long/permanent	Short
Thermal?	Yes	No
Mechanism of action	RPE HSP activation	Photoelectric

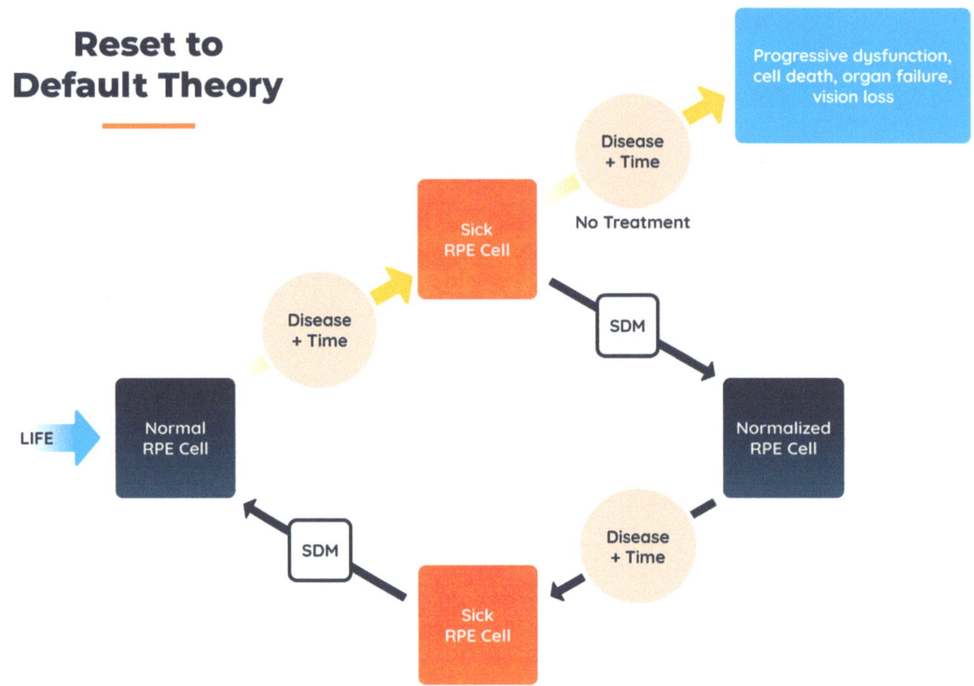

Fig. 6. Diagram of the reset effect of MRT and the basis of vision protection therapy (regular periodic SDM maintenance therapy). Note that by repeatedly interrupting disease progression with temporary reversals of disease severity the risks of irreversible dysfunction, apoptosis and visual loss are reduced by slowed disease progression.

it is clear that the therapeutic potential of retinal laser is directly proportional to the amount of affected RPE. Thus, in order of potential effectiveness we find MRT, RPC, PASCAL, SRT and then nanosecond laser. Note that this order of potential effectiveness is directly proportional to the pulse duration as shorter durations limit heat spread, with nanosecond laser being simply mechanically photodisruptive (MRT limiting heat spread to within a given cell, but not beyond in any notable degree). This is referred to as the *effective surface area* of retinal laser treatment (Luttrull and Dorin 2012, Chhablani et al 2018, Chang and Luttrull 2020) (Fig. 6).

Protein misfolding

Protein misfolding is the currency of cell dysfunction and death. The tertiary structure of proteins within the cell that gives them their essential function attributes wrests, from a nearly infinite number of potential conformations available to the average 100 molecule primary protein strand, the one single shape that confers the necessary functional capacity. Statistically, the probability of any one single protein strand, the primary structure of an enzyme, finding the correct shape by chance is effectively zero. Left to such chance, life would not exist. Instead, the sequence of amino acids is such that at various areas in the sequence the amino acids tend to be in groups that are either hydrophobic, or hydrophilic. Thus, within the aqueous cytosol of the intracellular gel, the hydrophilic polarized aqueous forces of the cytosol on the protein encourage, if not force it, to adopt a shape whereby the hydrophobic parts of the protein become oriented toward the inner part of the tertiary structure away from the cytosol, while the hydrophilic portions of the protein orient themselves toward the external parts of the protein toward the aqueous. While such forces are highly effective in aiding proteins to adopt their effective tertiary conformations, water wants to be everywhere it is not. Thus, the hydrophobic inner portion of the enzyme is under continual assault and stress from the external polar aqueous. Eventually, this leads to unfolding of the enzyme and loss of function. Eventually is not a very long time, as that typical half-life of most enzymes is on the order of just 90 minutes in healthy cells, decreasing to just 18 minutes in highly stressed dysfunctional cells (Banak et al 2019, Chang and Luttrull 2020).

Every disease state places unique stresses on cell function that reflect the primary disease process.

These might be age and environmental factors for AMD, metabolic dysfunction in diabetic retinopathy, or a genetic defect in retinitis pigmentosa. Each will stress the cell in a different but characteristic way, leading to a characteristic "menu" of enzyme misfolding and thus cell dysfunction. Initially, only the enzymes more intimately related to the underlying disease process will be affected. Eventually, as these fail and lead to secondary stresses and consequent dysfunction of upstream and downstream enzymes, virtually all the enzyme systems in the cell may become misfolded and nonfunctional. When this happens to a sufficient degree exceeding the cell's ability to compensate and maintain repair, apoptosis ensues (Luttrull et al 2015, Luttrull and Margolis 2016, Melo et al 2022).

From this point of view, every disease is as unique as the unique stressor, the underlying disease defect, and its unique menu of initial enzyme misfoldings. This is a "splitter" view. Viewed differently, as a "lumper," particularly in the retina, all can be viewed—and thus potentially treated—as they being essentially the same. First, despite the cause, all dysfunctions result from protein misfolding. Second, with little regard to the cause of this misfolding, for as long as the stressor lasts, its resultant protein misfolding and subsequent cell dysfunction both increase with time. All such time-driven retinal dysfunctions are property degenerations. Because the retina is central nervous system tissue, all chronic progressive retinopathies are thus neurodegenerations driven by protein misfolding. This is the basis for the therapeutic mechanism and benefits of MRT (Luttrull et al 2015).

Key point: MRT is the result of observations made in clinical practice. At every step along the way, science has validated those observations.

In the following discussion I am indebted to my late colleague and irreplaceable genius David B Chang, PhD, brilliant physicist, and unfailingly kind and humble man.

Heat shock protein activation
Key point: Our biology does not anticipate aging and the chronic progressive diseases that result. While we have powerful and effective means of repair and restoration, they are geared toward the existential threats of youth—trauma, exposure, infection. Aging does not get their attention. MRT does.

MRT elicited cellular repair and therapeutic immunomodulation is initiated by RPE heat-shock protein (HSP) activation and mediated via upregulation of the endoplasmic reticulum unfolded protein response (ER UPR) (Schroder and Kaufman 2005, Shpilka and Haynes 2018, Terrab and Wipf 2020).

Heat Shock Proteins
In the absence of LIRD and thus laser-induced alteration of local retinal anatomy, thermal activation of RPE heat shock proteins (HSPs) presented itself, by exclusion, as the most likely mediator of laser-induced therapeutic effects (Luttrull et al 2005). Mathematical analysis of the clinical effects revealed that the effects of SDM were temperature dependent. Temperatures lower that than elicited by various SDM treatment parameters used effectively clinically suggested that, at such temperatures—in the physiologic ranges, such as occurring from a fever—would result in spontaneous healing of various retinal disorders without treatment, something not observed. The effects of the calculated temperatures from various SDM treatment parameter combinations that had been used effectively clinically were studied in reference to model intracellular proteins, revealing only adiabatic responses, consisting of brief and inconsequential conformational perturbations—except with regard to RPE HSPs (Chang DB unpublished data 2016) The response of RPE HSP 70 to the same stimulus was found to both activate the HSP response and significantly alter HSP reaction kinetics.

Aging never used to be a problem

Reflecting their importance to normal cell function, HSPs constitute 40% or more of all intracellular proteins. Interestingly, HSPs have never registered much interest in ophthalmology. HSPs are highly conserved, little different in man, and the most primitive single celled organisms. This offers important insights into their roles in cellular repair and function restoration. First, such "conservation" indicates that HSPs are of fundamental importance to normal cell function (Kregel 2002). HSPs developed millions of years ago in the earliest forms of life. For those creatures, death came from being eaten, crushed, burnt, frozen, and so on. Nothing died from old age. Even if they did, death after reproductive activity was of little importance. The usefulness of the organism had been exhausted. Years of comfortable retirement pursuing all those activities that work and raising a family made difficult in earlier years is not a concern. Aging, and chronic diseases such as the CPRs is, in the big picture, a very new phenomenon that was unanticipated by biology.

MRT thermodynamics

Classified by their molecular weights, HSPs have a wide range of complex functions and interactions. As noted earlier, it is the 70 kDa HSPs that are of particular interest to MRT, as these are especially concerned with protein and enzyme repair and cell survival in response to existential threats. The HSP 70 family has two especially relevant portfolios: a maintenance/surveillance role; and a salvific role (Kregel 2002).

HSPs have essential functions in maintaining homeostasis via maintaining proteostasis. However, HSPs are also designed to respond to acute existential threats to the cell and thus organism—being bitten, smashed, heated, or frozen—by preserving cell function and thus life. The greater the acuity and severity of the stressor, the greater the response. Because the response is mediated by a living, not dead cell, the most effective stressor stimuli of HSP activation are those that are not only acute—a stab wound, perhaps?—but also sublethal to the cell (Richter et al 2010).

The best models for its operation contain 10 different molecular components, each with different rate coefficients (k_{1-10}) that interact with each other to keep the cell healthy (Rybinski et al 2013, Chang and Luttrull 2020). In these equations there are four sources of HSP in the cell:

(1) Induction of transcription and translation of new HSP via activation of HSP.HSF (heat shock factor) complexes; (2) HSP can be released by the cell's reservoir of HSP.HSF molecules; (3) HSP can be released from HSP that is attached to misfolded proteins after the misfolded proteins are repaired; and (4) HSP can be released from HSP that is attached to misfolded proteins even though the misfolded proteins have not been repaired.

Published equations for HSP activation describe a jump in temperature from normal body temperature to a constant higher temperature (Rybinski et al 2013, Szymanska and Zylicz 2018). Thus, the equations were modified slightly to describe the momentary laser-induced temperature rises produced by microsecond

pulsed laser treatment like SDM (Chang and Luttrull 2020). This means that the equations studied were for two different phases: (1) during the laser-induced higher pulse peak temperature, and (2) after the temperature has returned to body temperature, but during which time the HSP machinery is still active. Using the lowest energy SDM parameters documented to be clinically effective with an American National Standards Institute "Maximal Permissible Exposure" level (xMPE) of 18xMPE, calculations indicate the initial number of misfolded proteins to be decreased by $e^{-1} = 0.37$ (the equivalent of an Arrhenius integral =1) at an Arrhenius activation energy of 11.48×10^{-12} ergs (ANSI 2000, Luttrull et al 2005, 2008, Luttrull et al 2012, Rybinski et al 2013, Szymanska and Zylicz 2018, Chang and Luttrull 2020) (Fig. 7).

The concentrations of the HSP chaperone system as a function of time during the high temperature phase (assuming it lasts 0.2 sec) were determined. Assuming a diseased/dysfunctional state with an initial intracellular concentration of misfolded proteins 2X normal, the equilibrium concentration calculations show the following temperature effects on intra-RPE cell MRT elicited protein repair:

Temperature rise of 7.71 K: This is the calculated SDM elicited RPE temperature rise for the panretinal SDM laser parameters of spot size 1,000 um, wavelength 810 nm, power 2.0 W, duration 0.20 sec, DC 15% (18xMPE). In this case, HSP expression (transcription and translation of HSPs) hardly contributes, with the main source of HSP being the release of bound to misfolded and repaired proteins.

Temperature rise of 10 K: A much larger decrease in concentration of misfolded proteins is produced. At 0.2 sec, calculations show the concentration of misfolded proteins is 5.5% of the original concentration.

Temperature rise of 15 K: A much, much larger decrease in concentration of misfolded proteins. At 0.2 sec, the concentration of misfolded proteins is only 0.07% of the original concentration.

If short-term protein repair is so temperature sensitive, how do we explain the clinical effectiveness of lower energy, lower maximum temperature SDM laser parameters, such as those generating only 18xMPE reported to be effective for PDR? (Luttrull et al 2006). This is because the kinetics of HSP activation are catalytic. Once the HSP thermal activation threshold is exceeded, a maximal response will ensue which is largely independent of the degree to which the activation threshold is exceeded (Chang and Luttrull 2020). Thus, exceeding the RPE HSP activation threshold does not improve the therapeutic effectiveness. Further, the threshold for triggering the salvific HSP response is very low. Thus, ineffective subtherapeutic treatment is far less likely than supratherapeutic and potentially harmful treatment. Exceeding the threshold substantially may, however, thus be self-defeating, killing the RPE by exceeding the Arrhenius integral for cell death (Luttrull et al 2012, Luttrull AJO 2020) (Fig. 7).

Further study of the kinetics of thermal HSP activation shows that the increase in the concentration-free HSPs following treatment is actually fairly small. In part, this is because only a fraction of HSPs is available for activation at any one time, the balance being held in reserve (Rybinski et al 2013, Szymanska and Zylicz 2018, Chang and Luttrull 2021). This is consistent with *in vivo* and *in vitro* studies of laser RPE HSP activation which show small treatment associated increases in HSP staining (actually, of the HSP-promoter gene complex rather than free HSPs), which then increase dramatically once the temperature increase is sufficient to kill the cell causing extracellular extravasation of the normally intracellular HSPs following pyronecrotic cell rupture (Kern et al 2018). Instead, the main therapeutic effect of thermal

HSP activation is its influence on the final step in the HSP 70 thermal activation kinetics, $k_{10,}$ in which a temperature-dependent conformational change is induced in the free HSPs that accelerates the rate of protein repair by as much as 35% in highly dysfunctional cells with high concentrations of misfolded proteins. At the same time, normal cells, characterized by low levels of misfolded protein, are left unaffected (Chang and Luttrull 2020).

Key point: MRT activation of HSP 70 speeds intracellular protein repair to improve cell function.

The thermodynamics of the HSP response to SDM reveal an especially important attribute of microsecond pulsing; that is, by adjusting the treatment parameters appropriately, the Arrhenius integral for HSP activation can be easily achieved while remaining far below the Arrhenius integral for thermal cell death. Thus, MRT can be maximally clinically effective while precluding the possibility of thermal RPE cell death (Fig. 8). Note that for CW laser exposures, both inevitably vary in parallel. In other words, CW lasers become less safe as they become more effective. Microsecond pulsing allows thermal HSP activation to be effectively disconnected from thermal cell death, such that they can be constructed to vary inversely rather than in parallel. This allows for the creation of MRT parameters with vastly large therapeutic ranges, of 15 W and more in breadth, which allow effective treatment of all eyes without regard to individual variations such as media opacity, fundus pigmentation, or retinal thickness, with reliable safety while using identical treatment parameters in every eye (Table 3) (Luttrull and Dorin 2012, Luttrull et al 2012, Chhablani et al 2018, Chang and Luttrull 2020).

That these laser-induced effects on RPE HSPs occur only in dysfunctional cells and not in normal cells and in proportion to the level of dysfunction is a phenomenon well demonstrated by measures of retinal function, such as electrophysiology, in response to SDM MRT. In every disease setting thus far examined, linear regression analysis of treatment responses to SDM MRT find that the eyes with the greatest dysfunction prior to treatment improve to the greatest degree following treatment, while more normally functioning eyes remain proportionately unaffected by treatment (Karu 1989, Kregel 2002, Gao and Xing 2009, Richter et al 2010, Luttrull and Margolis 2016, Chang and Luttrull 2020).

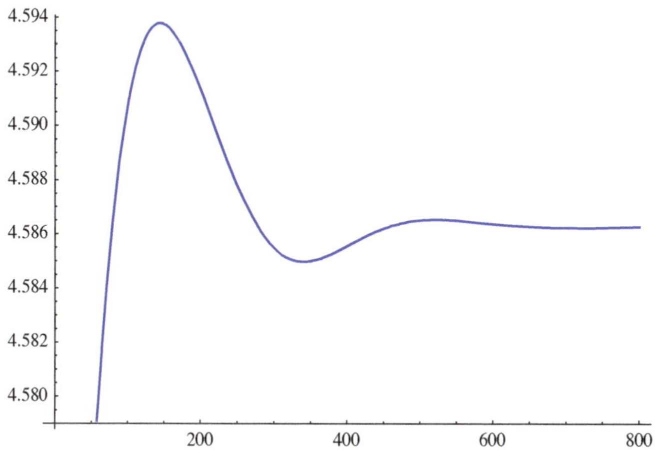

Fig. 7. Concentration of undamaged proteins [p] in arbitrary Rybinski et al (2013) units vs. time after SDM irradiation in minutes . . . SDM-induced changes in the rate constants appear to be the cause of SDM-induced improvement in the number of undamaged proteins in the cell. From: *Chang DB, Luttrull JK. Comparison of subthreshold 577nm and 810nm micropulse laser effects on heat-shock protein activation kinetics: Implications for treatment efficacy and safety. Transl Vis Sci Tecnol. 2020 Apr 28;9(5):23.doi: 10.1167/tvst.9.5.23. eCollection 2020 Apr.*

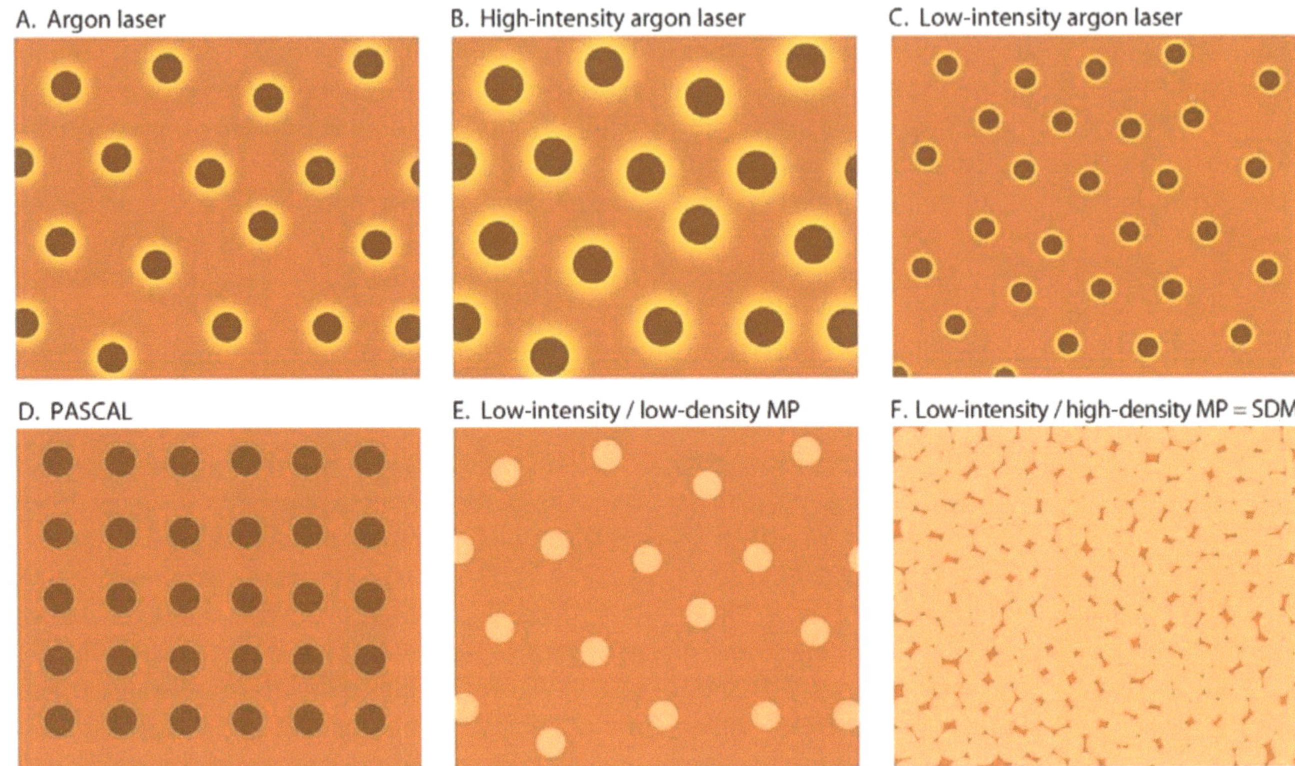

Fig. 8. A-F. Graphic representation of the "Effective Surface Area" of various modes of retinal laser treatment for retinal vascular disease. Vermillion = Retina unaffected by laser treatment. Brown = Area of retina destroyed by laser and inactive with respect to ability to produce extracellular cytokines. Yellow = Area of retina affected by the laser but not destroyed, able to contribute to the therapeutic effects of laser treatment via laser-induced alteration / normalization of cytokine expression. PASCAL = pattern scanning laser. MP = diode micropulse laser. SDM = "High density / low-intensity" subthreshold / subvisible diode micropulsed laser. From: *Luttrull JK, Dorin G. Subthreshold diode micropulse photocoagulation as invisible retinal phototherapy for diabetic macular edema. A review. Current Diabetes Reviews, 2012, 8, 274-284.*

Table 3. Comparison of Subthreshold (Sublethal) Diode Micropulse Laser Arrhenius Integrals, Therapeutic and Cell Death Thresholds for the Vujosevic et al.[45] 577 and 810 nm SDM Parameter Sets

Wavelength[45]	P (Treatment) Laser Power Watts	Arrhenius Integral for HSP activation	P (Reset) Watts	P (Death) Watts	TR Watts	SM Watts
577	0.25	2.59	0.16	0.45	0.29	0.20
810	0.75	0.84	0.85	2.67	1.82	1.92

P (Reset) = power required for the HSP activation Arrhenius integral to reach a value of unity; P (Death) = power required for the Arrhenius integral for damage to reach a value of unity, marking the upper limit of the therapeutic range, avoidance of RPE damage being a desirable end of treatment. TR = therapeutic range = P (Death) - P (Reset), or the width (expressed in laser power) of the nominal effective interval for SDM treatment sublethal to the RPE. The laser powers delineating the P (Reset) and P (Death) vary based on the particular combinations of each of the other laser parameters, including wavelength, duty cycle, pulse duration, and spot size. SM = safety margin = P (Death) - P (Treatment). The powers for the P (Reset) and P (Death) assume an Arrhenius integral for HSP activation of 1.0.

MRT is thus "pathoselective." Applied confluently over wide areas of the retina, MRT will improve and normalize the function of dysfunctional cells while leaving normal cells undisturbed (Luttrull and Dorin 2012) (Fig. 9). This is a valuable clinical attribute, as it makes precise identification, location, and characterization of dysfunction unnecessary, a key attribute of the "high-density" treatment paradigm of MRT.

Key point: MRT improves retinal function in proportion to its level of dysfunction.

HSP surveillance versus salvation

As noted earlier, in surveillance mode HSPs are vital to homeostasis—proteostasis to be more exact—

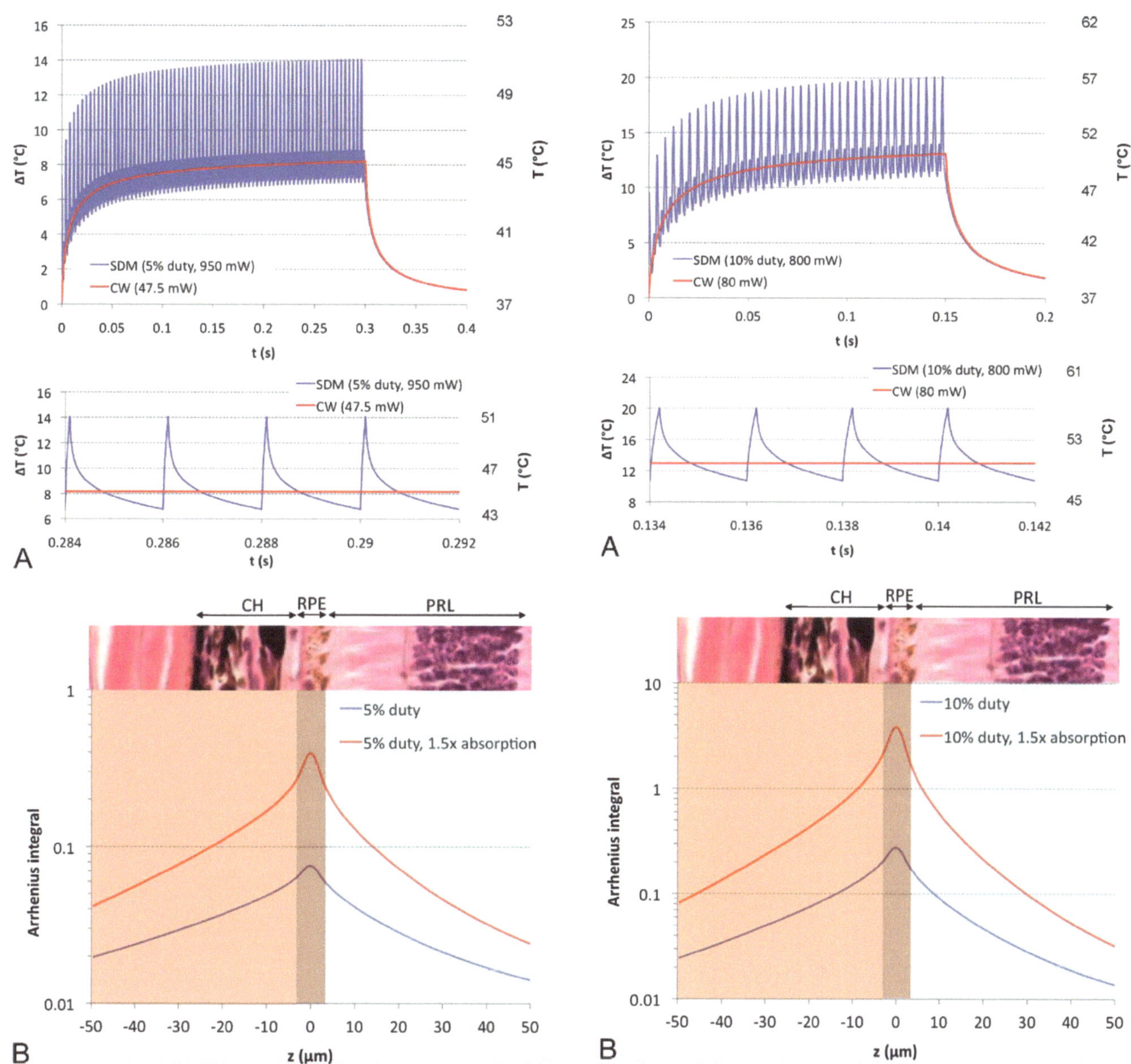

Fig. 9. Left side: A. Calculated temperature rise in the beam center at the RPE for low retinal burn risk SDM laser parameters (5% DC). Blue line corresponds to SDM, and red line depicts a continuous laser of the same average power. B. Arrhenius integral at low retinal burn risk SDM parameters, showing axial variation in the neural retina, RPE, and choroid. Traces corresponding to hyperpigmented RPE and choroid are shown in red. Peak value remains below the damage threshold V = 1, even in the case of hyperpigmentation. Right side: A. Calculated temperature rise at higher retinal burn risk SDM laser parameters (10% DC). Temperature rise is higher, reaching a peak of 57 C in the normal pigmentation case. B. Arrhenius integral at higher retinal burn risk SDM parameters. Maximum value of the Arrhenius integral in RPE does not exceed the damage threshold (V = 1) for the normal pigmentation case. With hyperpigmentation, the damage threshold is exceeded, which may lead to an ophthalmoscopically or fluorescein angiography–visible lesion. From: *Luttrull JK, Sramek C, Palanker D, Spink CJ, Musch DC. Long-term safety, high-resolution imaging, and tissue temperature modeling of subvisible diode micropulse photocoagulation for retinovascular macular edema. Retina 2012; 32 (2): 375-86.*

by monitoring, repairing, and removing damaged proteins from the cell. This prevents accumulation of toxic aggregates of misfolded proteins that would otherwise lead to progressive cell dysfunction and ultimately to cell death. Illustrating this function, Munk and associates described a case of nyctalopia that developed in a cancer patient treated with HSP blockers to potentiate chemotherapy. Once the HSP blocker was discontinued, the nyctalopia resolved (Munk et al 2014).

The response of HSPs to existential threats can be described as "salvific" or saving the cell from destruction. The salvific response is especially sensitive to the acuity and severity of the noxious stimulus, be it temperature, pressure, or chemical (Kregel 2002, Richter et al 2010). The cell temperature profile of SDM MRT shows that an average RPE cell hyperthermia of 6–8°C is achieved, with peak pulse temperatures of an additional 6–8°C on top of this average (Luttrull et al 2012). Both are sufficient to activate RPE HSPs, but the addition of the multiple recurrent pulse peak temperatures in series, abruptly, severe but still sublethal, are additional activators of the HSP salvific response (Dorin 2003, Richter et al 2010, Luttrull et al 2020, Rybinski et al 2019, Szymanska and Zylicz 2009, Baldwin 2007, Sramek et al 2007) (Fig. 8). Because the salvific response is designed to improve the cell's survival chances in the face of an acute, life-threatening crisis, the salvific response is immediate, robust, catalytic, and wide-ranging, triggering cascades of rapidly widely acting secondary protective, restorative, and reparative responses at the cellular, tissue, organ, and systemic level (Richter et al 2010, Luttrull et al 2012, Caballero et al 2017, Luttrull and Chang 2020). The net effect of activation of the HSP salvific response is a physiologic reset in the affected cell. "Reset theory" accounts for every observation of retinal laser effects from all laser modes and has allowed accurate prediction of all new retinal laser applications.

Key point: MRT resets and reprograms dysfunctional RPE cells to their "factory settings."

What does not kill me makes me stronger.

—Friedrich Nietzsche

MRT elicited hormesis: snatching life from death

It is the salvific function of HSPs that is therapeutically exploited by MRT (Sramek et al 2011, Luttrull et al 2012, Iwami et al 2014, Inagaki et al 2015, Lavinsky et al 2016, Caballero et al 2017, Kern et al 2018, Midena et al 2018, De Cillà et al 2019, Chang and Luttrull 2020, Luttrull AJO 2020, Frizziero, Calciati, Midena et al 2021). In the simplest sense, MRT works by making the RPE cell "think" it is going to die (Richter et al 2010). By so doing, all the protective, reparative, and restorative resources available to the cell are summoned in an attempt to preserve the cell and thus cell function. By activating and "waking up" the salvific HSP response in these settings, degeneration can be stopped, slowed, and even reversed, and chronic

inflammation diminished (Luttrull et al 2015, Luttrull and Margolis 2016, Chhablani et al 2018).

By providing an acute, severe thermal stimulus suprathreshold to RPE HSP activation but well below the threshold of thermal cell death, MRT activates the HSP salvific response to repair cellular damage, restoring and normalizing cell function, reducing chronic inflammation by activating reparative immunomodulation (Luttrull et al 2012, Caballero et al 2017, Midena et al 2018, De Cillà et al 2019). Improvement in health and function by applying sublethal stress to a biologic system is termed *hormesis*. Stress can also alter transcription, translation, and gene silencing or expression by inducing epigenetic changes. These include DNA methylation, histone modification and/or activation or inhibition of noncoding RNA (Dayeh et al 2016). Epigenetic alterations can be pathologic or homeotrophic, transient or permanent, and occur in response to virtually any stress. MRT is a stressor. The permanent reversals in DR severity following MRT, because of their duration, may reflect hormetic epigenetic changes induced by the stressor of MRT (Luttrull et al 2006).

Virtually any noxious stimulus can activate a hormetic HSP response. This includes any type of destructive retinal laser such as PC or photodisruption, such as produced by conventional and short-pulse CW lasers and nano-second lasers (Chhablani et al 2018). However, noxious stimuli damaging to the retina are also generally self-defeating, as the adverse effects of treatment—principally loss of functional tissue and excessive inflammation—reduce the net benefits of treatment (Figs. 1-4, 11-13). While any type of retinal laser exposure is potentially clinically effective, reliable safety is the unique province of microsecond pulsed lasers, epitomized by SDM. As mentioned previously, this is because while CW laser treatment becomes less safe as it becomes more effective, microsecond pulsing allows independence of safety from efficacy such that treatment can be tailored to be both more effective and safer at the same time (Luttrull and Sinclair 2014, Chhablani et al 2018, Chang and Luttrull 2020). Thus, very broad therapeutic windows and safety margins can be tailored to create "fixed" (nontitrated and universal) laser settings for use to treat all eyes of all patients safely and effectively for all appropriate indications, without regard for patient-specific factors such as diagnosis, lens status or media variations, retinal thickness, or pigmentation (Tables 3 and 4). Use of such fixed MRT laser

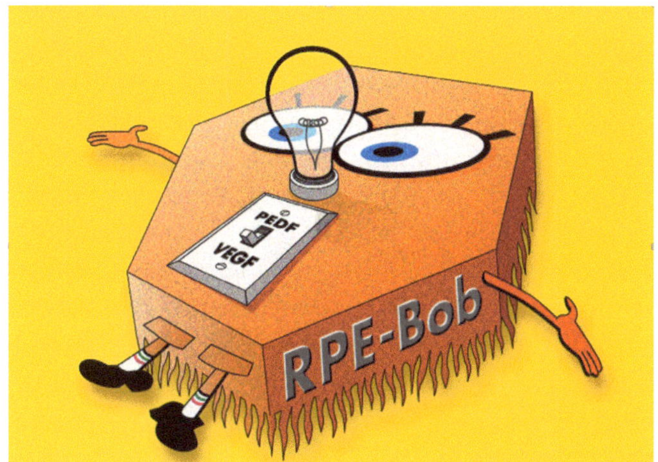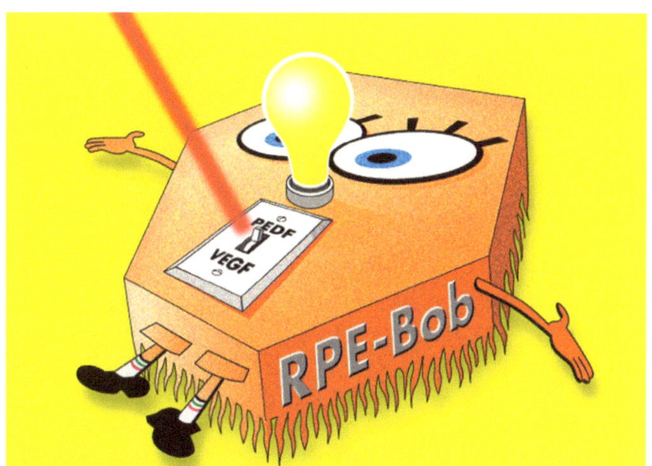

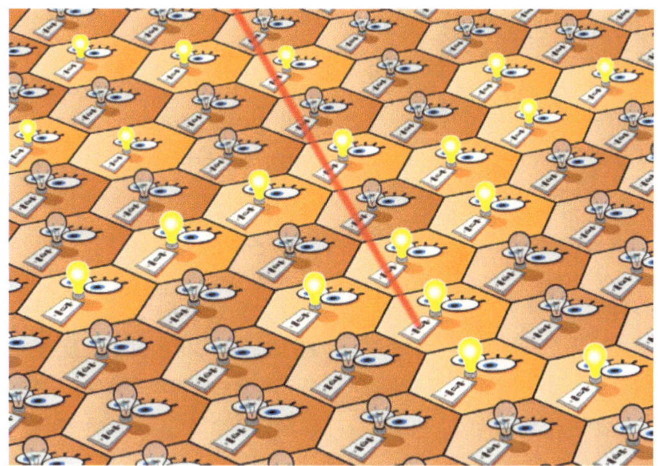

Fig. 10. Cartoon depiction of the low-intensity / high-density treatment strategy. "VEGF" denotes a dysfunctional RPE cell producing excessive vascular endothelial growth factor. "PEDF" denotes an RPE cell functionally normalized by SDM laser now favoring production of anti-angiogenic and neuroprotective pigment epithelial derived factor (PEDF). Note that the response to laser exposure at the cellular level is like switch, "on" or "off", and that the overall therapeutic effect of converting a single dysfunctional cell is minimal. Thus, while local treatment can improve the area exposed to MRT, there is little overall effect on the overall retinopathy, the influence of which may continue to fuel local disease such as DME. Therefore, MRT maximizes the therapeutic effects of treatment by confluent treatment over a wide area to recruit and convert as many dysfunctional RPE possible to optimize the clinical response by treating the retinopathy as a whole, like drug therapy. Because MRT has no effect on normal cells, the greater the area of retina directly exposed to confluent treatment, the greater the capture of dysfunctional retina and the greater the overall therapeutic effect, without adverse treatment effects.

parameters also minimizes the risk of retinal damage and visual loss from surgeon error, either from misjudgment or intentional use of inadvisable laser settings (Figs. 12 and 13). This facility represents another of the revolutionary, rather evolutionary, advances of MRT. By standardizing retinal laser treatment parameters, and as we will see, treatment techniques, MRT changes retinal laser treatment from a procedure dependent on surgeon experience and idiosyncrasy, to a standard "dose": uniform, predictable, and repeatable like drug therapy. This can only be described as an advance over the traditional approach to retinal laser therapy.

Key point: Any laser mode or other retinal stressor can be therapeutic. However, only microsecond pulsed laser administered as MRT is both reliably safe (sublethal to the RPE) and maximally effective.

Homeotrophy

While homeostasis describes that processes that maintain normal cell function, homeotrophy refers to restoring normal function from a prior state of dysfunction. This is the fundamental effect of MRT and the reset mode of action and hormesis (Luttrull et al 2015, Luttrull and Margolis 2016). Normalization of the RPE and thence the neurosensory retina in response to MRT thus results in predictable improvements and normalization of retinal function and the retinal milieu. Biologic changes following SDM-like

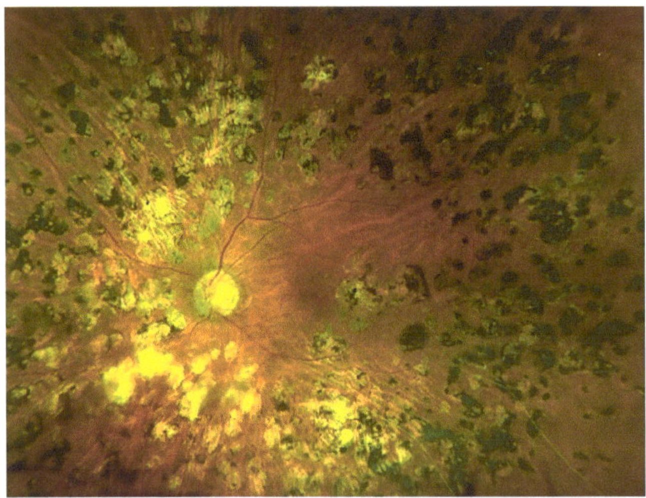

Fig. 11. 60 year old patient treated for diabetic retinopathy with conventional photocoagulation. Although effective, there is loss of visual field, mesopic visual acuity and night vision. Eventually, central vision may be lost due to progressive expansion of the macular laser burns into the fovea, or secondary choroidal neovascularization. MRT can inhibit both.

treatment reflecting such improvements have been identified *in vitro* and in animal and human studies as well. Some include normalized retinal cytokine expression, balance, and response; normalization of VEGF and pigment epithelial-derived factor production and equilibrium; and normalized glial fibrillary acidic protein (GFAP), inwardly rectifying potassium (Kir), and aquaporin (AQP) 4 expression (Midena et al 2018). Other effects include improved mitochondrial function and cellular metabolism, improved proteostasis and upregulation of the ER UPR, inhibition of apoptosis, reduced indicators of (degenerative) chronic and increased indicators of (reparative) acute inflammation; decreased reactive oxygen species and increased nitrous oxide and superoxide dismutase; improved retinal autoregulation; improved Mueller cell function and immunomodulation with local immune and stem cell activation and recruitment of systemic immune cells to the retina; and modulation of tissue matrix metalloproteinases (Karu 1989, Kegel 2002, Hattenbach et al 2005, Flaxel et al 2007, Beckham 2008, Sramek et al 2011, Iwami et al 2014, Inagaki et al 2015, Lavinsky et al 2016, Caballero et al 2017, Kern et al 2018, Midena et al 2018, De Cillà et al 2019, Wei et al 2019).

It is remarkable to consider that every response from effective photothermal stimulation sublethal to the

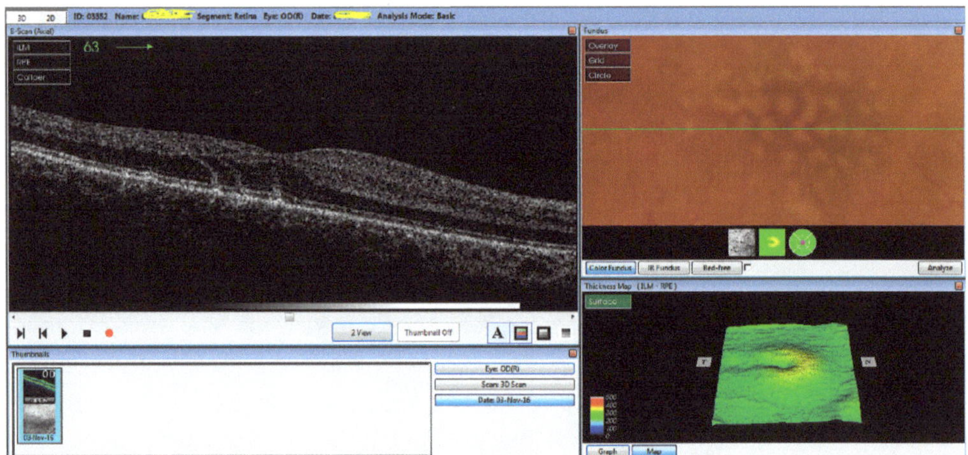

Fig. 12. Fundus photograph and optical coherence tomography (OCT) of eye after 577 nm micropulse laser treatment. The stated indication for treatment was macular edema due to a branch retinal vein occlusion. A titration algorithm was used to determine the subthreshold laser treatment parameters. A low-density conventional grid pattern of treatment application was employed, which traversed the fovea using a 5% duty cycle. The day following treatment the patient noted visual loss and multiple spots in his vision. One week postoperatively the fundus photograph demonstrates a grid of Q5 threshold macular photocoagulation lesions, including the fovea, and near-full thickness retinal damage at the foci of laser spot applications by OCT. From: *Chang DB, Luttrull JK. Comparison of subthreshold 577nm and 810nm micropulse laser effects on heat-shock protein activation kinetics: Implications for treatment efficacy and safety. Transl Vis Sci Tecnol. 2020 Apr 28;9(5):23.doi: 10.1167/tvst.9.5.23. eCollection 2020 Apr.*

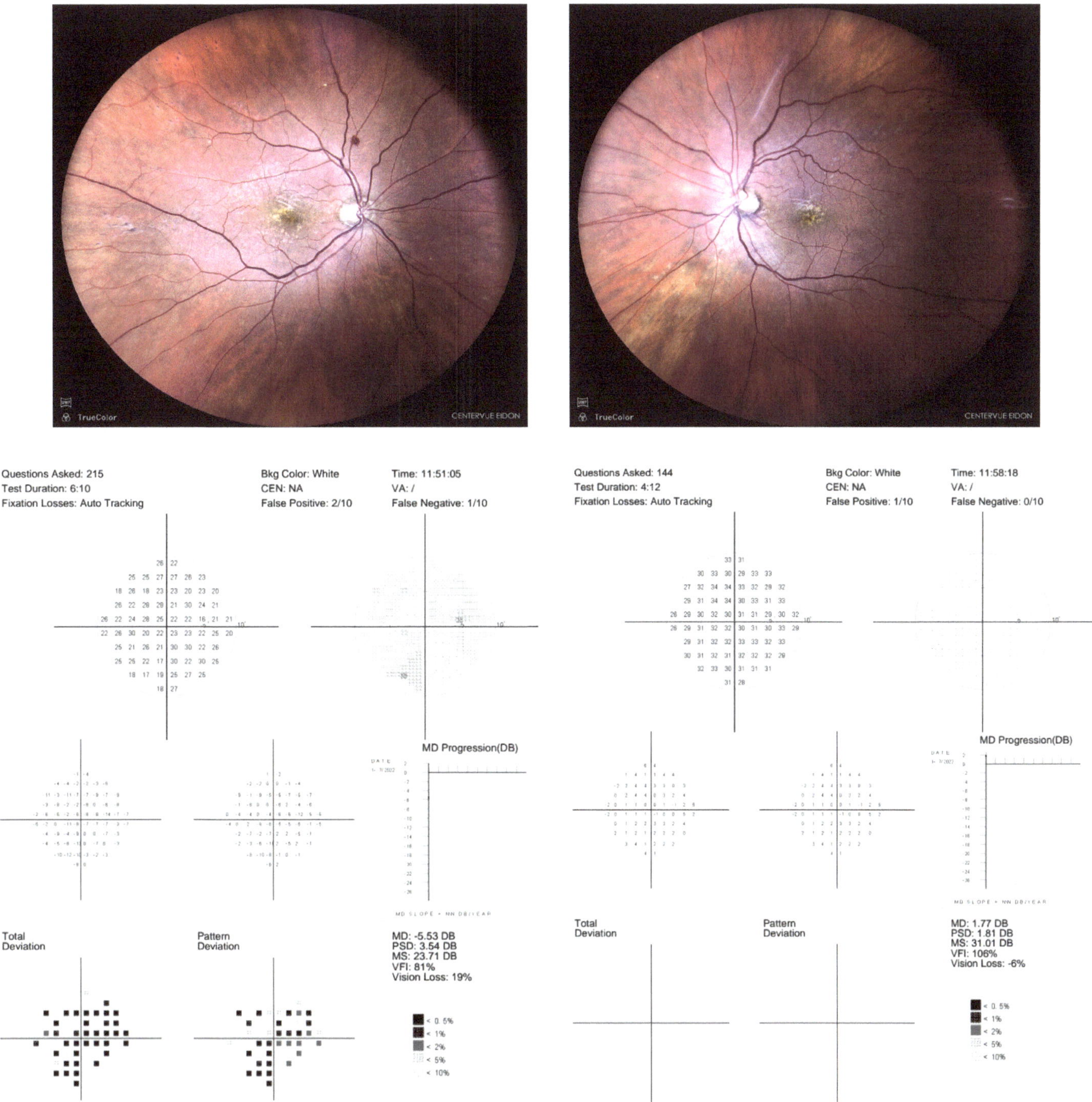

Fig. 13. Fundus photograph of both eyes taken August 2022 of an 82 year old woman who received vision protection therapy (VPT, regular periodic panmacular SDM MRT) for intermediate AMD OU beginning 2014. (A) Right eye, (B) left eye. In 2018 the patient moved to another state, where, at the patient's request, a retina specialist continued VPT using SDM laser parameters recommended by the author. Continuing to do well, in late 2019 he told her he was going to do a different laser treatment in her right eye because he "wanted to go deeper." At the time of treatment she noted many bright flashes of light, unlike her prior VPT. Immediately after treatment the patient reported a white-out of her vision with marked vision loss in the right eye lasting several weeks. Over a period of the next year the "white film" over the vision in her right eye gradually diminished, gradually replaced by the increasing notice of many small "spots" throughout her vision. At the time of this photograph in 2022, the patient continued to experience paracentral vision loss and the many point scotomata. In the fundus photograph of the right eye (A), note decreased drusen and incipient geographic atrophy above, temporal, and inferior to the fovea in areas occupied by multiple small focal laser burns. Note the titration burns in the temporal and superior periphery. (B) Shows intermediate dry AMD managed with VPT alone, without retinal laser burns. (C) Automated perimetry of right eye August 2022 showing visual field loss due retinal damage from visible wavelength photocoagulation titrated in an attempt to perform subthreshold treatment. (D) The visual field of the same date of the left eye managed by VPT alone demonstrating supranormal sensitivity.

Table 4. Example Treatment Parameters for Various Laser Modes and Settings and Effects on Therapeutic (Clinical Safety) Ranges

Laser Mode	Wavelength (nm)	Retinal Spot (um)	Power (Watts)	Duty Cycle (%)	Spot Duration (Seconds)	Therapeutic Range[g] (Watts)
Nano[a]	532	400	~24(mJ)[d]	CW	3×10^{-9}	0
Micro[b]	532	100	~ 0.117[d]	CW	0.00002	0.010
MP⁶[c,e]	577	105	0.250	5	0.20	0.29
MP⁶[c,e]	810	210	1.4	5	0.15	4[h]
MP[c,e,f]	810	525	1.7	5	0.30	15[h]

[a]Nanosecond continuous wave (CW).
[b]Microsecond CW.
[c]Micropulsed.
[d]Estimate, by titration.
[e]Fixed, published.
[f]Fixed, currently preferred; used in over 20,000 consecutive panmacular treatments (Luttrull, unpublished data 2020).
[g]Calculated difference between the laser power at given laser parameters required for reaching the activation threshold of 1.0 for the Arrhenius integrals of the therapeutic reset effect (lower limit of TR) and the 50/50 risk of thermal cell death (upper limit of TR).
[h]Note that the TR of these 810 nm laser parameters exceed the maximum available power of current retinal lasers allowing use in all eyes of all patients for all indications, safely and effectively.

RPE and retina ever reported has been therapeutic and restorative. No adverse effect has been identified in any experimental or clinical setting. It is difficult to think of another active intervention about which this can be said.

Key point: MRT is hormetic and homeotrophic, normalizing retinal function. This means it makes it more normal, not absolutely normal.

MRT and the endoplasmic unfolded protein response (ER UPR)

One of the critical relations in the process of maintaining and restoring cell function is the role of HSPs in the "unfolded protein response" (UPR) of the endoplasmic reticulum (ER) (Stella et al 2021, Terrab and Wipf 2020, Vitale et al 2019, Smith and Malluci 2016, Hetz et al 2020, Melo et al 2022). Proteostasis is essential to normal cell function and maintained by the ER. Within the ER, misfolded proteins are repaired or degraded, and toxic aggregates of unfolded proteins prevented and degraded. In disease, the concentration of unfolded proteins may exceed the ability of the ER UPR to process them effectively. When this happens the ER UPR triggers apoptosis, or an orderly programmed cell death. Apoptosis is a normal physiologic process whereby old, damaged, or misbehaving cells are removed with the least amount of collateral damage, to ensure and maintain proper tissue and organ function. The degree and pattern of disease-induced apoptosis generally defines the phenotype of the various CPRs (ADM, DR, IRDs, OAG, etc.) and the type and course of visual loss than typically ensues (Smith and Malluci 2016, Hetz et al 2020, Melo et al 2022). HSPs are critical to the ER UPR by virtue of their "chaperone" function. In this role, HSP 70 in particular, the main HSP activated by photothermal stimulation the RPE via MRT, identifies and collects misfolded proteins throughout the cell, including from the cytosol, the mitochondria, and nucleus, and protects them from further hydrostatic disorganization and damage from the aqueous cytosol, and ferries them (thus the "chaperone" function) to the ER membrane for transfer into the ER for reprocessing (Smith and Malluci 2016). Increased activity of the HSP chaperone function upregulates the ER UPR to increase its ability to respond to the increased demand of an injured or dysfunctional cell by increasing both protein transcription and translation within the ER, as well as repair and degradation of abnormal proteins and aggregates (Vitale et al 2019, Melo et al 2022). Hormetic upregulation of the ER UPR and the chaperone activity of MRT activated HSPs can thus inhibit apoptosis and enhance transport of proteins to the Golgi apparatus and the mitochondria (Melo et al 2022). Thus, one of the most important survival promoting therapeutic of MRT HSP activation commences within minutes of the thermal stress with stressor-induced upregulation of the endoplasmic reticulum (ER) unfolded protein response (UPR).). With the UPR, misfolded proteins are either rescued or diverted down the ER-associated degradation pathway (ERAD) and then shuttled to the cytosol for further degradation by the ubiquitin-proteasome system (UPS) (Almanza et al 2019, Friedlander et al 2000, Hiller et al 1996, Travers et al 2000). MRT activated HSPs can also direct cytosolic proteins towards an autophagy by facilitating the transport of proteins to lysosomal complexes, termed *chaperone-mediated autophagy* (CMA) or by upregulation of macroautophagy (Stetler et al 2010, Kiffin et al 2004, Majeski and Dice 2004).

Key point: MRT provokes a hormetic response in the retina. MRT works by making the RPE cell think it is going to die without harming it.

It takes time

The effect of HSP activation is "turning back the clock" on the disease process and revitalization of cell function. This is the critical attribute of the reset phenomenon triggered by MRT. Chronic disease requires both a primary defect and time. Only time allows the effects of that primary defect—such as insulin resistance, or a genetic defect in RP—to become manifest. This happens by progressive accumulation of unfolded proteins over time, failure of proteostasis, increasing cell dysfunction, immune failure, and ultimately cell death, and the chronic inflammation both resulting from and driving these degenerative changes. In AMD, the primary defect is time itself. Thus, the overarching effect of the reversal of these changes is literal reversal of cellular aging. In CPRs in general, upregulation of the ER UPR and associated processes by MRT-induced HSP activation reverses, at least for a time, the progress of the disease. By maintaining these reversals and renewing them on a timely basis by regular periodic retreatment, MRT can slow, stop, or reverse progression of chronic disease and reduce the resultant risks of functional losses. (Figure 6) Clinically, this is manifest by improvements in VA, visual fields, microperimetry, mesopic visual function, electrophysiology, reversal of retinopathy in diabetes, slower progression of disease and geographic atrophy, reduced vision loss and development of neovascularization in dry AMD, and reversal of anti-VEGF drug tolerance in dry AMD, to note a few (Luttrull et al 2005, 2006, 2008, 2015, Luttrull and Margolis 2016, Smith and Malluci 2016, Luttrull, Sinclair et al 2018, Luttrull, Samples et al 2018, Hetz et al 2020, Melo et al 2022, Luttrull and Gray 2020).

Key point: Vision loss requires more than the presence of an abnormality like defective gene or diabetes mellitus. It also takes time. Restoration requires turning back the clock.

Defining an injury: insights from wound healing on MRT mediated restoration
David Kent, MD
Liverpool School of Medicine,
Institute of Aging and Chronic Disease, Liverpool, England

David Kent has made an essential contribution to our understanding of the mechanism of retinal laser treatment by complementing our appreciation of the reset phenomenon with the dynamics of wound healing, inflammation, and tissue repair. In the following sections, Dr. Kent provides an overview:

To elucidate the possible mechanism of action of MRT, it is first of all necessary to understand that, irrespective of disease etiology (in this case CPRs), the response by any tissue in the body to injury (in this case the retina) is both stereotypical and generic (Clark 1996, Singer and Clark 1999, Kent 2015). In other words, MRT exploits this predictable tissue response for therapeutic purposes.

An injury may be defined as any process that induces tissue damage (Clark 1996). Biologically, the body deals with two types of injury, those arising from external trauma and those arising from normal biological processes within (metabolic). External or environmental injuries can be either acute (accidents, acute infection, surgery etc.) or chronic (smoking, chronic infections, chronic dietary/environmental/industrial toxin exposure etc.). Injury arising from within can be broadly understood as occurring from the "wear and tear" arising from normal cellular metabolism (Medzhitov 2008). This distinction is relevant here because in this context we can consider thermal retinal laser (MRL and conventional LPC) as a form of iatrogenic external injury (Chidlow et al 2013, Wood et al 2013, Caballero et al 2017). In contrast to external injuries which for the most part are undesirable, we can almost consider "wear and tear" injuries as physiologic or unavoidable in that they result from normal biological processes (Medzhitov 2008). Regardless of their "normality," these physiologic injuries still require repair and, in this context they are no different from external injuries (Xu et al 2009). As stated previously, the response by the body to injury is to launch the canonical reparative or stereotypical wound healing response (Medzhitov 2008). However, there is one other important difference to point out in relation to these two injury types: external injuries tend to be noxious in that they inevitably cause tissue destruction (and therefore trigger scarring/fibrosis; MRT is an exception to this biological canon) whereas the injury arising from normal metabolism can be considered to be occurring within the confines of the cell and though causing damage to intracellular organelles that require repair, this repair is not inherently destructive or pro-fibrotic.

Inflammation and repair

One of these stereotypical fundamentals to ensure repair is the generation of inflammation (Clark 1993, Singer and Clark 1996, Kent and Sheridan 2003, Xu et al 2009). This cannot be overstated. Without inflammation repair does not occur, a situation that is incompatible with life. Failure to heal from metabolic injury means failure to maintain cellular homeostasis and therefore gradual decline in cellular function and eventual activation of the cell death response (CDR), the molecular signature of all age-related neurodegenerative disorders, including CPRs (Stetler et al 2010, Almanza et al 2019). Therefore, at their most basic, age-related chronic disease can be considered to result from the progressive failure or inability to maintain cellular/intracellular repair (Kent 2015, 2021). To understand the pivotal role of inflammation in the maintenance of cellular health, it is necessary to take a closer look at the interactive roles of the various immune cells that coordinate the inflammation-repair axis.

As stated, everyday normal function produces "wear and tear" of tissue and generates waste, or "self-debris," such as damaged cells and macromolecules. Specific examples of this self-debris include unfolded or damaged proteins, fatty acids, amyloid, advanced glycation end-products and peroxidized lipids (Franceschi and Campisi 2014). This self-debris has a variety of fates: proteins or peptides, for example, can be repaired or be broken down into their constituent amino acids by the proteasome and then be recycled, other macromolecules can be dispensed through autophagy while others can be expelled from the cell into the extracellular matrix (ECM) (Almanza et al 2019). Self-debris in the ECM is antigenic and is referred to as

a damage-associated molecular pathogen or a DAMP (Roh and Sohn 2018). Its removal from the ECM is therefore immune-mediated and generates a basal, or physiologic, inflammatory response at local tissue level (Xu et al 2009). Resident macrophages and mast cells act as housekeepers in the removal of this self-debris (Medzhitov 2008). With time, this "housekeeping" immune function becomes less efficient due to aging (in effect the very beginning of immunosenescence) while another biological consequence of aging is increased generation of self-debris and indeed less efficient intracellular processing (Xu et al 2009, Fulop et al 2016).

The net result of the gradual decline in the performance of these various molecular pathways is the requirement for an increased inflammatory input to maintain cellular homeostasis (Medzhitov 2008, Xu et al 2009). In fact, this heightened but necessary immune state, may also trigger activation of the inflammasome. The inflammasome is a protein complex that is assembled in response to internal or foreign "danger signals" that ultimately leads to caspase-1-mediated maturation of pro-inflammatory cytokines such as interleukin(IL)-1β and IL-18 (Ambati 2013). Medzhitov coined the term *para-inflammation* to describe this heightened inflammatory state that is neither truly physiologic nor typical of what we consider classic inflammation (Medzhitov 2008). Moreover, with further aging, this para-inflammatory phase will eventually approach a stage of outright inflammation that can be measured clinically and in turn signifies that the inflammatory component required for homeostasis has escalated beyond a local tissue response to the harnessing of systemic immunity and includes the recruitment of additional leukocytes and the systemic expression of pro-inflammatory cytokines (Xu et al 2009).

Meanwhile, the aging clock continues to tick in both the tissues and in the immune system adding further to the inverse disparity between increasing self-debris and decreasing immune-driven reparative efficiency. Consequently, there is a transition from para-inflammation to full blown systemic chronic inflammation (*inflammaging*) as reflected by the presence of systemic inflammatory biomarkers (Franceschi et al 2000). In fact, we consider these biomarkers to be actual surrogates of this increased reparative demand rather than the conventional paradigm that their presence confirms that the pathogenesis of CPRs (and indeed all age-related diseases) is inflammatory mediated (Franceschi and Campisi 2014). We propose instead that the pathogenesis of these diseases arise instead due to an age-related decline in immune-based tissue repair (Kent 2021). It is important to emphasize that the foregoing outlines the normal process of repair arising out of the need for the maintenance of homeostasis. Age-related disease only ensues when this process is eventually overwhelmed, taking years or decades, in genetically predisposed individuals, usually in combination with environmental risk factors (Xu et al 2009, Kent 2021).In this context we consider diabetes to be a cause of an accelerated form of aging and therefore most of the complications arising from it, like DR, therefore arise because of the relentless reparative demands placed on the immune system, notwithstanding that chronic hyperglycemia also intrinsically interferes with the reparative functions of the immune system in its own right (Burton and Faragher 2008, Berbudi et al 2020).

Let us now briefly turn to what we might more intuitively understand as conventional wound healing and simply pose the question why do tissues heal following injury? To ensure the complete or adequate healing following any external injury, an acute inflammatory response is a fundamental necessity, and we believe it is this principle more than any other that explains the unique effect of MRT in the management of CPRs (Clark 1993, Singer and Clark 1999, Cabellero et al 2017). As stated earlier these CPRs are characterized by failure of repair (resulting from chronic and nonhealing metabolic injury) with the presence of chronic inflammation acting as a surrogate of this failure rather than being causal in pathogenesis (Kent 2021). Applying basic wound healing principles in this scenario, we postulate that the delivery of MRT, a brief and acute thermal tissue-sparing injury (stressor), will generate an acute inflammatory response and subsequently the promotion of the necessary molecular cascades that will induce healing and therefore preservation or recovery of retinal homeostasis.

MRT and the heat shock response and HSPs

As discussed earlier, MRT is a nonlethal thermal injury to the RPE activating HSPs via the heat shock response (HSR) in the RPE, that launches this necessary prorepair cascade (Richter et al 2010). Importantly, we further believe that it is the long-term effects of HSP activation (minutes to weeks) that is crucial to reset the cell towards homeotrophy and not just the instantaneous effects of the HSR in relation to misfolded proteins (Sramek et al 2011, Chang and Luttrull 2020). Moreover, it is HSP activation, acting as a gateway to a multitude of both intracellular and immune-harnessing proreparative pathways, as will now be outlined, that explains why MRT, delivered specifically to the RPE, has such wide-ranging therapeutic benefits, benefits that can extend well beyond the RPE to include the NSR.

MRT and the proteasome

The RPE HSR can be defined as a cytoprotective response that promotes stability of the proteasome following nonlethal injury (Richter et al 2010). Remember that most CPRs are characterized by a pathological accumulation of toxic misfolded proteins arising from either age-related excess, or failure of the proteasome to deal with this excess (de Pedro et al 2015, Ferrington et al 2016, Lynn et al 2017). This proteotoxic stress causes mitochondrial dysfunction that in itself results in excessive generation of reactive oxygen species (ROS) (Plafker 2010). Therefore, one of the most important prosurvival therapeutic benefits arising from MRL-induced HSP activation commences within minutes of the injury with stressor-induced upregulation of the endoplasmic reticulum (ER) unfolded protein response (UPR) (Mori 2000, Almanza et al 2019). With the UPR, misfolded proteins are either rescued or diverted down the ER-associated degradation pathway (ERAD) and then shuttled to the cytosol for further degradation via the classic ubiquitin-proteasome system (UPS) (Hiller et al 1996, Almanza et al 2019, Friedlander et al 2000, Travers et al 2000). Furthermore, HSPs can also direct cytosolic proteins towards an autophagic fate by either facilitating the transport of these proteins to lysosomal complexes, the so-called chaperone-mediated autophagy (CMA) or through an upregulation of macroautophagy (Kiffin et al 2004, Majeski and Dice 2004, Stetler et al 2010).

MRT and the antioxidant response

Another potential benefit of MRT-induced HSP activation is the multiple downstream cytoprotective effects resulting from the specific activation of the transcription factors heat shock factor protein 1 (HSF1) and nuclear factor erythroid 2–related factor (Nrf2), the induction of which is impaired in aging RPE (Akerfelt et al 2010, Sachdeva et al 2014, Dayalan et al 2015). Under basal conditions HSF1 is negatively regulated by tethering to both HSP70 and HSP90 in the cytoplasm, but following nonlethal injury (tissue-sparing MRT), it becomes activated, translocates to the nucleus, and binds to heat stress elements on its target genes (Akerfelt et al 2010). Similarly, Nrf2, normally regulated by Kelch-like ECH-associated protein 1 (KEAP1), similarly translocates to the nucleus and binds to antioxidant response elements (AREs) in its target genes (Kensler et al 2007, Suzuki et al 2013). Indeed, both transcription factors target overlapping protective genes, including those for the autophagy target protein p62, HSP70 and heme oxygenase 1 (HEMOX1) (Prestera et al 1995, Komatsu et al 2010, Wang et al 2014, Dayalan et al 2015). Yet another benefit of the MRL-induced HSR to HSF1 and Nrf2 in CPRs could be the promotion of a more reduced state in aging and/or diseased retina that likely contains potentially cytotoxic levels of oxidants (Sachdeva et al 2014, Xu et al 2014). Both transcription factors, but especially Nrf2 (through the action of the Nrf2-dependent enzyme glutathione reductase), have profound effects on levels of reduced glutathione (GSH) in the cytosol and the generation of mitochondrial superoxide dismutase (Yan et al 2002, Holmstrom et al 2013, Han et al 2020).

MRT and the inflammasome

If we consider that one of the characteristics of CPRs is persistent activation of the inflammasome (most typically the nucleotide-binding domain (NOD)-like receptor protein 3 (NLRP3) inflammasome), then it is reasonable to speculate that MRL, either directly through the HSR, or indirectly through the generation of an endogenous but 'therapeutic' danger signal (production of mitochondrial and cytosolic ROS), that results in triggering Nrf2 transcription, may modulate either inflammasome priming or activation in these aged and sick RPE or indeed in the NSR itself (Xu et al 2014, Davis and Ting 2010, Tschopp and Schroder 2010, Zhou et al 2011, Jhang and Yen 2017). The precise mechanism on how this is achieved is unknown but it may involve nuclear factor kappa B (NF-κB) transcrip-

tion (Pasparakis 2009, Hennig et al 2018). Of course, one of the pathological consequences of inflammasome activation in CPRs and neurodegenerations in general is cell death through pyroptosis (Celkova et al 2015). Activation of HSP70 has been demonstrated to be a negative regulator of inflammasome activation so this may be one mechanism by which MRL abrogates the CDR in RPE (MRL-induced neuroprotection) (Martine et al 2015). In this context, we contend that the acute 'injury' delivered by MRT, unlike the chronic metabolic injury associated with neurodegeneration, is therapeutic and must, by definition, promote inflammation because it launches a reparative cascade (Caballero et al 2017).

MRT and the cell death response

It is our further contention that the role of MRT in generating a neuroprotective HSR can also be extended to include abrogation of the UPR- and mitochondrial-mediated CDR (Stetler et al 2010, Almanza et al 2019). In the face of chronic overwhelming metabolic injury (neurodegeneration), the CDR is triggered by multiple and simultaneous upstream intracellular pathways that ultimately converge into a final common pathway which ends with apoptosis (Stetler et al 2010). The CDR includes the release of cytochrome c and apoptosis-inducing factor (AIF) from the mitochondria and their association with the proapoptotic B-cell lymphoma-2 (bcl-2) family in the cytosol, activities that can be either directly inhibited by HSP70 or indirectly prevented through inhibition of prodeath kinases such as c-Jun N-terminal Kinase (JNK) (Gabai et al 2002, Park et al 2002, Gotoh et al 2004, Stankiewitz et al 2005). In addition, HSP70 can also inhibit pro-caspase 3 formation and block assembly of the apoptosome by complexing with Apoptotic protease activating factor 1 (Apaf-1), and, by binding directly to AIF itself, sequesters it in the cytoplasm, thus preventing it from translocating to the nucleus (Selah et al 2000, Gurbaxani et al 2003, Komorova et al 2004). Meanwhile, HSP27 can also hinder the activity of members of the bcl-2 group by direct inhibition of Apoptosis signal-regulating kinase 1 (ASK1) and death-domain associated protein 6 (DAXX) while HSP90 inhibits caspase-2 activation and simultaneously prevents apoptosome formation (Pandey et al 2000, Charette et al 2020).

MRT and immunity

As outlined these MRT-provoked intracellular pathways (upregulation of the UPR, autophagy and antioxidant defenses together with inhibition of apoptosis) work in concert with the immune system to ensure cell survival in neurodegenerative conditions including CPRs. We believe that HSP activation is central to this role in accommodating cross talk between a cell and the recruitment of both innate and adaptive immunity and that such a mechanism may be a further potential therapeutic mechanism of MRL on RPE (Caballero et al 2017, Murshid et al 2019). Of course, this modulation of the inflammatory response may involve the inflammasome and proponents of the inflammatory hypothesis of age-related disease may suggest that inflammasome activation could potentially induce cell death rather than rescue. Yet, it must be acknowledged that inflammasome assembly is also pivotal in maintaining cellular homeostasis and these contrasting dual roles highlight the context-dependent dichotomy of various pattern recognition receptors (PRRs) and their role in both health and disease (Strowig et al 2012). In the context of neurodegenerative RPE (disease context), we speculate that the induction of MRT-induced acute inflammation (therapeutic context) may physiologically "reset" the inflammasome to promote homeostasis and trigger an appropriate innate immune response that supports neuroprotection, rather than promoting pyroptosis.

If MRT promotes homeostasis and neuroprotection, then it follows that it reverses the chronic and destructive "all or nothing" innate immune response that characterizes neurodegeneration and harnesses a nuanced and proportionate response by adaptive immunity which facilitates repair in CPRs. We realize this is provocative to proponents of the inflammatory hypothesis of chronic disease, but we believe the recruitment of systemic adaptive immunity (immunotherapy) should be central in the consideration of therapeutic neuroprotection (Schwartz et al 2010, 2020). HSP releases from cells, either in free form or through exosomes, is known to cause such adaptive recruitment and is, therefore, the potential mechanism whereby MRT recruits therapeutic adaptive immunity in the promotion of neuroprotection and repair (Murshid et al 2019). Free HSPs in the extra-cellular matrix can bind to scavenger receptors, such as oxidized low-density lipoprotein receptor-1 (LOX-1) and scavenger receptor class F member 1 (SCARF1)

expressed on both macrophages and dendritic cells (DCs) and be processed for antigen presentation to T lymphocytes that ultimately lead to activation of an adaptive immune response that contributes to tissue repair (Asea et al 2000, Facciponte et al 2005, Lancaster and Febbraio 2005, Mambula and Calderwood 2006, Li et al 2007, Chalmin et al 2010, Gong et al 2010, Murshid et al 2011, Tsen et al 2013, Guo et al 2018). Such a scenario is certainly exciting to consider as it introduces the novel concept of photo-vaccination as a genuinely viable therapeutic option, either alone or as an adjuvant, for a whole host of neurodegenerative conditions, including CPRs (Enomoto et al 2006, Gong et al 2009).

Finally, there is the potential contribution of bone marrow-derived hematopoietic stem cells to be factored into retinal repair following MRL, which again appears to be mediated by HSPs (Cabellero et al 2017). In an animal model evaluating the effects of MRT, it has been demonstrated that MRT generated an acute inflammatory response that led to not only microglial proliferation but also their migration to the outer retina along with neutrophilic, monocytic, lymphocytic, and bone marrow stem cell infiltration (Caballero et al 2017). Whereas the other cells were detected within hours to days, consistent with a "therapeutic" laser injury and the onset of acute inflammation, the presence of reparative progenitors was only detected some two weeks later. This coordinated, sequential arrival of these various immune cells is not only consistent with tissue repair but also supports the notion that the MRT effect is catalytic in nature and that the therapeutic benefits are more likely due to these longer term effects rather than the instantaneous effects of a modest increase in HSP expression and activation, our so-called concept of "lighting the fuse" (MRT-induced HSP activation) to set off a series of controlled and coordinated therapeutic "explosions" within the cell and beyond (Clark 1996, Chang and Luttrull 2020).

MRT and biological controversies

The foregoing regarding what we believe to be the possible mechanisms of action of MRT highlights a number of potential biologic incongruities in the literature. For example, as outlined earlier, does MRT activate the inflammasome and if so, could this promote pyroptosis? In contrast, if MRT is neuroprotective as we claim, then does this mean that MRT inhibits inflammasome activation? Could different HSPs have contrasting effects? For example, if HSP90 plays a role in NLRP3 priming in RPE, then could this mean that MRT-induced activation of this HSP promotes a CDR? (Piipo et al 2018). In contrast, MRL-induced activation of HSP70, a negative regulator of NLRP3 inflammasome activation, may have the opposite effect (Martine et al 2019). Similar contradictory conclusions can be made in relation to the role of the NF-κB family of transcription factors in inflammasome priming and activation. If MRT, as we propose, triggers an acute inflammatory reaction, then it is logical to assume that this involves NF-κB activation and as an extension of this logic, it can be argued that this once again promotes cell death. In contrast, it is also recognized that NF-κB signaling is not only central to the promotion of homeostasis but that its inhibition induces a state of severe chronic inflammation (Pasparakis 2009). There is also the whole aspect of the interplay between canonical and noncanonical pathways of inflammation/repair to be considered and how they may be affected by MRT.

On the subject of inflammation and various cellular pathways involved in inflammation, we prefer the term *modulation of the inflammatory response* rather than the binary nomenclature of a biological effect or intervention being either anti- or proinflammatory. Moreover, we believe it is the context of the inflammatory response that determines whether it is pathological and leading to neurodegeneration (CPRs) or physiological (MRT) and leading to neuroprotection, survival, and homeostasis (Doyle et al 2012, Kauppinen 2012, Tseng et al 2013, Tarallo et al 2012). This dichotomy further highlights the complex and often poorly understood interplay between various intracellular pathways, how they may vary from tissue to tissue, from one cell type to another, and even between identical cells in the same tissue (Davis and Ting 2014, Hennig et al 2018, O'Koren et al 2019). In addition, the context (physiological versus pathological or acute versus chronic) in which these pathways are activated or inhibited is similarly important (Hennig et al 2015). Finally, these diverse therapeutic pathways that are activated by MRT expose the challenges that are faced by pharmaceutical interventions in attempting to achieve these same therapeutic outcomes.

Resolution of these paradoxes certainly requires further investigation in general and, specifically in relation to MRT will form the basis of future studies. Nevertheless, bearing in mind our current level of understanding, we respectfully propose that it may well be the biological context that determines a cell's fate. In the context of neurodegeneration, we propose that it is the combination of a chronic pro-oxidative state, decreased antioxidant defenses, defective proteostasis and chronic inflammasome activation, which promotes the CDR while in the context of robust cellular health and homeostasis, activation of these same pathways promotes preservation and survival. In short, we believe that, regardless of the precise mechanism of action(s), MRT behaves as a catalytic switch that converts the neurodegenerative cellular phenotype to a neuroprotective one.

Summary of MRT mechanism of action

In summary, CPRs are characterized by age-related failure of immune-mediated repair due to a combination of ongoing lifelong cell injury and immunosenescence. A surrogate biomarker of this failure is the presence of chronic inflammation and immune cell infiltration in and around the Bruch's membrane/RPE complex while the RPE themselves are characterized by a dysfunctional proteasome, raised levels of oxidants and persistent inflammasome activation, hallmarks of a chronic neurodegenerative injury. We hypothesize that MRT, by activating the innate heat shock response, triggers a therapeutic cascade which involves multiple molecular pathways that result in the promotion of RPE homeostasis. Intracellularly, these pathways include upregulation of the antioxidant response, promotion of protein folding, activation of both the UPR and autophagy and downregulation of the canonical NF-κB pathway which results in inhibition of inflammasome assembly and ultimately abrogation of the CDR. Meanwhile, HSPs, released into the ECM, are processed by scavenger receptors on DCs and macrophages that ultimately leads to the recruitment of T cell-mediated adaptive immunity (photo-vaccination). This immunotherapeutic response is further enhanced by the mobilization of HSCs. The net result is a modulated acute inflammatory response that promotes a tissue repair phenotype and a return to cellular homeostasis. Finally, because MRT is by definition tissue sparing, it can be repeated at regular intervals to maintain cellular health in the face of ongoing chronic neurodegenerative-promoting metabolic injury.

Key point: Senescent local and systemic immune failure and the wound healing response shed important light on the manifold ways MRT can act to restore and normalize retinal function to prevent disease progression and visual loss.

Retinal glia and MRT

Immunoactivation has a generally negative connotation, because it is typically associated with immune dysfunction and the diseases that result, such as autoimmune diseases. Not so with MRT. Thus, the qualifier "therapeutic." Caballero and associates found local retinal activation of retinal immune cells in an animal model of SDM, as well as recruitment to the retina of bone-marrow derived immune cells to both eyes if only one eye was treated (Caballero et al 2017). Biomarkers of Muller cell activation have been identified in the aqueous of patients treated with SDM for DME (Midena et al 2020). Separately, HSP activation has been found to activate neurons and astroglia in neurodegenerations and stimulate cell proliferation (San Gil et al 2017, Gao and Xing 2009). As noted earlier, retinal micro- and macroglia, resident retinal immune cells, play key roles in both disease and healing. Retinal microglia are monocytic cells charged with surveilling the retina to provide neuroprotection in response to injury or threat. Microglia react to inflammation and tissue damage with amoeboid morphologic transformation, migration, inflammatory cytokine production, and proliferation that propagate and exacerbate neuroinflammation. Such changes are identified early in eyes with OAG in response to elevated intraocular pressure (IOP) and are implicated in GC loss. Microglial and Muller cell (macroglia) activation occurs in response to retinal cytokine signals, largely of RPE origin, the target of MRT (Kolomyer and Zarbin 2014, Wei et al 2019). HSP activation occurs in response to virtually any stimulus the cell perceives as an existential threat. This includes retinal laser (Kregel 2002, Richter et al 2021). HSP activation has also been shown in GCs in response to IOP elevation (Wei et al 2019). Axonal degeneration has been correlated with microglial activation in glaucoma and shown to precede GC death (Bosco et al 2012, Howell et al 2013). Activation of microglia may result in two distinct

phenotypes, referred to as "M1" and "M2," having antagonistic portfolios. M1 activated microglia predominate in neurodegeneration and are associated with neuroinflammation and are key drivers of glaucomatous degeneration. M2 activated microglia take on an opposite role, acting restoratively by reducing neuroinflammation and inhibiting apoptosis. The M2 microglial phenotype activity is thus neuroprotective. Thus, the Muller cell activation identified by Midena and associates following SDM for DME represents laser-induced M2 modulation (Midena et al 2020). By the same token, astrocytes, including macroglia such as retinal Mueller cells, also take on dual and opposing roles in response to specific cytokine signals, with the "A1" phenotype driving inflammation, complement fixation, promoting apoptosis, and neurodegeneration; while "A2" phenotypic astrocytes are neuroprotective, anti-inflammatory and improve and preserve retinal (and thus axonal and GC) function (Wei et al 2019). Thus, RPE HSP activation and normalization of retinal function includes normalized retinal cytokine expression and response leading to homeotrophic retinal microglia M2 and astrocyte A2 activation yet another important potential contributor to the homeotrophic reset response to MRT (San Gil et al 2017, Gao and Xing 2009). Finally, HSPs are also known to be key modulators of stem cell proteostasis, activity and function (Salimi et al 2018). Thus, in addition to RPE HSP activation and normalization of retinal function including normalized retinal cytokine expression and response leading to homeotrophic retinal microglia M2 and astrocyte A2 phenotype activation, immune cell mediated paracrine regeneration of preapoptotic cells and activation of resident and circulating and bone-marrow derived stem cells recruited to the retina may also contribute to retinal restoration in response to MRT. Like HSP activation, the effects of M2, A2, and stem cell activation are neuroprotective and agnostic to the underlying cause of the retinal dysfunction. In animal models of A2 and M2 activation in retinal degenerations, retinal function measured by electrophysiology is improved, similar to that demonstrated following SDM MRT in CPRs (San Gil et al 2017, Gao and Xing 2009, Otani et al 2004, Fukuda et al 2013, Moisseiev et al 2016). The general lack of success, thus far, of retinal stem cell therapy has much to do with technical problems associated with transplantation (Park et al 2017). It may be that *in situ* activation of resident retinal stem cells and recruitment of bone-marrow derived stem cells to the retina by stimulators such as SDM laser may offer an alternative to tissue transplantation. Recent clinical evidence suggests that MRT neuroprotection in CPRs may progress to neuroregeneration (see Chapter 12 "Glaucoma"). Activation of cellular immune restoration including MRT triggered stem cell activation could explain this observation (Luttrull and Bhavan 2022). This is just another of the endless opportunities for further research afforded by MRT, as per Information Theory (Cover and Thomas 2006).

Key point: MRT engages the full range of physiologic restorative processes available to improve retinal health and function.

A switch, not a dial

In nature, activators, enzymes, or other substances that speed reactions are far less common than inhibitors (Wang et al 2022). This fact is indicative of the value of MRT as an activator of restorative immunoactivation for retinal neuroprotection. The importance of MRT in this regard is underlined by the absence of any drug or biologic yet identified to do the same.

As a form of bioactivation (working by exceeding an enzymatic activation threshold, in this case RPE HSP 70), three additional key attributes are evident, following from the earlier mentioned text (Katsumata 1969). First, the response to treatment is always maximal. Rather than an adjustable, titratable response at the cellular level, like a rheostat, the response at the cellular level is a "switch" phenomenon, either "on" or "off." (Luttrull and Dorin 2012) (Fig. 9). As noted earlier, this is despite analyses of HSP activation kinetics showing that actual laser-induced increases in activated HSPs are relatively small, as reflected in *in vivo* and *in vitro* studies (Sramek et al 2011, Luttrull et al 2012, Iwami et al 2014, Inagaki et al 2015, Lavinsky et al 2016, Caballero et al 2017, Kern et al 2018, Midena et al 2018, De Cillà et al 2019, Luttrull AJO 2020, Chang and Luttrull 2020, Frizziero, Calciati, Midena et al 2021) (Fig. 4). As a catalytic threshold response, the treatment response cannot be increased by exceeding the activation threshold (Luttrull AJO 2020). However, if one thinks of HSP activation as a fuse, it is clear that the size of the fuse is less important than the bomb. This is the MRT-induced acceleration in HSP protein repair kinetics, constant $k_{10,}$ upregulation of the ER UPR, and local and systemic therapeutic immunoactivation

that follows (Chang and Luttrull 2020). Thus, second, for the same reason, the response to treatment cannot be improved by repeating treatment in the short-term in an attempt to increase the response by "stair-stepping" (Fig. 9). Third, the immediate effects of treatment wear off rather quickly (the half-life of normal proteins in normal cells only being about 90 minutes), although later and downstream effects may be long-lasting and even permanent (Chang and Luttrull 2020). The duration of MRT treatment effects is highly specific to, and characteristic of, the underlying disease process. In general, the more severe the dysfunction, the shorter the treatment half-life reflecting the severity of the stressor on protein folding and function (Luttrull and Margolis 2016, Luttrull 2018, Luttrull and Kent 2019, 2020). But, as the mechanism of action allows, once the clinical effects wane, because MRT is reliably sublethal and homeotrophic to the RPE, treatment can be repeated with reproduction of the same maximal treatment response, regardless of the number of retreatments, and over what period of time maintenance treatment needs to be continued. For most CPRs—with the possible exception of DR, as we will discuss later—maintenance treatment may need to be carried on for the lifetime of the patient to maximize treatment benefits and minimize the risks of vision loss (Luttrull and Gray 2022).

Key point: MRT works by bioactivation, exceeding the activation threshold of an enzyme system (HSPs). It is thus an "all or nothing" response.

Etiologic agnosticism

An especially interesting property of the actions of HSPs, following inevitably from the mechanism of action described earlier is that the actions of HSPs are agnostic to the cause and type of cell protein misfolding, and consequent cellular dysfunction (Kregel 2002, Richter et al 2010) MRT RPE HSP activation is thus a "non-specific trigger of disease-specific repair" (Luttrull and Dorin 2012). The importance, elegance, and utility of this property of MRT cannot be overstated. As this results in normalization of cell function, it is an example of a physiologic "reset to default" phenomenon (Luttrull et al 2015, Luttrull and Margolis 2016). Disease-specific repair means that each disorder will be improved and restored according to the particular nature and menu of protein misfolding induced by that particular disease stressor. Thus, while MRT will improve both AMD and DR, they will be improved in different and unique ways reflecting the different disease processes. These disease-specific responses to MRT are often easily seen clinically in reference to the disease process—resolving ME in DR and serous macular detachments in central serous chorioretinopathy (CRS), for instance. As we will discuss below, this specificity also extends to indices of visual and retinal function, including characteristic disease-specific improvements in electrophysiology following MRT, different, for instance, in AMD, IRDs, and OAG in specific ways (Luttrull and Margolis 2016, Luttrull, Samples et al 2018).

Key point: MRT acts as a nonspecific trigger of disease-specific repair.

See the world with new eyes, or just through different lenses, and 'presto!'—a whole new world.
—John Steinbeck

Aging, the chronic progressive retinopathies, and MRT

As noted, the most important causes of irreversible visual loss are the chronic progressive retinopathies of AMD, DR, OAG, and the IRDs. Visual loss from each requires two key ingredients: a stressor, and time. Viewed in this way, visual loss from each of the main CPRs can be thought of as an aging problem, and the problem of aging as the accumulated effect of unaddressed biologic stressors (Lu et al 2014, Meusser et al 2005, Morimoto 2020, Walther et al 2015, Wang-Michelitsch and Michelitsch 2015). Thus, the problem of treatment of the CPRs is not different than the quest for longevity and prevention of aging, increasingly thought of as a disease process in its own right (Brandvold and Morimoto 2015) (Fig. 10). Along such lines it is interesting to note that a meta-analysis of AMD prevalence found a decreasing prevalence of AMD since 2006, attributed to generally improving health (Colijn et al 2017). Competing with this trend is, for the same reason, increasing longevity leading to increasingly larger numbers of people with AMD.

Diabetes can be seen as an accelerated form of aging with the neurodegeneration of DR resulting from the relentless reparative demands placed on the immune system, compromised by chronic hyperglycemia interfering with the normal reparative functions of the immune system (Sinclair and Schwartz 2019, Berbudi et al 2020, Burton and Faragher 2018, Pillar et al 2020). A biomarker of such failure is the presence of chronic perineurovascular inflammation and immune cell infiltration in DR, and around the Bruch's membrane/RPE complex in AMD. Within the RPE itself is a dysfunctional proteasome and elevated reactive oxygen species (ROS), both hallmarks of a chronic neurodegenerative injury (Stetler et al 2010, Roh and Sohn 2018, Almanza et al 2019, Friedlander et al 2000, Tschopp and Schroder 2010). All these abnormalities are amenable to hormetic immunomodulation from MRT (Sinclair and Luttrull 2022) (Fig. 13).

The question arises, "If HSPs are so effective, how is it that cells and thus tissues can become so thoroughly dysfunctional in chronic progressive disease? Why don't HSPs prevent progressive dysfunction, degeneration, aging and loss of function?" The simplest answer appears to be that the HSP system does not respond well to chronic diseases such as CPRs, because in an evolutionary context, senescence is sufficiently rare as to be unanticipated, and postreproductive survival of little concern (Kregel 2002, Baldwin 2007, Beckham 2008, Richter et al 2010). Primitive simple early organisms in which HSPs developed were generally short-lived, or died "young" from trauma or disease. Thus, the HSP developed to respond to acute, severe, life-threatening events of reproductively capable organisms, rather than the insidious degradations characteristic of chronic progressive diseases and aging. The slowly accumulating dysfunctions of chronic disease develop and progress largely "under the radar" of the HSP system, failing to trigger a salvific response, such that the end stage of many chronic disease states of many organ systems is often characterized by failure of the HSP system itself (Xu et al 2012, Lu et al 2014, Srivastava et al 2016, Luttrull and Kent 2018).

Key point: MRT elicits an acute inflammatory response in the absence of injury to reduce or eliminate chronic inflammation. It is the absence of injury that unleashes the therapeutic potential of MRT.

5. Pillar II of Modern Retinal Laser Therapy: High-Density Treatment

If I'm not doing much, I'd better do a lot of it.

—The author

The therapeutic effects of conventional RPC and other modes of retina-damaging laser treatments arise entirely as side-effects of laser exposure. They are indirect, not direct, effects of treatment. Thus, as all direct effects of RPC and other damaging laser modes are adverse, they are contraindicated as complications of treatment. As a practical effect of LIRD is the fact that treatment density must be limited to prevent both immediate and late treatment-associated visual loss. This limitation on treatment density represents a significant limitation on treatment effectiveness and optimization as it results in—at best—only partial treatment.

Because the therapeutic responses of MRT arise from retina directly exposed to treatment but not killed, a "high-density" treatment strategy of MRT can be employed to maximize the therapeutic effects of low-intensity treatment sublethal to the RPE, optimizing the clinical benefits of treatment by *en masse* recruitment of dysfunctional RPE to the restorative and functionally normalizing process. This is accomplished by confluent treatment of large areas of dysfunctional retina. For macular disease, this is panmacular treatment. For generalized retinopathies, peripheral retinal treatment is added to achieve total retinal treatment, as is done with drug therapy (Keunen et al 2020) (Figs. 6 and 9). Because high-density treatment requires a high number of laser spot applications, patience is required. Patience is hard.

Most CPRs are generalized retinopathies wherein the retina is diffusely affected and abnormal. In the predominant maculopathies, such as AMD, the same can be said about the posterior retina. In the worst case, every RPE is abnormal and thus so is retinal function. In the "best" case—the earliest preclinical disease in the extreme—for instance, just one RPE is affected. Which one? But, because we are considering the case of CPRs, which are by definition progressive, only time separates the best and worst case. Medically, we want to intervene early, when treatment is most effective and thus the course of disease affected the most. If we must intervene late, we want to intervene as effectively as possible, again, to alter the disease course in the most favorable way possible despite the advanced condition. This means the ideal therapy should be equally applicable and optimized for both situations. Via the property, again arising from the reset mechanism, of "pathoselectivity," MRT is such a therapy (Luttrull et al 2015, Luttrull and Margolis 2016).

As previously noted, a fundamental property of the reset mechanism of MRT is that dysfunctional cells (those with high percentages of unfolded proteins) are improved by direct treatment and improved in proportion to the degree of dysfunction. This is because the more misfolded proteins there are, the more proteins that will be repaired as the result of treatment, and the more cell function that will be improved. By the same token, normal cells with little to no (excessive) protein misfolding will not be affected in any significant way by treatment, both in the percentage of misfolded protein present—already well regulated and maintained at physiologic levels by efficient ER UPR proteostasis, and thus with respect to resultant cell function. Normal cannot be made more normal. In an eye with diffuse dysfunction, completely normalizing the function of a single cell would clearly have no notable clinical effect. The clinical effect of treatment is thus clearly proportional to the number of dysfunctional cells treated and normalized. Because the target RPE is a monolayer, this translates to area of treatment coverage.

MRT uniquely exploits the pathoselectivity of the reset phenomenon to optimize and maximize the clinical benefits of treatment by allowing functional transformation of the dysfunctional retina to be maximized. With currently available technology, it is impossible to identify which cells in the retina are dysfunctional and to what degree. Ideally, one should treat them all to achieve the greatest clinical benefit. By virtue of the safety of low-intensity MRT, identification and localization of dysfunctional cells is unnecessary. One merely needs to treat all the retina in the area of concern (the macula in AMD, all of the retina in DR). By so doing, all dysfunctional cells will be included in treatment and the normally functioning cells will be left undisturbed. Note that anything less than confluent coverage of all retina of concern will be incomplete and necessarily less than maximally effective. In the RPC, this limitation was accepted in order to limit inherent treatment-associated visual loss. In the era of MRT and drug therapy, both retina-sparing treatments, such a compromise is no longer necessary, and thus no longer acceptable.

Treatment responses in CSR are illustrative of the importance of the high-density treatment paradigm. In eyes with CSR, low-intensity (sublethal to the RPE) low-density (avg. 110 applications of a 125-um spot size) has been shown to be ineffective in chronic CSR, and marginally effective in acute CSR (Malik et al 2015, van Rijssen et al 2019); while low-intensity/ high-density treatment (avg number of 700, 200 um spots) was found to be uniformly effective in both acute and chronic CSR (Luttrull 2016). While the one cannot really compare a large RCT to smaller studies, the poor results of the "PLACE" trial run counter to wider experience (Luttrull 2016, Battaglia-Parodi and Iacono 2019, Luttrull AJO 2020).

Treatment area, density, and the PLACE trial. Why people think MPL does not work

The PLACE trial is an excellent illustration of the importance of understanding what one is doing and why. It is not the only study to fail in this regard, just the most recent relevant to this discussion. In this case, the "what" and "why" are an understanding of the mechanism of retinal laser and employing the consequent principles of MRT. More is required for a good, meaningful, and useful study than prospective randomization and good statistical methods. To paraphrase a popular aphorism, you only get out of something the quality of what you put into it. In the PLACE study design, we see the all-too common mistake

of combining treatment concepts held over from the RPC era applied to the use of a microsecond pulsed laser "subthreshold" treatment (Battaglia-Parodi and Iacono 2019, van Rijssen et al 2019, Keunen et al 2020, Luttrull AJO 2020).

The PLACE trial compared half-dose photodynamic therapy to a microsecond laser for chronic and diffuse CSR, employing laser protocol of an 810 nm diode laser at 1.96 W, 125 um spot size, 5% DC, with average 110 applications (van Rijssen et al 2019). In a testament to the safety of 810 nm at a 5% DC, the PLACE trial did not report any case of LIRD, despite using a laser power at essentially maximum for the laser devices employed, and over twice the power previously reported for the spot size and other parameters. Thus, treatment met the definition of "low-intensity," by being sublethal to the RPE, despite use of an unnecessarily high power. Why was nearly 2.0 W employed when, for this spot size, 0.78 W had been reported to be highly effective? (Luttrull et al 2005, 2012, Chang and Luttrull 2020). According to the PLACE authors, this unprecedentedly high power was chosen to improve therapeutic effectiveness. Despite trying to perform "subthreshold" treatment, drawing on their experience with RPC, and in the absence of experience with microsecond pulsed laser, SDM, or MRT concepts, the authors stated that they believed efficacy would parallel (subthreshold) treatment intensity. This error led to a second (almost inevitable) error, the authors stating that this high laser power would overcome the planned low treatment density and small treatment area to achieve effective treatment (van Rijssen et al 2019). Thus, the authors mistakenly believed that laser treatment sublethal to the RPE would result in lateral heat spread to the retina surrounding the laser spots such as that produced by suprathreshold conventional RPC. The problem is that microsecond pulsing sublethal to the RPE produces no biologically significant collateral heating or heat spread outside the spot directly irradiated (Fig. 8). This has been demonstrated and confirmed theoretically, in the lab, and clinically. The thermal effects are limited entirely to the spot directly exposed to the laser beam (Sramek et al 2011, Chhablani et al 2018, van Rijssen et al 2019, Chang and Luttrull 2020) (Figs. 8-10). Thus, the PLACE trial employed the least effective of all retinal laser strategies: low-intensity (no burns were noted) combine with low-density;

with either high-density treatment localized to a small area (a kind of low-density treatment), or a low-density noncontiguous grid treatment spread over a wider area, leaving most of the area untouched. The study is unclear on this point except to say that an average of only 110 125 um spots were applied per eye per treatment. However, either approach would be expected to be largely ineffective. Compare this to the 400 500 um spots often employed in panmacular SDM MRT (Fong et al 2007, Luttrull and Dorin 2012, Keunen 2020) (Fig. 6). Long experience teaches that insufficient treatment *area and density* is by far the most common reason for novice failure when learning the use of MPL.

For surgeons accustomed to placing 5, 10, or even 20 small low-density spot applications for typical macular photocoagulation treatment, the hundreds of confluent spot applications in the macula necessary to maximize the treatment effects of MPL seems otherworldly, if not frightening. Such thinking fails to appreciate, as did the PLACE authors, that at the cellular level, the sublethal laser response is a threshold phenomenon occurring in only those cells directly exposed to the laser (Battaglia-Parodi and Iacono 2019, van Rijssen et al 2019, Keunen et al 2020, Luttrull AJO 2020, van Rijssen et al 2020). Below this level, treatment is biologically ineffective (< 1xMPE). Fortunately, that level is very low and this is seldom an issue clinically (Chang and Luttrull 2020). As an activation threshold phenomenon, exceeding the HSP activation threshold will not increase the therapeutic response. However, it will increase the likelihood of cell death if the Arrhenius integral for cell death is also exceeded. Further, as the effect of RPE HSP activation is a constant for the area directly exposed to laser, MRT dosimetry is primarily a function of treatment density and area rather than treatment intensity. Because the reaction to thermal RPE HSP activation is catalytic, any effective activation will result in a maximal response at the cellular level and thus in the area directly irradiated. Thus, the clinical response from a given area and density of dysfunctional retina will be a constant, "on" or "off," and not a gradient (Fig. 9). Only increasing the area of confluent treatment will increase the clinical treatment response (Luttrull and Dorin 2012, Luttrull et al 2012, Chang and Luttrull 2020) (Fig. 7).

Sometimes more is better

The PLACE trial illustrates the importance of adequate treatment density and area very well, although not intentionally. Consider the following thought experiment: (1) Any localized retinal treatment that is sublethal to the retina must necessarily work by treatment-induced therapeutic normalization of retinal cell function (We do not really know how PDT works, but for the sake of this experiment, it is reasonable to assume that this is the end result) (Luttrull 2007). (2) The clinical effect of normalizing the function of a single cell is minimal. (3) The clinical effect of normalizing the function of every dysfunctional retinal cell is maximal. (4) Therefore, for any treatment of the retina that is both therapeutic and sublethal to the retina, the clinical effect will be largely dependent on the thoroughness of the functional transformation achieved by treatment. Since each individual cell exposed to treatment is maximally transformed, this thoroughness is a function of treatment density and area. So, let us compare the difference in treatment area of the various sublethal retinal treatments in question: the PLACE trial MPL protocol area (avg 110 spots × 125 um spots = 1.4 mm^2); a typical 3 mm PDT spot (7.1 mm^2); to the area of panmacular SDM MRT and the International Retinal Laser Society guidelines for subthreshold laser (~36 mm^2) for treatment area ratios of 1/5/26 (PLACE MPL/PDT/MRT). Thus, in the PLACE trial, the area of treatment covered by half-dose PDT exceeded the retinal treatment area of the PLACE MPL by 5X. Not surprisingly, PDT worked better (Chang and Luttrull 2020, Keunen et al 2020, Luttrull AJO 2020). What difference would a 26X increase in treatment area with MRT make over the PLACE MPL protocol? According to the PLACE authors, none. However, employing MRT principles the author has yet to experience a CSR treatment failure, clearly different from the PLACE results. As one would predict based on this obvious difference alone, the PLACE microsecond laser protocol was ineffectual and inferior to half-dose PDT, paralleling the area of high-density treatment.

Thus, instead of comparing the effectiveness of MPL to half-dose PDT, what the PLACE study actually compared was a simple standardized procedure which did not require practitioner skill or experience (PDT) to a different procedure requiring some skill and experience, performed by practitioners apparently inexperienced with MPL and MRT concepts using an ill-conceived treatment protocol destined to fail (Battaglia-Parodi and Iacono 2019, van Rijssen et al 2019, Luttrull AJO 2020). Such undertreatment (inadequate treatment area and density) is by far the most common cause of novice failure with MPL for all indications. This reflects application of traditional high-intensity RPC thinking and techniques to low-intensity treatment. The low-intensity/low-density laser treatment protocol employed in the PLACE trial is the least effective of any retinal laser treatment strategy for any type of laser mode for any indication. The trial results speak for themselves (Fong et al 2007, Luttrull and Dorin 2012, Lavinsky et al 2011) (Figs. 6 and 9).

The chief causes of human errors is to be found in the prejudices picked up in childhood.

—Rene Descartes

Key point: The most common novice error for those learning MRT is undertreatment, the result of thinking in terms of RPC and manifest by placing too few laser spots over too small a retinal area in too low a density.

6. Targeted versus Nontargeted Therapy: Fragility versus Antifragility

There is nothing that can't be made more complicated.

—The author

An idea is always a generalization, and generalization is a property of thinking. To generalize means to think.

—GWF Hegel

While science tends to think of itself as binary, the reality of biology—and thus medicine—is analog. There are no zeros and ones, no "always" and "nevers." The possibilities are endless and on a continuum. As noted earlier, it is thus interesting to reflect that effective treatment with MRT via the reset phenomenon requires minimal understanding of the underlying disease process. While this may sound like MRT has no real scientific basis or that the users of MRT are uninformed, this is actually quite a good and advantageous property for any treatment to have, due to the analogous nature and complexity of biology. It is impossible to imagine developing a single drug that could do all of the things that MRT does in all of the disparate conditions it does them in. This places MRT in the realm of the "antifragile" (Taleb 2012). A brief digression should serve to illustrate:

Antifragile describes processes that actually become more effective in the context of uncertainty or chaos. Are there such things? Why is this important and what does it have to do with MRT?

It is helpful to consider "fragile" processes first. A fragile process is one that requires a very precise knowledge and highly accurate assumptions and very specific conditions to be effective or successful. An example of a fragile process is targeted drug therapy. For targeted drug therapy to work, one must first select the right target. Next, one must effectively target the therapy. Finally, the beneficial effects of treatment must outweigh any adverse treatment effects. While this may sound simple and straightforward, it is in fact prohibitively difficult and unlikely. Why?

Math. There are approximately 2,000 different types of molecules in the typical cell. All interact to some degree. Thus, altering anything within a cell eventually alters everything within the cell (the "butterfly effect") (Kellert 1993). These 2,000 different types of molecules have 10^{680} possible and thus eventual interactions (DB Chang, personal communication 2016). As if such numbers were not daunting enough, recent studies suggest that almost half of intracellular proteins remain unidentified, and thus their actions and interactions are unknown (Quin et al 2021). At a femtosecond pace, the universe is not old enough to allow the time necessary to run through all the interactions of all the molecules in a single cell resulting from a single perturbation. These kinds of numbers have implications. For practical purposes, the effects of any therapy targeting a process within a cell may as well be infinite. Such a vast number and variety of potential interactions arising from any targeted intracellular manipulation are thus, certainly in a practical sense, impossible to predict, and impossible to control.

Key point: MRT is antifragile and thus robust and useful.

Strategic Studies is an academic discipline that is self-describing. Following on von Clausewitz, the motto of Strategic Studies is "No plan survives implementation." Targeted therapies are examples of highly planned strategies (Clauswitz 1832). How can anything go wrong?

First, even if one successfully targets the desired molecule or process effectively, the downstream effects of that perturbation rapidly lose any relation to the initial intended alteration, as these effects rapidly expand exponentially away from the point at which the pebble hits the pond. This means that most of the effects of any targeted drug therapy are unknown and impossible to predict, simply due to their number. Further, this means that unanticipated and thus likely unintended consequences exceed by far the intended effects of any targeted therapy. Broadly, there is one intended and desired effect of targeted therapy while there are a near infinite number of unintended and potentially undesirable effects.

Second, effective targeted therapy typically requires a precise set of conditions to be met for the targeting, and its hoped-for therapeutic effects, to be achieved. These might range from simply taking the medication, to interactions with other drugs or medical conditions, patient age, sex, correct dosage, and timing, and so on. Common sense suggests that reliance on the ideal is a poor plan, as perfection is seldom encountered.

Against such odds, what is required to create a new effective and safe targeted therapy? First, the conditions for effective therapy and the desired interaction and effect have to be right, if not perfect. Rare. Second, the correct target must be chosen from the vast number of possibilities. Third, the target must be affected in the desired way to achieve the hoped-for effect. Fourth, the innumerable unanticipated and unintended adverse effects must be either fortuitously therapeutic, or sufficiently benign that they are tolerable when weighed against any benefits arising from the attempt at effective targeting. Unintended consequences are the only certainty in targeted therapies. Therefore, it is most likely that the overall effect of any targeted therapy will be dictated by unanticipated and unintended consequences making selection of the ideal target almost irrelevant. Consider for a moment how many of our most important drugs were originally intended for a purpose for which they failed, only to discover an unexpected and valuable therapeutic effect completely unrelated to the intended purpose. Thus, at the end of the day, the likelihood of developing safe and effective targeted therapy amounts to little more than chance.

Is this assessment of targeted therapy too sanguine? Certainly not in light of the probabilities. Consider another example from real life: A recent meta-analysis of randomized clinical trials (RCTs) leading to FDA approval of the leading oncologic chemotherapies found that none actually worked by effectively targeting as claimed. Instead, the effectiveness of these leading cancer chemotherapies was solely attributable to the fact that they were simply so toxic that they preferentially killed cancer cells over normal ones. Do chemotherapies work by effective targeting, or by causing vomiting, diarrhea, and hair loss? Apparently, the latter. In this they have much in common with RPC (Lin et al 2019).

Consider further the case of the targeted therapies we use to treat the visually threatening complications of the most important CPRs, VEGF inhibitors. They are highly effective and have revolutionized the treatment of, particularly, neovascular AMD (Solomon et al 2019). The success of these agents and the financial rewards for the manufacturers have created an understandable gold-rush mentality about new drug development in ophthalmology. But is this reasonable? First, realize that the task of binding extracellular factors, such as VEGF in the retina and vitreous, is vastly simpler than therapeutically altering cell function (described earlier). Anti-VEGF therapy is an example of a relatively antifragile process because it is generally effective and minimally dependent on circumstances. All that matters is the presence of VEGF. Anti-VEGF therapy represents the "low-hanging fruit" of targeted drug therapy. Targeting cell function, on the other hand, is a highly fragile proposition.

Moore's Law has accurately predicted the exponential increase in computing chip processing power since the 1960s. Eroom's Law (Moore spelled backwards) is the targeted therapy correlate to Moore's Law, but describes an inverse relation. Eroom's Law states that the development of safe and effective drugs is decreasing exponentially with time, while the costs of these increasingly unsatisfactory drugs will increase exponentially at the same time (Hall et al 2018). This is because, as described earlier, successful target therapy discovery is dictated by Murphy's Law. The modest results and high rate of adverse effects thus far associated with target therapy discovery complement inhibitors for age-related geographic atrophy (ARGA) are illustrative (Halawa et al 2021). Because public demand for cures and shareholder demand for industry profits are high, regulatory approvals continue apace. One need look no further than approvals for Luxturna for Leber's amaurosis and brolucizumab for neovascular AMD for examples. The underappreciated phenomenon of "regulatory capture" takes the process a step further. Nowhere is this better exemplified than in the approval of Aduhelm for Alzheimer's disease (Dal Bó 2006, Karlawish and Grill 2021, Enríquez et al 2021, Mendell et al 2021). Noteworthy is the fact that not a single new (non-VEGF inhibitor) drug or biologic for retinal disease has been approved since the introduction of anti-VEGF therapy with pegaptanib in 2004 (date of this writing, July 2022) (Holz et al 2018, Blau and Daley 2019). The reason? Fragility. The need for safe and effective targeted drug and biologic therapies is massive and we will almost certainly soon have approved targeted therapies for retinal diseases. Will they be both highly effective and very safe? Eroom's Law suggests it is not likely.

In the midst of chaos, there is also opportunity

—Sun-Tzu

Great results can be achieved with small forces.

—Sun-Tzu

The point of the preceding discussion is not to bash targeted therapies. We need them. They are simply extraordinarily problematic and difficult to develop and thus cannot be relied on to meet our needs to the degree that most expect. Instead, it is to praise the properties of MRT. MRT shares virtually none of the foibles and limitations of targeted therapies. As such, it is a far more promising and useful treatment approach. The property of antifragility is an enormous advantage that nontargeted therapies like MRT have over targeted therapies. Antifragility describes the ideal system or intervention. Instead of being vulnerable, conditional, tenuous, or one that depends on one or more conditions or assumptions being in a particular state, stable and/or ideal for its success, an antifragile process is one that continues to be effective, or is actually even more effective, in the face of the unexpected or chaos (Taleb 2012). An ideally antifragile treatment works, no matter what. For a fragile process to work, everything has to be perfect. Perfect is rare (Fig. 14 and 15). By acting on the universal currency of cell dysfunction, protein misfolding, MRT is applicable to almost any retinal

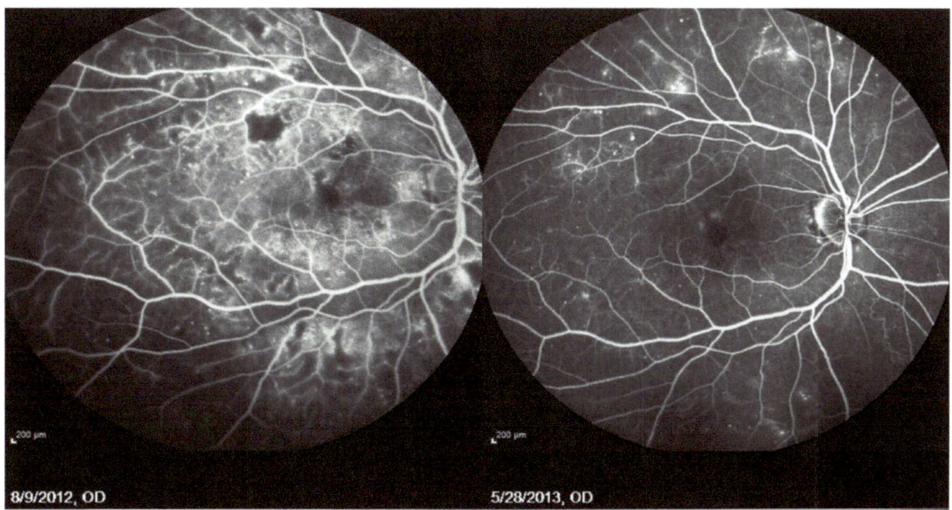

Fig. 14. FFA of eye with severe non proliferative diabetic retinopathy before (left) and 9 months after (right) total retinal SDM MRT. Prior to treatment, note diffuse micro and macrovascular leakage consistent with chronic neurovascular inflammation. Note focal areas of capillary non perfusion. Note resolution of vascular leakage and reperfusion of ischemic retina after treatment. Once reversed, the DR will not again worsen or pre-progress. (Note: photographic timer is in error. Actual post injection time for each photograph is approximately 10 minutes). From: *Chhablani J, Roh YJ, Jobling AI, Fletcher EL, Lek JJ, Bansal P, Guymer R, Luttrull JK. Restorative retinal laser therapy: Present state and future directions. Surv. Ophthalmol 2018 May - Jun;63(3):307-328.*

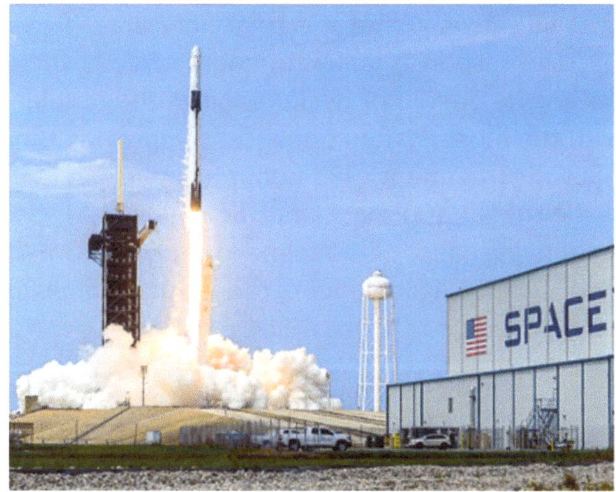

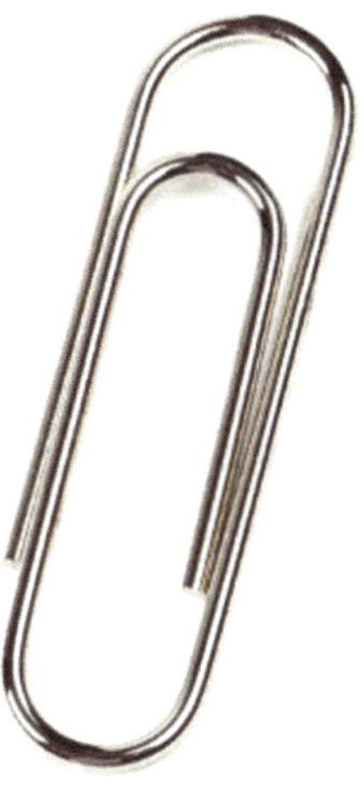

Fig. 15. Examples of fragility (left) and anti-fragility (right). One always works, the other often fails.

dysfunction from almost any cause, and every CPR. Because of the mechanism by which dysfunction is addressed, initiation of proteostasis and functional normalization by RPE HSP activation, MRT will be effective—that is, result in the intended biologic effect—in every clinical setting (such things as retinal detachment excepted) excepting two: either complete normality, or such severe end-stage dysfunction such that the HSP system itself fails and becomes nonresponsive and inactive. This is a common characteristic of end-stage disease in many organ systems (Dudega et al 2009, Xu et al 2012, Wang-Michelitsch and Michelitsch 2015, Wu et al 2018). Thus, MRT is scientifically elegant, a radically simple yet powerful conceptual approach and clinical application at odds with the complexities of the vast majority of targeted therapies.

One for all and all for one

The *reductio absurdum* of therapeutic targeting is the concept of "personalized" or "precision" medicine (Martin et al 2021). Such terminology echoes the ethos of our time. Me. But is it a good idea? Personalized medicine envisions treatments that are narrowly tailored to a particular disease process in a particular individual. The effect of such precision is to create as many diseases and treatments as there are people. Theoretically, such "precise" treatments would have no value to any other person or for any other condition. Personalization is a targeting goal breathtaking in its complexity and inefficiency. It is fragility by design. The alternative? *Non*-personalized medicine. While this term has less emotional appeal, it describes a more sensible goal: of a single, safe, and effective treatment that is curative for all ills, in all people, at all times: the "silver bullet" (OED 1989). Antifragile, acting by activating rather than attempting to alter normal physiologic processes—this is the genre to which MRT aspires. MRT is not alone in this regard. Other promising treatment approaches in the MRT genre include drugs and biologics that improve cell function generically to slow senescence, maintain health, and even extend longevity. Remarkably, it may be easier to reduce aging

than to independently cure cancer or heart disease. But by inhibiting aging, all the consequences of aging can be reduced as well, including most of the diseases amenable to MRT. Let us hope that what can be done in mice can be done in humans as well (Selvarani et al 2021).

Key point: Target therapies like drugs and biologics are highly fragile, limiting their usefulness.

Summary

While at odds with popular perceptions, the complexities of targeted drug and biologic therapies render these approaches the least promising therapeutic solutions for the task of preventing visual loss from the CPRs currently (Brooks 1896, Hall et al 2018). Rather than attempting to target and manipulate specific intracellular processes, MRT seeks to simply improve cell function broadly in a nontargeted fashion by triggering a biologic "reset" via activation of RPE HSPs. A rising tide floats all ships. This response is catalytic and leads to cascades of reparative and restorative reactions including upregulation of the ER UPR to normalize and improve retinal function and inhibit apoptosis, to stimulate local and systemic therapeutic immunoactivation. The effectiveness of treatment clinically directly parallels the degree of adherence to the twin pillars of MRT: "low-intensity" treatment that exceeds the Arrhenius integral for RPE HSP 70 activation while remaining far below the Arrhenius integral for thermal cell death; and "high-density" treatment consisting of confluent treatment of broad areas of clinically relevant retina to achieve *en masse* recruitment and functional transformation of all dysfunctional RPE cells within the treatment area (Figs. 6 and 9). The response to treatment is directly proportional to the degree of dysfunction at the cellular level, with the most dysfunctional cells improving the most following treatment. MRT is thus a pathoselective nonspecific trigger of disease-specific repair, agnostic to the underlying cause of the retinal dysfunction. MRT is thus highly antifragile, lending it an unusually high clinical utility.

Section III. General Clinical Considerations of Modern Retinal Laser Therapy

7. Neurodegeneration, Neuroprotection, and Neuroregeneration

A penny saved is a penny earned.

—Benjamin Franklin

Neuroprotection and neuroenhancement

In the context of chronic progressive disease, not losing form and function can be counted as gain. The fundamental effects of MRT are neuroprotection (preventing degradation) and neuroenhancement (improving function) (Stella et al 2021, Johnson et al 2022). The concept of neuroprotection in ophthalmology is so closely associated with glaucoma that it is easy to forget that it applies equally to the retina, and particularly with reference to the CPRs. As noted, MRT normalizes dysfunctional retina via the reset effect with little regard to the underlying cause of dysfunction. The retina is central nervous tissue, and the most common causes of irreversible visual loss are the degenerative retinopathies of AMD, DR, OAG, and the IRDs. Thus, all CPRs are neurodegenerations. As such, despite different etiologies and phenotypes, they share many, if not most important features in common. By improving retinal function, MRT is, by definition, neuroprotective.

The results of neuroprotection in the various CPRs reflect the characteristic abnormalities associated with each. Thus, retinal neuroprotection and neuroenhancement in OAG looks like improved visual fields and mesopic visual function, improved ganglion cell and optic nerve function, and either stopped or slower progression of glaucomatous optic neuropathy. In diabetes, retinal neuroprotection and neuroenhancement manifests as reversal of retinopathy severity, resolution of DME, and regression of neovascularization (NV). In AMD, retinal neuroprotection and neuroenhancement looks like improved visual function, slowed disease progression, slowed progression of ARGA, and reduced risks of visual loss including macular neovascularization and so on. In each, the effects of MRT elicited neuroprotection are disease-specific reduced future risks of visual loss, normalized retinal function, and decreased chronic inflammation. Note that we talk in terms of "retinal" neuroprotection even for OAG, because it is MRT treatment of the retina that produces the neuroprotective effects in all cases, including OAG, thus identifying the retinopathy of open-angle glaucoma (ROAG). Evidence of neuroprotection and neuroenhancement from MRT have been demonstrated in every CPR. These will be presented and discussed in detail in Section IV on "Clinical Applications."

Might effective neuroprotection do more than improve and maintain function and slow down disease progression? Anatomic improvements following neuroprotective MRT are easily observed in DR, with resolution of DME, regression of NV, reperfusion of areas of retinal ischemia, and resolution of micro- and macrovascular leakage. In AMD, the anatomic effects of MRT neuroprotection manifest primarily by slowing progression and preventing neovascular conversion (Luttrull, Sinclair et al 2018, Luttrull et al 2020, Luttrull and Gray 2022). Might these changes reflect more than neuroenhancement? (Johnson et al 2022). Can MRT-stimulated neurotrophy improve retinal neuroanatomy? A recent study suggests that MRT may be more than neuroprotective and neuroenhancing. It may also be neuroregenerative (see Chapter 12 "Open Angle Glaucoma and the Role of MRT").

Key point: All chronic progressive retinopathies are neurodegenerations. MRT is neuroprotective.

Diagnostic testing and modern retinal laser therapy

Functional versus anatomical markers

While the author will argue that MRT has as many uses as there are caues and types of macular dysfunction, by dint of social and economic impact, application of MRT to the most common CPRs—AMD, DR, OAG, and IRDs—is most important (Bourne et al 2019). As noted, all are neurodegenerations. Because MRT improves retinal function it is retinotrophic and thus neurotrophic and neuroprotective (Luttrull and Kent 2019). Intracellular molecular damage and cellular dysfunction always precede clinical disease and visual loss (Luttrull and Margolis 2016). This dysfunction, as noted, is due to a disease-specific menu of protein misfolding induced by and reflecting the particular stressor(s) of the primary disease process that will, with time, lead to disease-specific cellular and retinal dysfunction that characterize the clinical syndrome due to failure of proteostasis (Luttrull and Margolis 2016, Friedlander et al 2000). While intervention may occur at any point in the course of disease, it is this preclinical, purely physiologic, stage of dysfunction that is most amenable to treatment, allowing visual loss to be prevented—a critical consideration in that restoration of normal visual function, once lost, is difficult and rare (Luttrull and Sinclair 2014).

Physiologic dysfunction does not lend itself to most current modes of diagnostic testing, consisting predominantly of imaging of retinal structure and anatomy (Luttrull and Margolis 2016). In these earliest stages of disease most amenable to treatment, patients are asymptomatic. Retinal anatomy is generally grossly unremarkable and visual function is usually clinically normal. Thus, identification of the presence of disease and a risk of future vision loss requires retinal function testing, rather than structural imaging. In the same way, standard methods of visual testing employing high contrast photopic chart acuity and photopic visual field tests are more likely to miss the subtle first signs of visual dysfunction, than are more sensitive measures of visual function such as mesopic visual function testing (MVFT) (Arden et al 1982, Riggs 1986, Katz et al 2010, Lahav et al 2011, Feigl et al 2011, Puell et al 2012, Jackson et al 2014, Gutstein et al 2015, Stringham et al 2015, Luttrull and Margolis 2016, Luttrull and Kent 2019, Hirji et al 2021). As cardiologists are well aware, if you want to find out how well something is working, stress it. This is MVFT.

Key point: Retinal imaging is for advanced disease. Retinal function testing is for early diagnosis.

Retinal function testing

The following observations are based on years of experience with clinical methods for early detection and evaluation of the disease process in CPRs. These include measurement of the degree of baseline dysfunction; assessment and characterization of the response to MRT; temporal monitoring; and finally, confirming and characterizing the responses to retreatment (Luttrull and Margolis 2016, Luttrull and Kent 2019). It is key to remember that the biophysics of MRT is such that treatment will virtually always improve the function of dysfunctional retina (Chang and Luttrull 2020). Only complete normality or complete organ failure with failure of the HSP system would result in no treatment response. In the normal clinical setting, therefore, retinal function testing will generally detect both baseline retinal physiologic dysfunction, as well as the treatment response, in eyes with otherwise clinically normal vision and normal morphology, down to eyes with very limited—hand motions or worse—visual function and highly deranged morphology. Electrophysiology, such as pattern electroretinography (PERG) and the visual evoked response (VER) have proven especially useful in this regard (Luttrull and Margolis 2016, Luttrull, Samples et al 2018, Luttrull and Kent 2019). Because the PERG depicts the function of the full-thickness retina, and not only the photoreceptors as does the ERG, PERG can provide additional information that allows identification of characteristic disease-specific electrophysiologic dysfunctions and treatment responses. The PERG generally provides useful information even in eyes with RP that may have a flat, nonrecordable ERG.

The PERG responses in the CPRs are generally logical, reflecting disease characteristics, topography, and severity. In AMD, a low-contrast macular PERG has been shown to be most sensitive and informative. This reflects the fact that loss of contrast sensitivity is one of the earliest visual abnormalities in eyes with AMD. In RP, often unmeasurable by ERG, early disease PERG shows greatest dysfunction outside the macula where the disease is most manifest; while in late RP, and in macular IRDs such as Stargardt's disease and cone degenerations, macular dysfunction predominates. These differences can be seen using PERG protocols that distinguish peripheral (24⁰) from more central (16⁰) visual responses (Luttrull and Margolis 2016, Luttrull 2018). The electrophysiologic dysfunction of the main primary retinopathies is most apparent in measures of signal latency, which demonstrate delay. In contrast, the PERG and VER treatment response signatures in OAG, shown to also be a CPR due to its responsiveness to SDM/MRT revealing the presence of ROAG, demonstrate

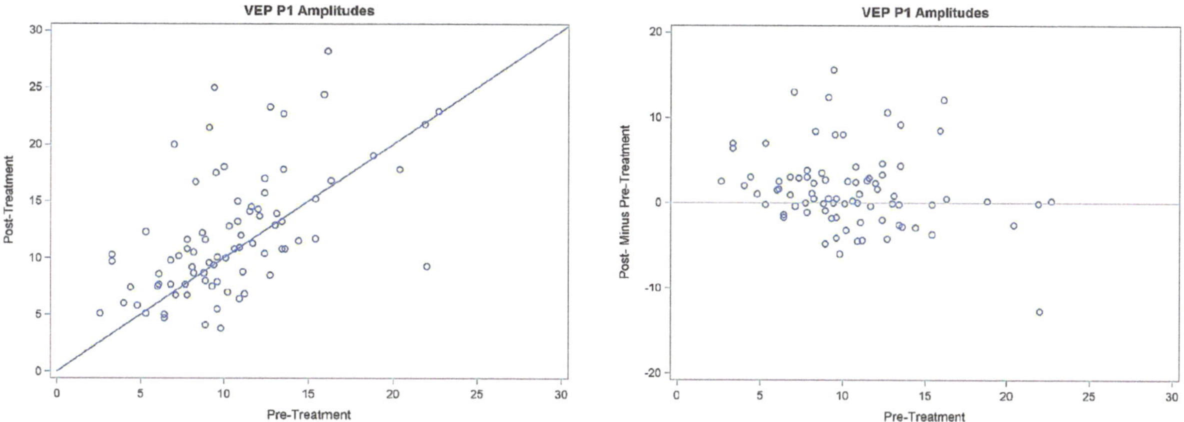

Fig. 16. Left: Scatter graph of VEP P1 amplitudes (in microvolts) before and after SDM treatment. Note significant improvements in VEP P1 amplitudes after SDM treatment. Right: Comparison of post- to pre-treatment VEP P1 amplitudes (in microvolts). Note significant improvements in VEP P1 amplitudes after SDM treatment. From: *Luttrull JK, Samples JR, Kent D, Lum BJ: Panmacular subthreshold diode micropulse laser (SDM) as neuroprotective therapy in primary open-angle glaucoma. Glaucoma Research 2018-2020, pp. 281-294 Edited by: John R. Samples and Paul A. Knepper © 2018 Kugler Publications, Amsterdam, The Netherlands*

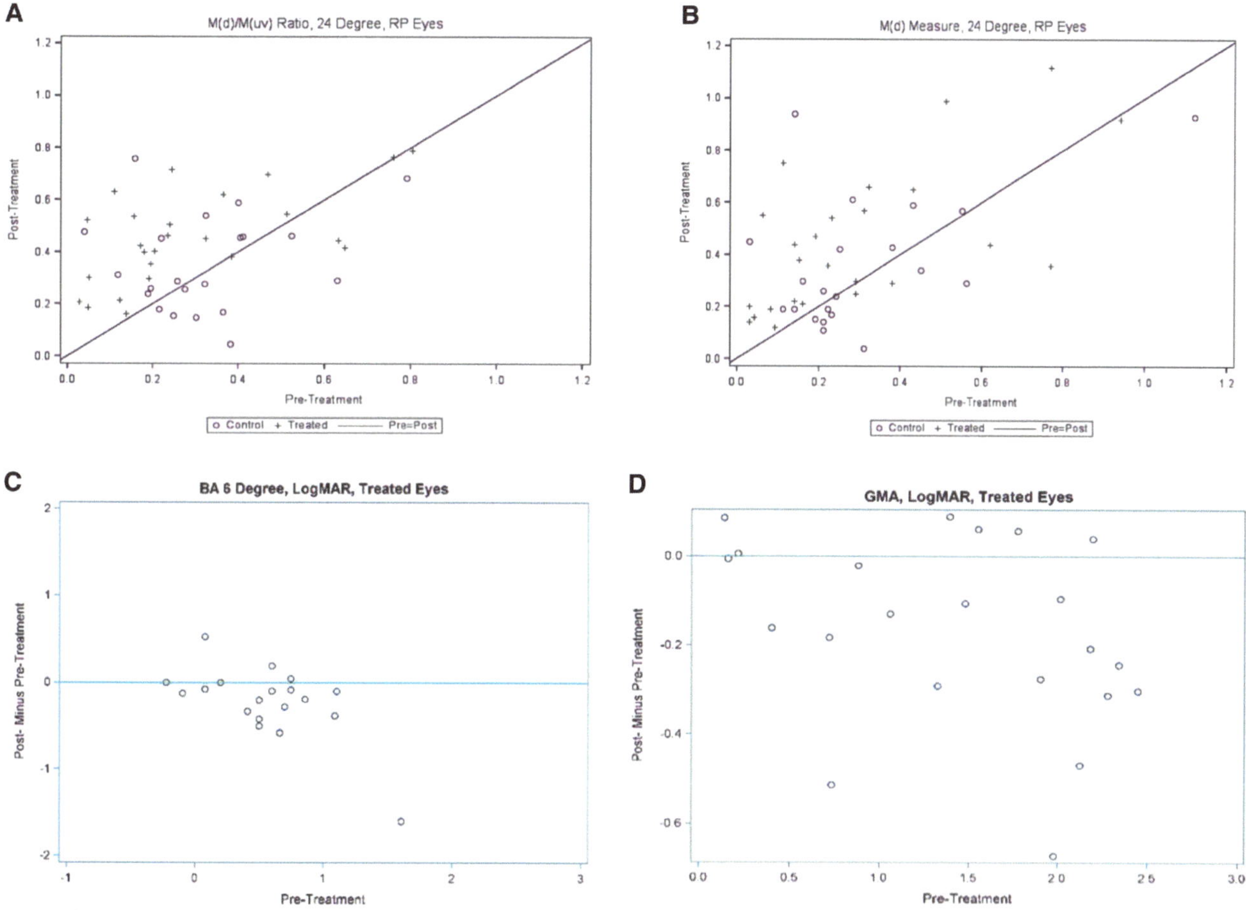

Fig. 17. (A) Scatter plot of pre vs. post treatment pattern electroretinography (PERG) MagD(µV)/Mag(µV) ratios (*in retinitis pigmentosa*). +=treated eye. O = control eye. (B) Scatter plot of pre vs. post treatment MagD(µV) amplitudes. +=treated eye. 0 = control eye. (C) Plot of post—pre treatment ORP BA six values. Values below the line represent improvements after SDM treatment; above the line worsened after treatment. (D) Plot of post—pre treatment ORP GMA values. Values below the line represent improvements after SDM treatment; above the line worsened after treatment. From: *Luttrull JK. Improved retinal and visual function following subthreshold diode micropulse laser (SDM) for retinitis pigmentosa. Eye (London) Feb 2018 PAP open access https://doi.org/10.1038/s41433-018-0017-3*

improvements in signal amplitudes more than latencies. The reason for this difference is unclear, but it is helpful in distinguishing the relative contributions of disease in patients with comorbidities, such as both AMD and OAG (Banitt et al 2013, Luttrull and Margolis 2016, Luttrull, Samples, et al 2018) (Figs. 15-17). It is interesting to note that in eyes with both AMD and OAG, the OAG PERG signature of amplitude improvement predominated over the AMD signature of latency improvement following SDM MRT (Luttrull, Samples et al 2018).

As will be discussed later, the electrophysiologic responses to SDM MRT have helped identify the fact that a fundamental part of OAG is a previously unrecognized retinopathy of open angle glaucoma (ROAG) characterized by treatment-responsive reversible hyponeurotropia (Figs. 16-18). Unlike the other CPRs, the only evidence of ROAG is glaucomatous optic neuropathy and its associations, and the tendency for this to progress, along with visual loss, despite IOP lowering (Luttrull, Samples et al 2018, Luttrull and Kent 2019). Reversal of this failure of retina-derived neurotrophy by MRT suggests MRT may help reduce the risks of visual loss in glaucoma by maintaining neuroprotection over time (Luttrull and Kent 2019). The author has not studied electrophysiology and its treatment responses in DR, as the clinical responses to treatment are so easily appreciated by exam, photography, OCT, and FFA.

Promising new methods of retinal function testing include retinal hyperspectral imaging and use of visible markers of cell function. Hyperspectral photographic imaging may provide new *in vivo* indicators of disease characteristics and treatment response with respect to specifics of cellular function, metabolism, and immunologic status at various levels within the retina. Cell viability markers, such as fluorescent staining of preapoptotic cells, may offer direct graphical assessment of the severity of disease dysfunction and the treatment response. Both could also be used to monitor disease progress and indicate the need for retreatment (Mordant et al 2011, Mazzoni et al 2019).

Key point: Retinal function testing identifies disease prior to clinical manifestations. MRT improves all measures of retinal function safely.

Visual function testing

Of the more commonly performed visual function tests, chart visual acuity, generally done under photopic conditions, is the least sensitive measure of both visual dysfunction and an MRT treatment response. Conventional automated perimetry can also be a useful test of both visual dysfunction and the MRT treatment response in preclinical and clinically manifest disease, although possibly less sensitive to such changes than mesopic visual function testing (MVFT). The more sensitive the test, the better. Thus, automated perimetry programs focusing on macular function, such as the 10-2, are generally more sensitive, and best. In some devices, the perimetry parameters can be modified to be made more sensitive by adjusting the background luminance to mesopic levels (generally 38 dB). In the same way that whispering is more likely to identify a hearing deficit than shouting, specific tests of MVFT (engaging both rods and cones by reducing background illumination to "indoor" ambient levels), such as Omnifield Resolution Perimetry (ORP, Sinclair Technologies, Salt Lake City Utah) has have proven far more sensitive and thus more useful than chart acuity and even subjective reporting for early detection of disease. Like retinal function testing, visual function testing often shows consistent post MRT improvements even in the absence of subjective improvements. The effects of early, preclinical, retinal dysfunction can also be detected by visual function testing (Fig. 19-23). In dry AMD, dark adaptometry (DA) is also useful both as an identifier of preclinical disease, and to demonstrate and monitor the effects of MRT (Jackson et al 2014). Consistent with the long-appreciated early dysfunctions in contrast acuity and mesopic visual function, it is dysfunction of the perifoveal rods (blue light respondent), rather than red and green cone sensitivity, that is primarily affected in AMD, and which is most responsive to MRT function restoration. Thus, the blue light DA response is the most useful detector of both age-related macular dysfunction, as well as the MRT treatment response. In fact, all visual function tests thus far employed have demonstrated both disease related baseline abnormalities, and improvements following MRT. These include microperimetry and contrast visual acuity testing (Katz et al 2010, Lahav et al 2011, Feigl et al 2011, Puell et al 2012, Jackson et al 2014, Gutstein et al 2015, Stringham et al 2015, Luttrull and Margolis 2016, Luttrull and Kent 2019, Sinclair and Luttrull 2022) (Figs. 18-23).

Key point: MRT improves visual function. More sensitive measures are more informative.

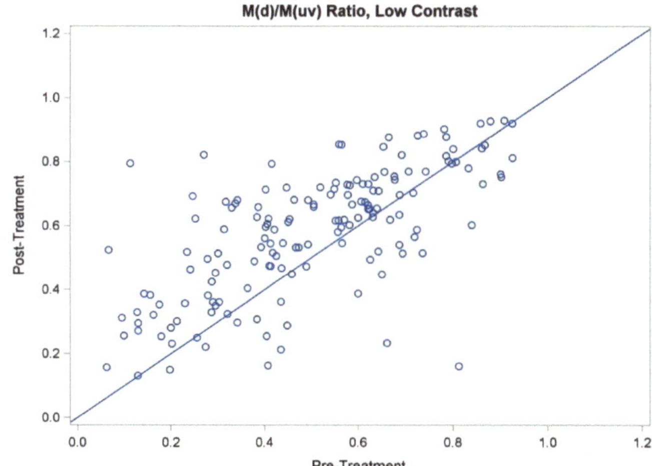

Fig. 18. Scatterplots of AMD PERG low-contrast MagD(lV)/Mag(lV) ratios (*in dry AMD*) before and after SDM treatment. From: *Luttrull JK, Margolis BWL. Functionally guided retinal protective therapy as prophylaxis for age-related and inherited retinal degenerations. A pilot study. Invest Ophthalmol Vis Sci. 2016 Jan 1;5 7(1):265-75. doi: 10.1167/iovs.15-18163.*

Subjective responses to MRT

Treatment of maculopathies associated with various forms of macular edema, be it cystoid (CME) associated with retinal vascular disease or inflammation; or solid macular thickening associated with current or prior epiretinal membrane (ERM) and/or tractional maculopathy; or subretinal fluid (SRF) associated with central serous chorioretinopathy (CSR), should be approached with the expectation of improving chart VA with treatment. These improvements may be fairly rapid in eyes with pseudophakic CME and CSR, but take longer in eyes with DME or ERM-associated thickening (Luttrull et al 2005, Luttrull 2016, 2018). Such gradual VA improvements often go unnoticed by the patient. In eyes with any type of ME, VA improvement following MRT will often precede and exceed reduction in macular thickening. Eyes with dry AMD and IRDs, disorders absent macular edema, may or may not note improvement. This is because visual function, photopic in particular, may already be good, or be irreversibly compromised due to death of visual elements.

Overall, about a third of patients with nonexudative macular disease, such as dry AMD, OAG, and so on, will report subjectively improved visual function. This is far fewer than demonstrating post MRT improvements in retinal and visual function testing. Most reported improvements are immediate (hours, days after treatment).

Long-term subjective visual improvements are also often reported following MRT. For instance, it is not uncommon for patients treated for AMD to report, after 1 to 2 years of treatment (VPT), that they realize they no longer note metamorphopsia, are again able to read the fine text at the bottom of TV news reports, can read more easily, or that they no longer need or use glasses as they did before for near or distance (More on this later.). It is important to keep in mind that simple prevention of vision loss by slowing disease progression in a retinal degeneration may be considered an "improvement" compared to the inexorable worsening of visual function absent treatment (Luttrull and Gray 2022). In eyes with scotomata due to AMD, retina vascular disease, OAG, or optic atrophy, patients often report fading and/or shrinking of the scotoma following MRT (Fig. 20) (Luttrull and Kent 2019). With time, as the treatment effects begin to wane, patients may report gradual recurrence of the scotomata.

However, by far the most common subjective response to MRT in virtually any setting is the report of brighter, more vivid, and clearer vision almost immediately after treatment. Colors are often reported to be more vivid as well. Recall that this was the frequent subjective report from the first patients treated with SDM for DME that seemed so remarkable, compared to the usual worsening that patients experienced following RPC. Such reports encouraged continuation of SDM for DR in the early days of treatment before the clinical effects became apparent (Luttrull et al 2005, 2008). This may be thought of as "high-definition" vision. One does not necessarily see more (lines on the eye chart); one just sees it "better." By analogy, consider the differences in picture quality between the most modern television screens and those of just 5 years ago. Having had SDM MRT 20 times in each eye over the last several years for his own OAG, the author can attest that MRT "updates your screen." Interestingly, while this subjective improvement may be not associated with improved chart acuity, it is consistently associated with improvements in other measures of retinal and visual function.

Another very frequent subjective report from patients receiving vision protection therapy (regular periodic panmacular SDM as maintenance therapy, VPT) is that their previous floaters either disappear, or become markedly diminished. The author has no explanation for this at this point, but the frequency of this report suggests it is real. If so, it is almost certainly the result

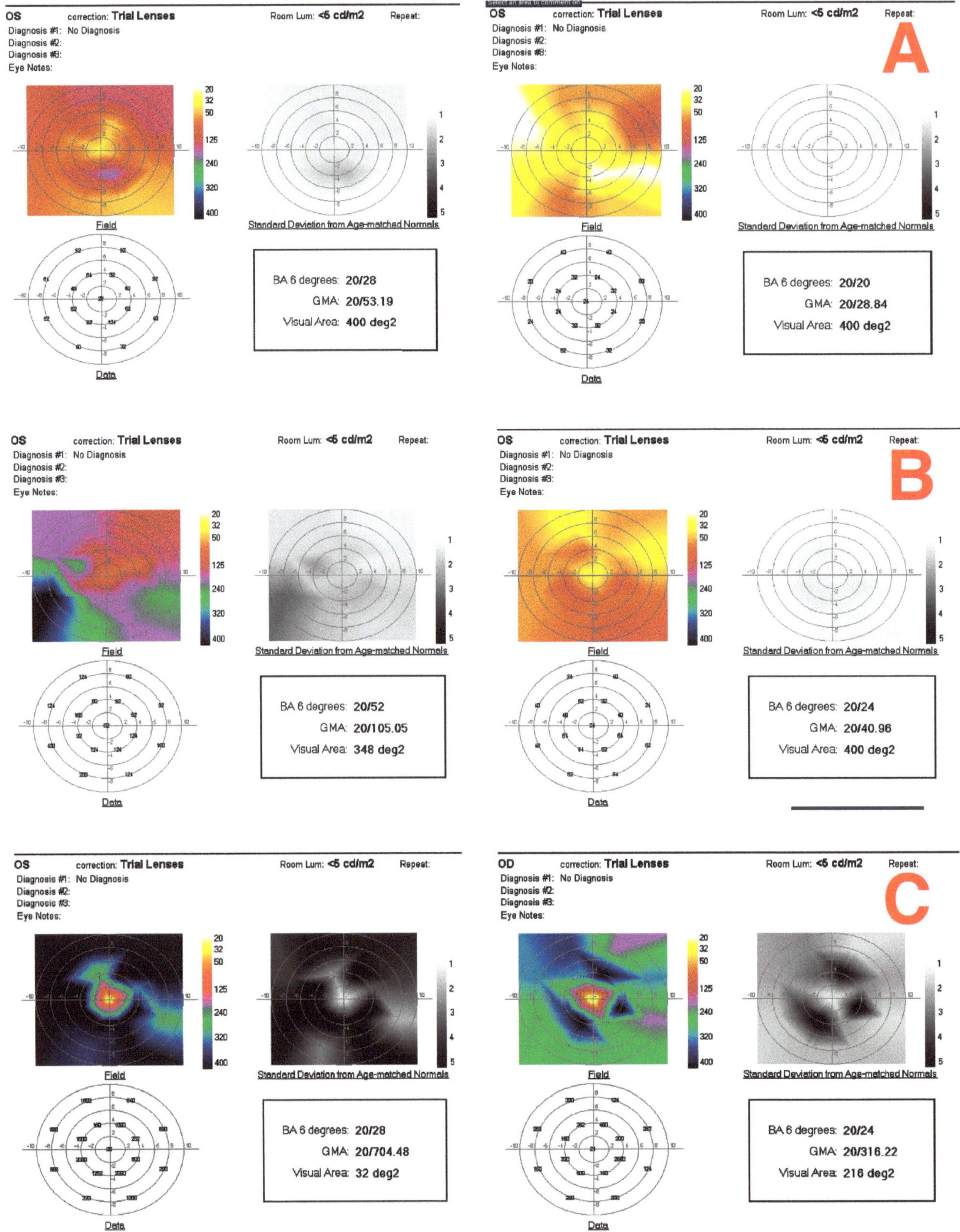
OS   correction: Trial Lenses   Room Lum: <5 cd/m2   Repeat:
Diagnosis #1: No Diagnosis
Diagnosis #2:
Diagnosis #3:
Eye Notes:
Field
Standard Deviation from Age-matched Normals
BA 6 degrees: 20/28
GMA: 20/53.19
Visual Area: 400 deg2
Data
A
OS   correction: Trial Lenses   Room Lum: <5 cd/m2   Repeat:
Diagnosis #1: No Diagnosis
Diagnosis #2:
Diagnosis #3:
Eye Notes:
Field
Standard Deviation from Age-matched Normals
BA 6 degrees: 20/20
GMA: 20/28.84
Visual Area: 400 deg2
Data
B
OS   correction: Trial Lenses   Room Lum: <5 cd/m2   Repeat:
Diagnosis #1: No Diagnosis
Diagnosis #2:
Diagnosis #3:
Eye Notes:
Field
Standard Deviation from Age-matched Normals
BA 6 degrees: 20/52
GMA: 20/105.05
Visual Area: 348 deg2
Data
OS   correction: Trial Lenses   Room Lum: <5 cd/m2   Repeat:
Diagnosis #1: No Diagnosis
Diagnosis #2:
Diagnosis #3:
Eye Notes:
Field
Standard Deviation from Age-matched Normals
BA 6 degrees: 20/24
GMA: 20/40.96
Visual Area: 400 deg2
Data
C
OS   correction: Trial Lenses   Room Lum: <5 cd/m2   Repeat:
Diagnosis #1: No Diagnosis
Diagnosis #2:
Diagnosis #3:
Eye Notes:
Field
Standard Deviation from Age-matched Normals
BA 6 degrees: 20/28
GMA: 20/704.48
Visual Area: 32 deg2
Data
OD   correction: Trial Lenses   Room Lum: <5 cd/m2   Repeat:
Diagnosis #1: No Diagnosis
Diagnosis #2:
Diagnosis #3:
Eye Notes:
Field
Standard Deviation from Age-matched Normals
BA 6 degrees: 20/24
GMA: 20/316.22
Visual Area: 216 deg2
Data

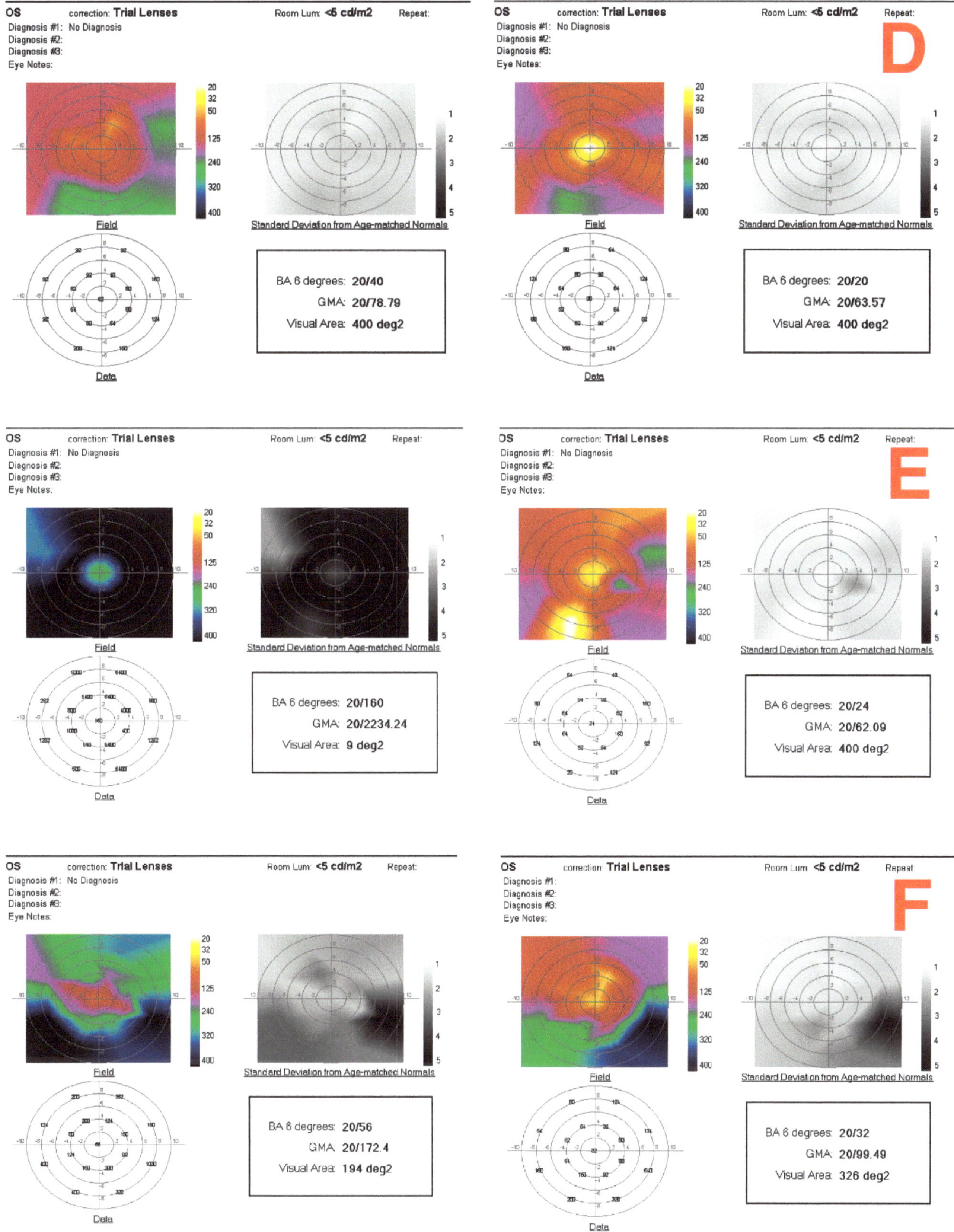

Fig. 19. Mesopic visual function, left before; right after, panmacular SDM MRT. Rows: (A) intermediate AMD, (B) retinitis pigmentosa, (C) Stargardt's disease, (D) macular telangiectasis, (E) retinitis pigmentosa, and (F) open angle glaucoma.

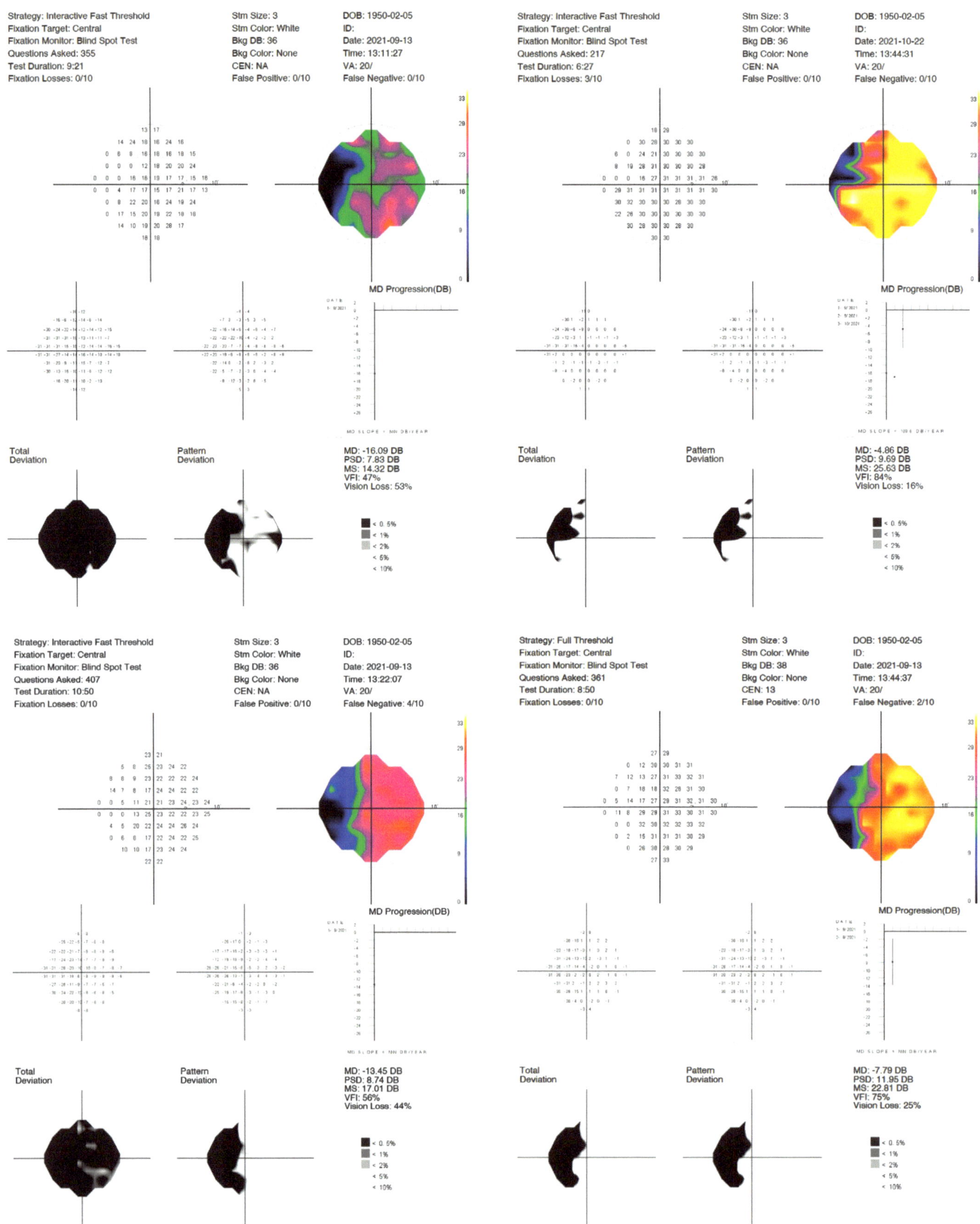

Fig. 20. 71 yo man with left homonymous hemianopsia, early dry AMD, and OAG. 10-2 automated perimetry (Micro Medical Devices, Calabasas, California) with false color mapping display. (Left) before and (right) after panmacular SDM MRT. (A) right eye (B) left eye. Note improvements following treatment.

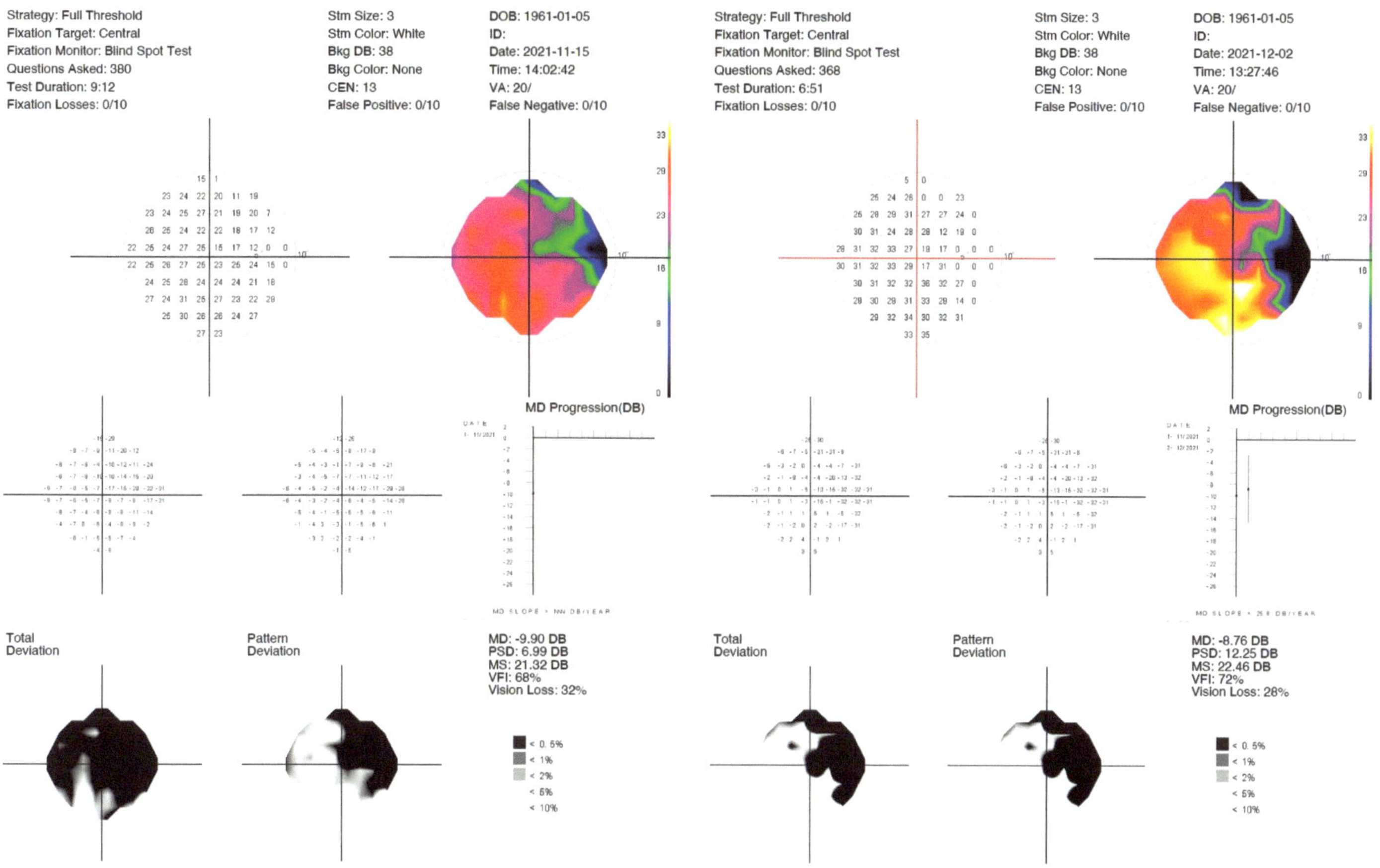

Fig. 21. Pre (left) and post panmacular SDM (right) mesopic 10-2 automated perimetry of the same left eye shown above in Figure 11 with post extensive conventional macular and peripheral retinal PC for PDR and DME, with macula threatening PC scars. Panmacular SDM to slow progression of RPC lesion expansion in the macula. Note improved visual function, indicating improved retinal function, following panmacular SDM MRT.

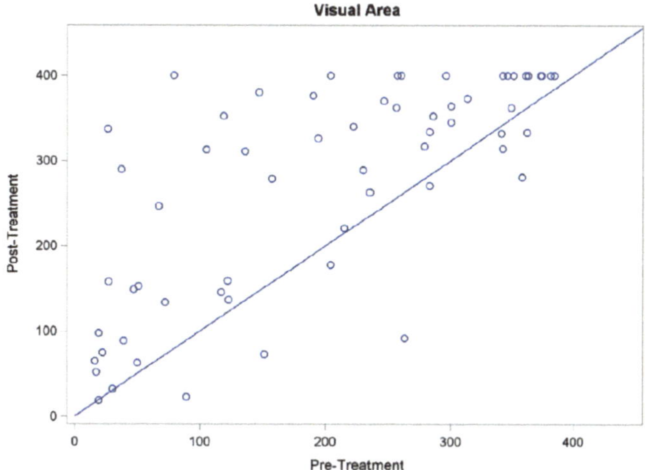

Fig. 22. Mesopic visual function, visual area better than 20/80, before (left) and after (right) panmacular SDM MRT for open angle glaucoma. Note significant improvements following treatment. From: *Luttrull JK, Samples JR, Kent D, Lum BJ: Panmacular subthreshold diode micropulse laser (SDM) as neuroprotective therapy in primary open-angle glaucoma. Glaucoma Research 2018-2020, pp. 281-294 Edited by: John R. Samples and Paul A. Knepper © 2018 Kugler Publications, Amsterdam, The Netherlands*

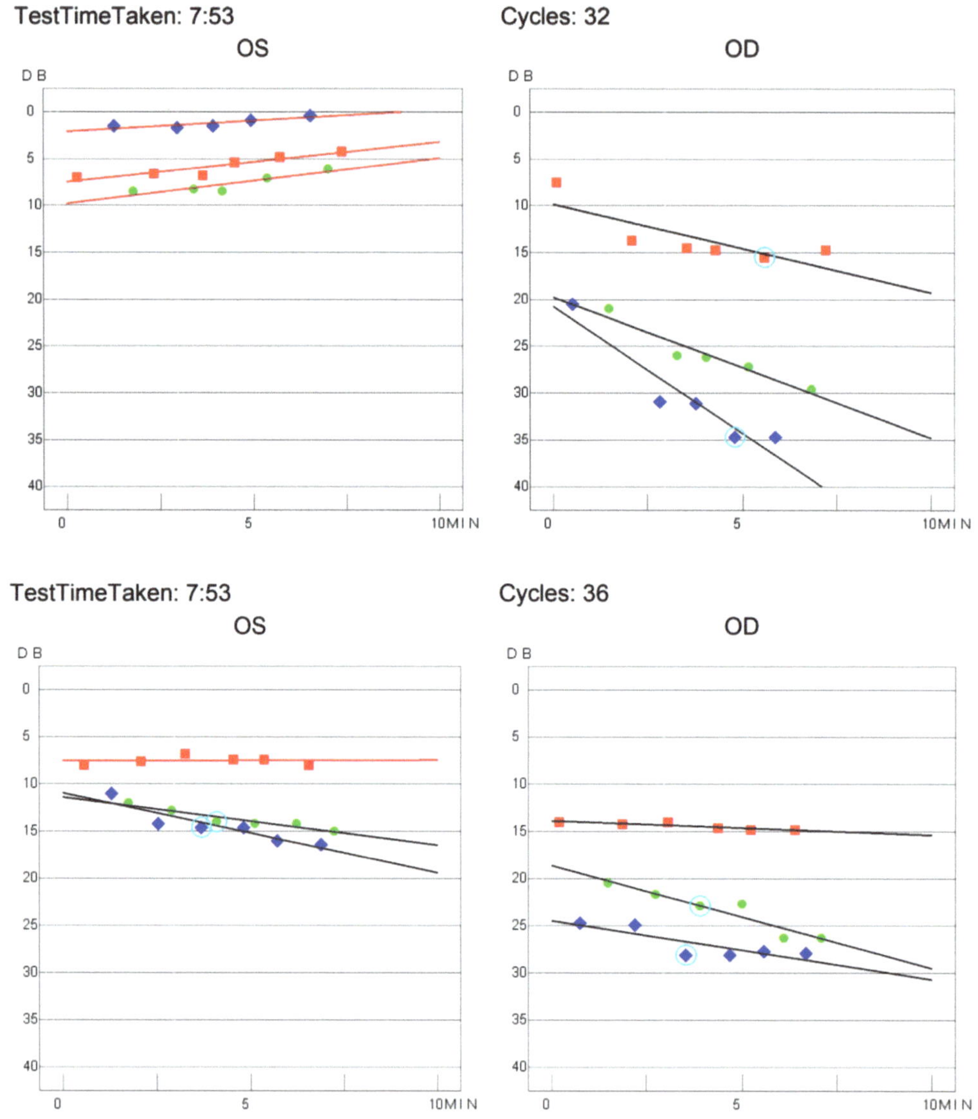

Fig. 23. Dark adaptometry (DA) in bilateral intermediate AMD (A) before and (B) one week after panmacular SDM in the left eye only. Note improvement indicated by a steeper slope in the left eye after treatment, particularly in the blue response arising from the parafoveal rods. Experience with DA in AMD indicates that the blue rod response is the most responsive to treatment, consistent with the long noted clinical finding of early decreased scotopic and mesopic acuity in eyes with AMD. Because MRT improves dysfunction, it is the blue, parafoveal rod response that is most moved by MRT treatment.

of MRT induced changes in visual function rather than an actual diminution in vitreous opacities.

For practical reasons, regular clinical testing of patients in the early postoperative hours and days following MRT has not been done except in rare circumstances. However, in a few tested patients, post SDM MVFT and PERG improvements have been documented as early as 4 hours post treatment (Luttrull and Kent 2019). Patients generally report that the experience of vivid vision is transient, lasting only days to weeks. This may cause some distress, seeming to suggest that the therapeutic effects of treatment are fleeting, and therefore inconsequential. This is a mistake. As will be seen in the following discussion, the effects of MRT are nothing if not significant and long-lasting. Retinal and visual function testing following SDM MRT, such as MVFT and PERG, consistently show that the improvements in retinal and visual function persist and are robust in most disorders through at least 3 to 4 months (shorter in IRDs such as RP) prior to gradually returning to baseline (Luttrull and Kent 2019). Rather than rapid waning of the initially striking visual improvements, what appears to be happening in most cases is adaptation. The improvement becomes the new normal. Further evidence suggesting adaptation is that patients will often note subjective diminution of visual function again, months later, often shortly prior to their scheduled retreatment, and understand this later diminution as an indication of their need for retreatment.

The duration of treatment effects in IRDs, such as RP, is shorter than AMD and DR. This likely reflects the severity and mechanism of the underlying disease process. As with other nonexudative macular disorders, about a third of IRD patients, including RP and Stargardt's disease, report visual improvements, sometimes within hours, even driving home following treatment. Some of these experiences can be fairly dramatic, such as regained color vision, improved peripheral vision, renewed ability to drive at dusk, or the ability to ambulate safely in a less than fully illuminated house. In some cases, these regained functional abilities had been lost for 10 years or more prior to MRT. In no case do patients report worsened vision following MRT.

In light of the above, treating surgeons are best advised to hope for, but not promise, improvements in VA or visual function following MRT. What can be promised with confidence is that retinal function will be improved, and that this should slow disease progression and reduce the risks of visual loss; and that visual function should be improved to the greatest degree possible in the context of their pretreatment retinal status. Any improvement in VA or other visual function will be a welcome, although not an expected, benefit of MRT.

Key points: While objective improvements in retinal and visual function are the norm, subjective improvements are less common and should not be promised.

MRT and reversal of CPR progression

The results of objective retinal and visual function testing are clinically useful and provide important insights into certain disease processes. As usual, these insights are generally understandable and predictable in the context of the mechanism of MRT action. PERG, MVFT and DA have long been known to be both abnormal in the early, preclinical phases of CPRs; and to predict the likelihood of disease progression—and thus visual loss—years later (Katz et al 2010, Lahav et al 2011, Feigl et al 2011, Puell et al 2012, Banitt et al 2013, Jackson et al 2014, Stringham et al 2015). The ability of MRT to improve visual function measured by these responses

provides three important bits of information. First, that MRT is able to reverse, not just slow, disease progression, reducing the risk of visual loss (provided treatment is suitably maintained). This reflects the neuroprotective effect of MRT in CPRs (Luttrull et al 2005, 2008, Luttrull and Dorin 2012, Luttrull et al 2012, 2015, Luttrull and Margolis 2016, Luttrull 2018, Luttrull, Sinclair et al 2018, Luttrull, Samples et al 2018, Luttrull and Kent 2019, Chang and Luttrull 2020, Luttrull et al 2020, Luttrull and Gray 2022) (Fig. 10). Second, that retinal cells may be sufficiently sick that they have no detectable function prior to treatment but are restorable to measurable and useful visual function by MRT (Fig. 16-23). This reflects the ability of MRT to inhibit apoptosis via HSP activation to revitalize the cell and restore function, effectively reversing the disease process (Luttrull and Margolis 2016, Luttrull and Kent 2019). Retinal function studies reveal that there is virtually always measurable retinal function indicative of bioactive, and thus functionally modifiable retinal tissue, even in the midst of severe disease, such as within areas of ARGA (Luttrull 2018, Luttrull and Margolis 2016). MRT revitalization of this nonfunctional but surviving preapoptotic tissue is easily demonstrated by visual field testing, where MRT can restore visual function to previously unrecordable areas; and by PERG, which demonstrates improved retinal function even within large areas of ARGA following MRT (Luttrull and Margolis 2016, Luttrull and Kent 2019) (Figs. 16-22). Third, while the degree of measurable dysfunction generally parallels disease severity, linear regression analysis shows that, by all measures and in all settings, eyes with the worst baseline function show the greatest degrees of improvement following MRT. This again reflects the mechanism of action of MRT on RPE HSP protein repair kinetics, improving the most abnormal cells most (Chang and Luttrull 2020). Finally, as noted earlier, improvements in long-term trends of nerve fiber layer (NFL) and ganglion cell complex (GCC) thickness in eyes with AMD and OAG managed with vision protection therapy (VPT) (SDM performed on a regular basis over time to maintain treatment effects) suggest that the neuroprotective effects of MRT may be neuroregenerative as well as neuroprotective and neuroenhancing. Neuroregeneration would represent the most extreme example of disease progression reversal (Luttrull and Bhavan 2022).

If one hopes to improve the long-term prognosis of a chronic progressive retinal disease, a logical prerequisite is to improve and normalize retinal function early in the treatment process and maintain this improvement over time. Improvement in retinal function must always precede improvement in visual function. This is the basis for the use of any surrogate indicator of reduced event risk. These include some of the most common interventions in medicine, such as blood pressure reduction to prevent stroke, and blood glucose reduction to prevent complications of diabetes. Retinal and visual function testing in CPRs in response to MRT have proven highly predictive of significant improvements in long-term outcomes, such as slowed progression of GA and low neovascular conversion rates in AMD (Luttrull and Margolis 2016, Luttrull et al 2018, 2020, Luttrull and Gray 2022).

Long-term studies of experimental therapies for CPRs are sometimes embarked upon that have not included near-term testing of the effects of treatment on retinal function. Vast amounts of resources in time, money, and expectation might be saved if early retinal function testing was used routinely to determine if the treatment had any actual promise. Typically, an effective treatment should show prompt improvements in retinal function, within days to weeks at most, if longer term benefits are to be hoped for. These can be objectively tested for and measured. With MRT, such improvements can usually be demonstrated within days, and sometimes just hours, after treatment. Treatments that do not improve retinal function, or especially worsen it, would likely have little to no chance of producing long-term benefits, allowing the trial to be discontinued prior to the expenditure of more resources. Of course, the reverse is true as well, that treatments of any kind found to improve retinal function should be investigated as a potential therapy.

Key point: The improvements in clinical findings, retinal function, and visual function following MRT represent reversal of disease progression in CPRs.

Fellow eye effects

Treatment of one eye with MRT very often results in measurable improvement in the untreated fellow eye. Such bilateral improvements following unilateral MRT are frequently observed with electrophysiology, MFVT, and DA. Usually, the fellow eye response is less robust than the primary eye, but not always. In the past it has been theorized that such occurrences may reflect local factors elicited by treatment, such as RPE-derived cytokines, reaching the fellow eye through the peripheral circulation. However, Caballero et al found therapeutic systemic immunoactivation following MRT, indicated by recruitment of bone marrow-derived immune cells to the retina of both eyes in mice following SDM treatment of just one eye (Caballero et al 2017). Thus, systemic immunomodulation may be the actual cause of such fellow eye improvements, illustrating the catalytic and expansive cascading nature of the response to MRT.

Key point: Fellow eye effects are commonly detected by retinal function testing.

Effective patient communication

In medicine, it is a challenge to communicate and illustrate the value of treatments to patients who do not experience any notable or prompt improvement in symptoms or function. Consider the perennial problem of glaucoma medication compliance. However, since most patients treated with MRT do not experience any immediate changes after treatment, and the goals of treatment are to slow disease progression and prevent future vision loss (a distant abstraction for many), it can be very helpful to be able to show patients graphic demonstrations of the immediate positive treatment effects of MRT on retinal and visual function that they may not otherwise appreciate. A clear graphic illustration showing "This was you before treatment; this is you after treatment. Can you see the difference?" is worth the proverbial thousand words. If they can see the difference (as is usually the case), much has been achieved. The author has found that modification of report formats, such as replacement of the gray scales of automated perimetry with bright false-color mapping, can be extremely helpful by creating a more accessible, intuitive display, that is more easily apprehended by patients (Figs. 18, 19, and 21).

Key point: Intuitive illustrations of treatment effects and improvements are appreciated by patients and aid compliance.

8. Laser Parameters for Modern Retinal Laser Therapy

General concepts of MRT dosimetry

The critical requirements of MRT laser parameters are to provide a threshold stimulus to RPE heat shock protein activation while at the same time maximizing the therapeutic range such that it is broad enough to preclude the possibility of LIRD in any eye, regardless of fundus pigmentation or other individual ocular variation (Luttrull and Dorin 2012, Luttrull et al 2012, Chang and Luttrull 2020) (Figs. 9). Scaling law analysis of laser parameters shows that each parameter, including spot size, wavelength, power, pulse frequency (duty cycle), and spot duration, make separate contributions to both efficacy and safety (proprietary data, Ojai Retinal Technologies, LLC) (Luttrull et al 2012, Luttrull and Sinclair 2014, Chang and Luttrull 2020, Keunen et al 2020). The potential parameter combinations are nearly infinite, but their relations are limited with regard to the ends of MRT for reliable safety and effectiveness. The contributions to retinal safety and efficacy of each parameter of microsecond pulsed lasers have sufficient degrees of freedom that exact formula calculations in Mathematica (http://www.mathematica.org/) require several days to solve on most current computers (circa 2022). Fortunately, a simpler approximate formula derived from the exact formula gives much the same results for every day calculations (Ojai Retinal Technologies, LLC, proprietary data). As it happens, most of the parameter contributions are intuitive, but others are not.

As noted elsewhere, virtually any laser wavelength and treatment strategy may be therapeutically effective. However, microsecond pulsed lasers are best suited to achieving reliable safety, making them ideal for MRT (Chhablani et al 2018, Chang and Luttrull 2020). For CW lasers, including PC, short-pulse CW, and nanosecond CW, safety and efficacy vary inversely, treatment becoming less safe as efficacy increases. For appropriately constructed microsecond laser parameters, safety and efficacy can be made to vary in parallel; treatment becoming safer and more effective at the same time. This special facility of microsecond laser pulsing is fundamental to MRT, making all else possible (Dorin 2008, Luttrull and Dorin 2012, Luttrull et al 2012, Chhablani 2018). As wavelength is not a determinant of efficacy, longer wavelengths such as 810 nm are preferred as they are less energetic and less absorbed in the retina and RPE, and thus less likely to cause inadvertent retinal damage, being less influenced by individual variations in pigmentation and pathology, and enjoying broadest therapeutic windows and thus greatest safety margins while remaining highly effective thermal activators of RPE HSPs. For this reason, shorter, more energic better absorbed wavelengths should be avoided as reliable safety cannot be guaranteed and the added risk of damage comes at no added therapeutic benefit (Luttrull and Sinclair 2014, Chang and Luttrull 2020) (Figs. 4, 5, 11-13). This is because as wavelengths narrow the therapeutic window and safety margins shrink exponentially (Chang and Luttrull 2020, Keunen et al 2020). For instance, 577 nm is 4× more energetic than 810 nm and 2× more absorbed by the RPE (Chang and Luttrull 2020). Thus, for a given set of parameters, the therapeutic/safety range of 577 nm is 88% less than for 810 nm. For 532 nm, it is even less. Because the reliable safety of MRT makes all else possible, this is not a trivial concern. A simple example is illustrative: it is virtually impossible to create a retina burn with a 5% duty cycle (DC) with 810 nm; it is very easy with 577 nm; and difficult to avoid with 532 nm (Fig. 5, 9, 12-14). Only Laursen et al (2004), using a small spot size and very long 3 sec exposure durations, has reported even mild LIRD from an 810 nm laser at a 5% DC (Dorin 2003, Laursen et al 2004, Luttrull et al 2005, Luttrull and Sinclair 2014).

The infinite gulf between always and usually

Why is wavelength selection so important for MRT? It is because the gulf between always safe and usually safe is not incremental; it is infinite. Use of 810nm makes the goal of MRT certain, always reliably safe (absent surgeon error). Every patient can be assured of safety from correctly performed treatment, and any treatment indication can be entertained with the knowledge that the condition will not be worsened in any way even if treatment is ineffective. None of this can be said for "usually" safe treatment, such as that using 577nm (and certainly not for unsafe shorter wavelengths). No patient can be assured of safety, and treatment-induced worsening of the treatment indication due to inadvertent LIRD can never be guaranteed. The difference in "always" vs "usually" is a difference in kind, the difference between always and never. Only laser parameters that are always safe and never cause LIRD are thus appropriate for MRT and unlock the unique and key abilities of MRT over any other laser treatment and most drugs: transfoveal treatment, ad lib repeat treatments, application to indications particularly vulnerable to aggravation from LIRD such as AMD, glaucoma and IRDs.

Given that the object of microsecond pulsed laser (MPL) and MRT is to avoid retinal damage, why has 577 nm become by far the most prevalent wavelength in practice? As with most mysteries, follow the money. The MPL 810 nm was never commercially patented, reducing the potential for exclusivity and financial gain by manufacturers. Further, early in the history of MPL, practitioners continued to think in terms of RPC and wanted a laser that was highly effective at burning the retina and "closing" microaneurysms (Neely et al 1998), and 577 nm fit the bill. Thus, even though the goal of MPL is to avoid retinal damage, in order to appeal to the market, shorter wavelengths like 577 um and 532 nm, highly effective at burning the retina and thus inappropriate for MPL and MRT, were marketed by manufacturers over 810 nm, which made retinal burning much more difficult (a good thing). The cognitive disconnect between the goal of treatment and the tools provided to achieve the goal is profound. Unfortunately, most practitioners assume that laser manufacturers are knowledgeable and expert in retinal laser therapy. They make and sell retinal lasers, after all. Practitioners trust that, because laser manufacturers offer and even recommend 577 nm and 532 nm for MPL, these must be the wavelengths medically best suited to the task. In fact, experience shows that the manufactures of retinal laser devices have little to no understanding of retinal laser treatment, the biophysics of treatment, the mechanism of action, and so on (JK Luttrull, unpublished data). At best, their understand-

ing is rooted in the RPC era, which has virtually nothing in common with MRT (Table 1). But most importantly, their main concern is market-driven, about product sales and not medicine. This should surprise no one. All currently available retinal laser systems have been approved by the FDA on 510K applications. This means that the basis for FDA approval is that they are essentially equivalent to the argon lasers first approved for RPC. Thus, current laser systems are not inherently suited to MRT. They must be made suitable for MRT by use of appropriate treatment parameters and treatment techniques. One such basic adjustment is to employ wavelengths that maximize, rather than minimize, treatment safety—a fundamental goal of treatment. Thus, the retinal laser manufacturers have done a great disservice by saturating the market with unnecessarily risky visible wavelength microsecond pulsed lasers.

Key points:
1. CW lasers are not appropriate for MRT
2. MRT is a particular application of microsecond pulsed laser (MPL)
3. Thus, not all MPL are suited for MRT
4. Unlike MPL, MRT is safe by definition, always sublethal to the RPE and thus harmless

The evolution of SDM MRT macular laser parameters and dosimetry

No man ever steps into the same river twice. For it's not the same river, and he's not the same man.

—Heraclitis

There is nothing new under the sun.

—Solomon

The author's current parameters for SDM MRT are the result of over 22 years of clinical use and refinement in over 50,000 (and counting) treatment sessions. As such, they represent an evolution and reflect the understanding of the mechanism of retinal laser treatment gained in that time, and how laser parameters can be constructed to optimize treatment by maximizing treatment safety and efficacy. As an evolution, the reader should understand the current parameters do not represent metaphysical perfection. They are not the end. They are just the best and most useful at this point in time.

The initial MPL laser parameters chosen on April 19, 2000 were wavelength: 810 nm, spot size: 125 um, power: 0.78 W, DC: 5%, spot duration: 0.30 sec with a Mainster macular contact lens (magnification factor 1.05) (Ocular Instruments, Bellvue, Washington). At the same time, the high-density treatment strategy was implemented in hopes of making the low-intensity treatment clinically effective. Because it was effective as well as safe and without any evidence of RPE damage, use of these treatment parameters continued essentially unchanged for several years (Fig. 5). However, the area and thus number of contiguous laser spots placed continued to increase, from the early average of 600 spots per session, to over 1,200 spots per session for DME and ME due to retinal vein occlusions (RVO). 600 spots were already tedious, and 1,200 even more so. So, after several years, different parameters were tried with the hope of maintaining efficacy and safety, while increasing the speed of treatment. This was done both intuitively, and with information from the ANSI xMPE standards (American National Standards Institute 2000) (Fig. 24). To speed treatment, a larger spot size was employed of 200 um. At the time, it was felt that small spot sizes were most ideal (scaling law analysis reveals this to be incorrect). In addition, shorter spot durations were used to place more spots more quickly. Without a precise understanding of MPL biophysics, the DC was increased to 10% and 15% hoping to make up for the larger spot size and shorter pulse duration, again, in order to speed up treatment.

As noted previously, to learn something new you have to do something different. To develop good judgment, you first have to make mistakes and then, ideally, learn from them. The subsequent changes in the laser parameters were undertaken about 4 to 5 years into the use of SDM for DME and other ME, and another 5 years before the author had sufficient confidence in the safety of treatment to attempt transfoveal treatment. This was a good thing. In several patients, unexpected LIRD occurred. Fortunately, these were all patients treated for DME outside the fovea and despite the LIRD, the DME resolved and their vision improved. All damage occurred at DCs of 10% or more (Dorin 2003, Luttrull and Dorin 2012, Luttrull et al 2012). Even at a 15% DC, however, macular LIRD was rare. But unexpected retinal damage was disturbing enough that DCs over

5% were abandoned in favor of reliable safety. A retrospective review of cases up until that time revealed that DCs above 5% indeed significantly increased the risk of LIRD (Fig. 9) (Luttrull et al 2012). In retrospect, this should have come as no surprise as 15% DCs were the rule in the literature at that time, and LIRD was common in such studies. Further, a better understanding of the impact of increased DCs on cell heating would have strongly recommended against this approach as well (Dorin 2003). While an increase from a 5 to 15% DC sounds minor, this change decreases the interpulse cooling interval time by 75%, causing even 810 nm MPL at 15% to behave clinically like CW laser (Dorin 2003, Luttrull et al 2012). 577 nm at 15% would be comparable to 810 nm at a 60% DC.

For many years, the preferred parameters for macular treatment became wavelength: 810 nm, spot size: 200 um, power: 1.4 W, DC 5%, spot duration: 0.150 sec. This slight increase in spot size and shorter spot duration made high-density treatment, evolving to panmacular treatment, more tolerable, requiring ~ 800 spots per session. Treatment was effective and, with 810 nm and a 5% DC, reliably safe. No cases of LIRD were ever seen with treatment parameters employing a 5% DC, either in the first days, or with this parameter set.

It is important to understand that all of the above parameters were undertaken in virtually complete ignorance of the mechanism of action, other than that treatment somehow normalized retinal function; and consequently, complete ignorance of the biophysics of the effects of the various contributions of each of the fundamental laser parameters of wavelength, power, spot duration, DC, and spot size. However, in 2014 the author began a collaboration with physicist David B Chang, PhD. Through his son Steven D Chang, MD, a corneal specialist and referring physician, Dr Chang had developed an interest in SDM. Using the information gained from long clinical experience with SDM to inform his investigations, in collaboration with Dr Chang the basic mechanism, thermodynamics, and kinetics of the reset mechanism of retinal laser treatment were elucidated and developed. Interestingly, in many cases the physics alone led to obviously incorrect predictions and results. However, by basing the physics and mathematical analyses on real-world observations, a highly predictive model was developed, as were formulas for calculating the effects of treatment which included all retinal laser parameters as variables (proprietary data Ojai Retinal Technologies, LLC). This "reset" model predicted novel applications for retinal laser treatment that had not been previously imagined. These included treatment of IRDs, neuroprotection for OAG, reversal of anti-VEGF drug tolerance in wet AMD, slowing of ARGA in dry AMD, and inhibition of neovascular conversion in dry AMD. Each was subsequently confirmed clinically (Luttrull et al 2015, Luttrull and Margolis 2016, Luttrull 2018, Luttrull, Samples et al 2018, Luttrull, Sinclair et al 2018, Luttrull et al 2020, Luttrull and Gray 2022).

Since that time, SDM MRT laser parameters have continued to evolve, this time informed by the above analyses. As noted previously, there are an almost infinite number of potential parameter combinations that can achieve the goals of MRT. However, by imposing practical constraints of treatment time, laser platform limitations, and so on, the list narrows. The priorities for parameter selection were, in the following order: safety, efficacy, patient comfort/treatment time. This led to use of the following parameters: wavelength 810 nm, spot size: 500 um, DC 5%, power 1.8 W, spot duration: 0.30 sec. Use of the larger 500-um spot speeds treatment by reducing the number of spots required for thorough panmacular treatment to approximately 400 spots. This, and all of the above parameter sets, assumed use of a Mainster macular contact lens with a magnification factor of 1.05%. While the 50/50 retinal burn risk for the original SDM parameters was approximately 2 W, and approximately 4 W for the above parameters using a 200-um spot size, the above parameters using a 500-um spot increased the 50/50 burn threshold to 15 W. Although inadvertent burns had never been seen with 5%DC parameters in the author's experience, this 15 W TR represents an immense safety cushion. Because the range of reported human RPE pigment variation is only approximately 2×, none of the above 5% DC parameter sets would be expected to result in LIRD in any patient, consistent with years of clinical observations. With a 15 W-wide therapeutic range that exceeds the maximum power of the typical 810 nm laser by over 7×, the risk of inadvertent LIRD in any eye of any patient is effectively nil (Chang and Luttrull 2020, Keunen et al 2020).

As noted, patient comfort is a key consideration in the choice of laser parameters. This is because many of the patients who are candidates for MRT have "treatment fatigue," such as is commonly exhibited by patients with diabetes mellitus due to many years of medical encounters and procedures; or will require long-term maintenance therapy requiring many treatment sessions over time. Compliance is critical to the success of any treatment regimen, especially long-term and preventative treatment regimens. Thus, maximizing treatment comfort and minimizing treatment time is an essential aid toward this end. Because MRT is not painful, this is not an issue. The shorter the treatment time, the better. Current MRT treatment techniques take patient comfort a step further with elimination of the contact lens, elimination of pupillary dilation (for panmacular treatment) and elimination of slit lamp illumination—as will be described in the following text.

Current treatment parameters for panmacular MRT

Currently, the author's approach to macular disease is panmacular treatment performed in the following fashion: No dilation or topical anesthetic is employed. A 90D lens is used. With only the laser pointer beam for fundus illumination, turned down very low to avoid inducing miosis, the aiming beam is used to orient treatment by identifying the optic nerve and thus major arcades. Panmacular treatment is then performed by slowing scanning horizontally up and down across the panmacular region between the major vascular arcades. At the end of each horizontal scan the optic nerve is revisualized to ensure proper orientation within the desired panmacular treatment field. The entirety of the panmacular area is scanned with confluent treatment spots approximately three times. This is intentional "overtreatment." Intentional overtreatment is done to ensure complete confluent coverage of the panmacular area, and to avoid undertreatment, which is the most common novice error with MPL/MPT and most common mistake that adversely affects clinical outcomes. This requires ~ 400 spot applications. The laser spot counter is used to make sure that sufficient treatment has been performed, as the tendency is to want to end treatment prematurely. In this way panmacular MRT is performed without eye drops, dilation, or contact in a little over 2 min. The laser parameters for this noncontact approach are: 90D lens (mag 1.32×), wavelength: 810 nm, spot size: 300 um (396 um retinal spot), power: 1.7 W, DC: 5%, spot duration: 0.30 sec. With a little practice, this approach is very quick and easy, and as pleasing to the doctor as the patient. Because the MRT treatment strategy (given in the following text) does not employ focal or local treatment, targeting aided by detailed visualization of the fundus, such as is afforded by dilation and slit lamp illumination, is unnecessary (Fig. 25).

Peripheral retinal treatment

Treatment of the peripheral retina is essential for generalized retinopathies such as diabetic retinopathy, other proliferative retinopathies, and some IRDs such as retinitis pigmentosa. Thus far, treatment of the peripheral retina has been approached slightly differently than the macula, primarily because the retinal area that needs to be covered with confluent contiguous spots is vastly greater than the macula, thus requiring many more spots; and because rare LIRD in the peripheral retina is inconsequential, while it can be visually devasting in the macula.

On the same first day of SDM April 19, 2000 patients with PDR were also treated with the SDM strategy of low-intensity/high-density treatment. It was clear that the parameters chosen for macular treatment could not be used in the peripheral without treatment taking literally hours. Therefore, guess-timation, intuition, and divine intervention were again employed to come up with SDM parameters for peripheral retinal treatment. A wide-field contact lens (magnification factor 2×) was used along with the maximum 500 um laser spot size (1 mm retinal spot). Because of the large spot, maximum laser power (2.0 W) was employed. Because of the very large retinal spot, chosen to speed treatment to a tolerable duration, it was felt that a higher DC was needed to achieve effective irradiance. Therefore, a 15% DC was employed. In another attempt to speed treatment, a 0.20 sec spot duration was chosen.

What is remarkable about the above early peripheral retinal SDM parameters is that they worked very well. This is remarkable because they represent the lowest irradiance parameters used clinically in SDM, of just 18×MPE, and reaching only about 25% of the maximum Arrhenius integral for RPE HSP activation (American National Standards Institute 2000, Luttrull et al 2012).

(Figure 24) This served as a very important indicator of the low-end SDM MRT treatment threshold, illustrating the power of the catalytic nature of RPE HSP activation. In darker pigmented eyes, pain could occur with these parameters, and rarely, retinal burns in the very thin retina just behind the ora serrata. The pain threshold was always lower than the burn threshold, allowing the treatment to be adjusted to maintain comfort and at the same time avoid retinal burns. If pain occurred, the first adjustment was to shorten the spot duration as this would also speed treatment. If reducing the spot duration did not alleviate pain, the DC was reduced to 10%. More adjustment was never required. Peripheral retinal SDM was generally performed in two sessions of approximately 1,000 spots each, 1 to 2 months apart. A review of the results of peripheral retinal SDM for PDR from 2000 to 2003 revealed that treatment appeared to be at least as effective as standard RPC PRP, but with better visual results. Peripheral retinal SDM reduced progression from severe nonproliferative retinopathy to proliferative from an expected 50% to just 8% (p<0.001).

The above approach for peripheral retinal treatment remained unchanged from 2000 to 2020, in light of the power and time constraints of peripheral treatment, and the fact that peripheral treatment was required far less often than macular treatment lessening the impetus for modification (Fig. 23).

Current treatment parameters for peripheral retinal MRT

Since 2020, a contact lens for peripheral retinal treatment has been eliminated in favor of noncontact treatment with a 90D lens. Such noncontact treatment is much preferred by patients, and easier for the doctor as well. In an undilated eye, the same technique and parameters employed for panmacular treatment can be used to treat as far as the equator with little difficulty. For more peripheral treatment, dilation is necessary. Currently, the author tends to perform peripheral treatment of both (dilated) eyes on the same day, with application of approximately 700 to 800 spots in each eye circumferentially. Fundus illumination and retinal focus confirmed only by the aiming beam is usually sufficient, and much preferred by patients over slit lamp illumination, which is bright and uncomfortable. Peripheral treatment is then repeated in both eyes a second time about one month later, resulting in approximately 1,500 spot applications per eye. The one-month interval between peripheral treatment sessions is informed by animal studies indicating that the complete initial response to SDM ends at approximately 3 to 4 weeks post treatment in recruitment of bone marrow immune cells to the retina. The thought is that it may be best to let the treatment response to the prior treatment run its course prior to performing additional treatment.

The current treatment parameters for peripheral retinal SDM MRT are, lens: 90D, wavelength: 810 nm, spot size 500 um (retinal spot 660 um), DC 10%, spot duration: 0.20 sec, power 2.0 W. As with the original contact lens parameters, patients with darker pigmentation may experience pain, especially over the long posterior ciliary nerves at the horizontal meridians. No LIRD has been noted. If pain occurs, reducing the spot duration to 0.15 sec is usually effective, and speeds treatment.

Perspective on MRT dosimetry and application

Human nature is unchanging. Thus, the enduring relevance of the Book of Job, Shakespeare, Dostoyevsky, and The Far Side. Technology, on the other hand, is always changing (Barnes 2014). The current parameters and techniques for reliably safe and effective MRT described earlier are largely dictated by the fact that all current retinal laser systems are repurposed systems designed to perform RPC, little changed since the 1960s. Thus, they are not ideal and do not exploit the unique properties of MRT. When technology does not change, it should concern us.

The author has created a new retinal laser system designed to address the earlier cited problems. Called SAPRA™ (for Safe Pulse™ Retinal Activation™) (Retinal Protection Sciences, LLC, Los Angeles, CA) this will be the first retinal laser system designed with the express intent to deliver only optimized MRT. SAPRA™ will be the first retinal laser device without any potential for harm under any circumstance, including precluding the possibility of surgeon error.

9. Modern Retinal Laser Therapy Treatment Strategies

No local or focal treatment targeting

RPC was conceived of as a torch well suited for finely controlled thermal ablation of the retina and related localized structures such as microaneurysms, small tumors, and retinal and choroidal neovascularization. Because such focal and local treatment was often ineffective, such as in PDR, widespread photothermal retinal ablation was employed. Widespread retinal ablation was not an informed response based on a good understanding of retinal laser effects and the nature of the disease process. Instead, it was an extreme response to the lack of such understanding, addressing it by simple retinal reduction. No retina, no problem.

If one thinks back to focal treatment of microaneurysms in the era of the Early Treatment of Diabetic Retinopathy Study (EDTRS), those with experience in that era remember that even white suprathreshold retinal burns generally failed to actually infarct and close the targeted microvascular lesion, whether it was a microaneurysm or neovascularization. After focal ETDRS treatment of microaneurysms one was generally left with patent aneurysms and multiple photocoagulation burns (Fig. 10). Thus, focal RPC simply resulted in a nonaesthetic nonuniform grid treatment. It is no surprise, therefore, that the ETDRS found that focal and grid treatments were equally effective and that focal and local lesion targeting—generally employing higher treatment intensities—were associated with more frequent SAEs (ETDRS 1985).

MRT recognizes that the CPRs are extensive and often panretinal disorders for which targeted therapy is inappropriate. This includes diabetic retinopathy. Instead, disease reversal by complete treatment and transformation from dysfunctional to functional retina, along with preservation of maximal retina to achieve this end, is the preferred, most effective, and maximally visually preserving approach to treatment. This is the basis of the low-intensity/high-density treatment paradigm of MRT (Fig. 25).

Titration? Non

Titration of suprathreshold burn intensity was standard practice in the RPC era. This reflected two important considerations. First, the very high energy of argon laser producing wavelengths of 488 and 514 nm had the potential to rupture retina, Bruch's membrane, and even expose bare sclera beneath the retina if the treatment intensity was excessive. Secondly, as LIRD was thought to be essential for a therapeutic effect, the treating surgeon wanted to verify a desired level of retinal cautery before proceeding with the planned treatment. Because visible laser wavelengths are subject to eye-specific variations in laser uptake influenced by fundus pigmentation, retinal thickness, and media opacity, every eye—and in fact every part of every eye—had to be assessed by titration using test burns to fine-tune the desired level of LIRD intended for treatment.

Remarkably, titration remains standard practice today, despite transition to MPL and low DCs intended to avoid retinal damage (Chhablani et al 2022). RPC thinking dies hard. This is problematic, as there are no objective and scientifically evidence-based algorithms on which to base titration decisions, and certainly none that have any relevance to MPL or MRT (Luttrull and Sinclair 2014, Keunen et al 2020). If one reviews the literature, one will find as many titration algorithms as there are authors (Luttrull and Sinclair 2014, Chhablani et al 2018). Because titration algorithms lack any basis in objective science (all rely on subjective judgments), they perversely increase rather than decrease the risk of inadvertent LIRD by giving the surgeon a false sense of security that he or she has taken adequate measures to avoid retinal burns (Figs. 11, 12, and 22).

The "endpoint management" (EpM) algorithm is an example of the titration fallacy. ANSI industrial safety xMPE data and laboratory studies demonstrate that the therapeutic range—from no effect to a 50/50 burn

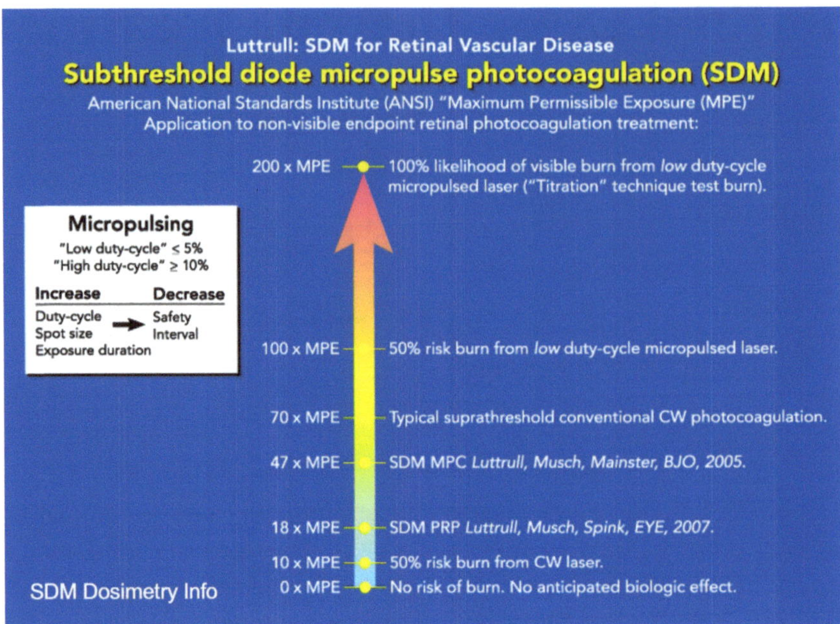

Fig. 24. Relative levels of retinal damage risk with MPL and CW lasers according American National Standards Institute (ANSI) Maximal Permissible Exposure (MPE) levels. Note that the original SDM parameters fell well within the range of biologic effect and low risk of retinal damage. Note that reducing the power of typical RPC according to most titration algorithms to try to perform non-damaging treatment still leaves one above or at the laser burn threshold for CW laser.

risk—for CW lasers is 0.010 W in breadth (American National Standards Institute 2000, Lavinsky et al 2016) (Fig. 24). EpM instructs the user to first create a barely visible retinal burn, then reduce the laser power by a fixed amount according to the EpM, which is nothing more than a titration algorithm, to perform retina-sparing treatment and avoid LIRD. Let us examine EpM, as it typifies the use of titration. First, and most problematic, is reliance on the subjective interpretation of retinal burn intensity in a given eye by any given surgeon. This alone forfeits any claim of scientific objectivity and practical reliability. One man's barely visible burn is another's suprathreshold burn. Second, let us consider the size of the "target" that titration with EpM is supposed to hit—a target that is only 0.010 W in breadth. Such a small target is sufficiently narrow that, even if the surgeon were to guess the test burn intensity correctly and implement the algorithm perfectly, the chances of then performing treatment—especially across a wide region of the macula where variations in pigment and retinal thickness are common—is remote at best. Note that the EpM algorithm was developed in rabbits, not humans (Lavinsky et al 2016). Rabbits have a uniform, homogeneously pigmented RPE. The melanin distribution in the human RPE, on the other hand, is very irregular and heterogenous from one point to the next (Marmor 1975).

In a rabbit, the laser uptake in one spot is predictive of the uptake in the adjacent spot. In humans, with CW one might create a sublethal spot in one location, and a full-thickness retinal burn 200 um away despite using exactly the same laser settings (Figs. 4, 12, and 13). Safe treatment employing titration algorithms, even EpM, is a theoretical possibility but a practical improbability. This translates directly to "Don't worry Mrs. Smith, this treatment may not blind you." Mrs. Smith deserves better. This is to say nothing about attempting to titrate CW to MPL or translating one MPL duty cycle to another. There is simply no evidence-based support for titration to achieve the goal of clinically *reliable* LIRD avoidance in any setting or by any technique or algorithm. Thus, MRT is defined, in part, by the use of fixed laser parameters and the absence of titration (Luttrull and Sinclair 2014, Chhablani et al 2018, Keunen et al 2020).

Key point: If what you are doing requires titration, you should not be doing it.

Use of fixed laser parameters

Absent eye-specific titration of laser parameters, what does one do to achieve laser parameters that will be both safe and effective? The answer is simply to use MPL laser parameters known to be both safe and effective in large numbers of patients and in numerous published studies. Some of these have been listed earlier. Why is this a more reliable and sensible approach? Because rather than a therapeutic range of 0.010 W for CW laser, even the most modestly safe SDM parameters listed earlier have a therapeutic range of at least 2.0 W—200 times broader; and more recent parameter sets up to 15 W—1,500 times broader than any CW laser (Tables 3 and 4).

If by this the practical importance of the difference is not sufficiently obvious, imagine a 15 × 15 m wall. In the middle of that wall is a fly. With CW laser and the aid of a titration algorithm such as EpM, your job is to stand 5 m away from the wall with your bow and arrow and hit the fly. Possible, if you are Robin Hood. But not likely. With known safe and effective SDM parameters for MRT, you only have to hit the wall. Easily done.

In the context of retinal laser treatment and the conceptual hangover from the RPC era, use of identical (fixed) laser parameters in every eye sounds odd, if not irresponsible. Understanding the above discussion will hopefully help. However, how many of us who use intravitreal anti-VEGF medications aim the needle at the macular edema, and adjust the anti-VEGF dosage on a patient-by-patient basis guided by our personal impressions of the patient?

Key point: Virtually every concept taught about retinal laser treatment during the photocoagulation era was wrong because it was based on a false premise. You may need to examine your thinking.

I bought a 577 / 532 nm microsecond laser. What do I do now?

After calling your laser sales representative to register your displeasure at having been misled, there are things you can do. Unfortunately, if you purchased a 532 nm laser for MPL, do not use it except to treat retinal tears. It is too dangerous for MRT.

However, if you are like most people you would have purchased a 577 nm MPL laser. While 577 nm is less safe than 810 nm due to its higher energy and higher melanin absorption, 577 nm can still be used with a high degree of safety provided one applies MRT principles by avoiding titration and using the fixed parameters that have been shown to be safe and effective and published by those highly experienced in this area. In the author's

estimation, the best sources for information regarding 577 nm SDM MRT at this time (September 2022) are the Italians, who have published extensively on 577 nm applying MRT principles for many years, including Midena, Vujosevic, Battaglia-Parodi, and others (Bandello et al 2001, Lanzetta et al 2001, Parodi et al 2006, Vujosevic et al 2010, 2013, 2015, Vujosevic et al 2018, Midena et al 2019, Vujosevic, Gatti et al 2020, Vujosevic, Toma et al 2020, Frizziero, Calcati, Torresin et al 2021) (Table 3) (Fig. 12). Safe fixed 577 nm parameters have also been published by LIGHT: The International Retinal Laser Society along with comparisons of the therapeutic ranges and safety margins of various other retinal laser modes for reference (Keunen et al 2020) (Table 4) (Figs. 4, 12, and 13). The most commonly used power setting for fixed parameter 577 nm SDM has been 0.25 W. However, a study of HSP activation kinetics suggests that 0.16 W would be just as effective, but significantly safer, by broadening the safety margin by about 30% (Chang and Luttrull 2020).

Summary: modern retinal laser therapy dosimetry

Visible wavelengths and DCs over 5% increase the risk of inadvertent and unpredictable retinal damage that limit treatment indications and usefulness. The number and size of retinal spot applications are an index of treatment density and area, the main determinant of treatment efficacy. More is better. Titration of treatment intensity increases the risk of inadvertent retinal damage and should be avoided. Instead, use of published treatment parameters from trusted sources known to be safe and effective based on extensive clinical experience, and supported by scaling law analyses of the thresholds of RPE HSP and thermal cell death Arrhenius integral activation. Use of fixed MRT treatment parameters known to be safe and effective is the best insurance against harm and minimizes the only remaining risk of retinal laser treatment, that of surgeon error.

Key point: You are not smarter than over 22 years of clinical experience with MRT, over 50,000 MRT treatments, and physics. Do not try to reinvent the wheel. Use published laser parameters for MRT proven to be safe and effective.

MRT treatment fields

MRT treatment strategy reflects both the mechanism of action and the specific nature of the disease process. While this latter point may sound contradictory to the etiologic agnosticism ascribed to MRT, it is not. Etiologic agnosticism refers to the mechanism of action at the cellular level, rather than to clinical application of MRT. While the treatment approach to MRT is tremendously more generic than conventional RPC, there are simple, important, and rational allowances to be made for different disease processes. For example, treatment of AMD should reasonably include the entire macula, as visually significant pathology outside the macula in AMD is uncommon and generally of little consequence. Peripheral retinal treatment in AMD does not appear to be important. As protection of the macula, and the fovea in particular, is central to the treatment of all retinal disorders, "panmacular" treatment is the most basic and essential MRT treatment application (Fig. 25). The safety of MRT allows direct treatment of the fovea in the same way that is routine with drug therapy but prohibited with destructive laser modes. In disorders that involve the entire retina in a clinically relevant way, panmacular treatment is then logically complemented by treatment of the balance of the (peripheral) retina outside the major vascular arcades to address the entire disease process, the "retinopathy" as a whole (Fig. 25). In this way, the entire retina is treated with MRT to maximize treatment benefits and optimize the clinical outcome, in much the same way that intravitreal drugs treat not just the macula, but the entire retina. CPRs where total retinal treatment (TRT) is particularly useful are diabetic retinopathy and earlier stages of retinitis pigmentosa, for instance, when the peripheral retina is still functional and viable (Luttrull et al 2006, Luttrull 2018). Thus, clinical application of MRT employs only two treatment fields: "panmacular" treatment for all disorders; and the addition of peripheral retinal treatment to accomplish "total retinal treatment" (TRT) for the generalized retinopathies (Figs. 25 and 26). Thus, this simplification of the clinical treatment strategy reflects both the mechanism of action, and the nature of the disease process.

Compound interest is the 8th wonder of the world. He who understands it earns it…he who doesn't, pays it.
　　　　　　　　　　　　　　　　　　—Albert Einstein

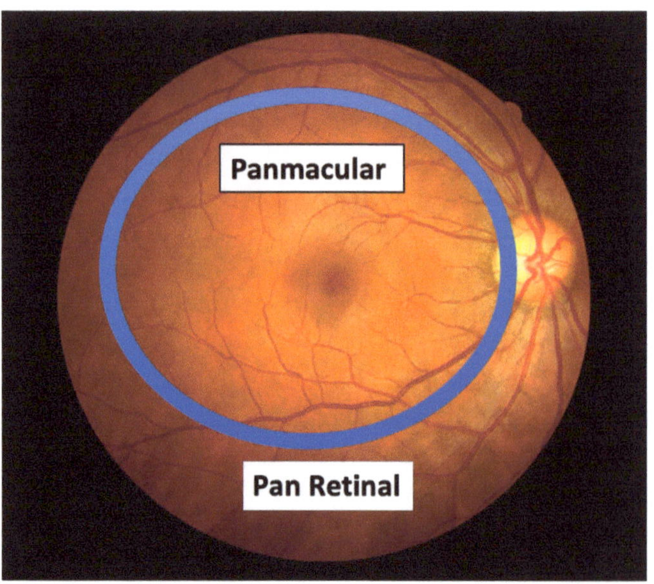

Fig. 25. Standard MRT treatment fields. The panmacular field is the default field for diseases with macular involvement. For generalized retinopathies extending significantly beyond the macula, panretinal treatment is added to achieve "total retinal treatment" (TRT) to maximize therapeutic effectiveness by addressing the entire retinopathy.

Treatment timing

Even small improvements achieved early can result in enormous long-term benefits (Fig. 27). It is important to consider the timing and periodicity of treatment in hopes of maximizing the therapeutic effects of treatment, and for optimal maintenance of treatment benefits. The absence of adverse treatment effects with MRT makes it the ideal first line treatment for many disorders, and the only reasonable preventative treatment for all CPRs (Luttrull 2017). Some disorders, such as central serous chorioretinopathy (CSR) or DR, may require only a single treatment (Luttrull 2016). Others, like AMD, OAG, and IRDs, require periodic retreatment in the form of maintenance therapy (VPT) to sustain clinical effectiveness and maximize treatment benefits (Luttrull, Samples et al 2018, Luttrull, Sinclair et al. 2018, Luttrull et al 2020, Luttrull and Gray 2022). The frequency of retreatment is dictated by the nature and severity of the disease process, with more severe and rapidly progressive disorders, such as autosomal recessive retinitis pigmentosa for example, requiring more frequent retreatment, as often as every 6 weeks (Luttrull 2018). As a rule, the earlier the intervention is begun, the greater the long-term benefit. Compounding

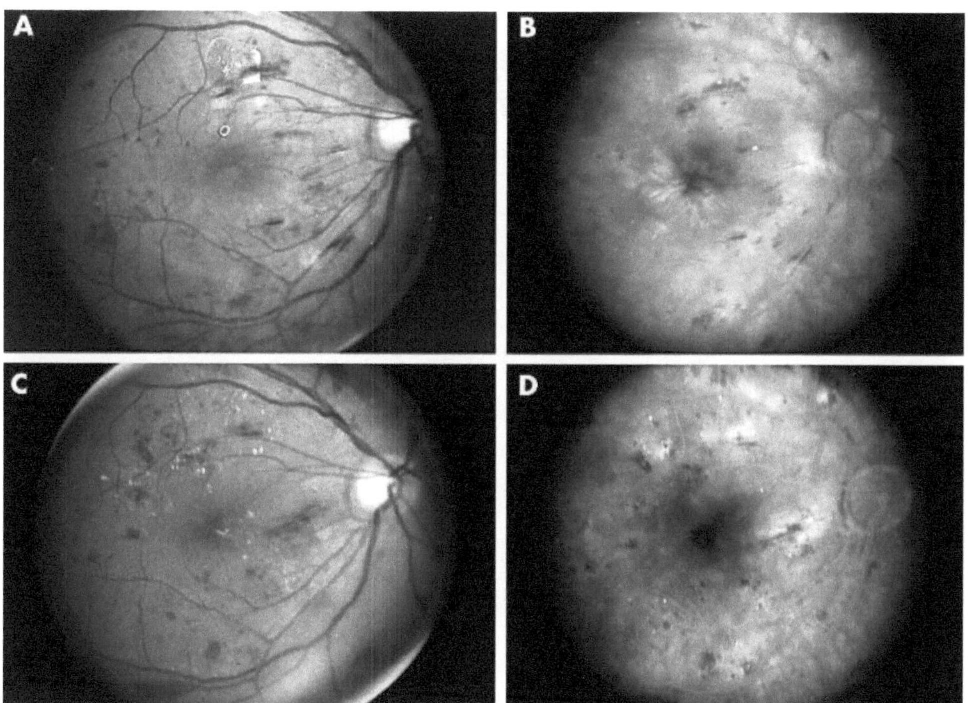

Fig. 26. (A) Preoperative red-free fundus photograph of patient with diffuse clinically significant diabetic macular oedema and foveal cysts. (Note film development artefacts superior to fovea and at temporal edge of photograph.) (B) Late phase preoperative intravenous fundus fluorescein angiogram of diffuse clinically significant diabetic macular oedema. Note cystoid leakage pattern in fovea. This patient was treated with 602 applications of SDM photocoagulation in a nearly confluent grid pattern throughout the macula extending to the edge of the fovea circumferentially. (C) Red-free fundus photograph 8 months following SDM photocoagulation. Note marked reduction in macular oedema without visible chorioretinal scarring or pigmentary disturbance. (D) Postoperative intravenous fundus fluorescein angiogram. Note marked reduction in diffuse and cystoid leakage. Note absence of angiographically visible pigmentary disturbance or chorioretinal scarring following SDM macular photocoagulation. From: *Luttrull JK, Musch MC, Mainster MA: Subthreshold diode micropulse photocoagulation for the treatment of clinically significant diabetic macular edema. Br J Ophthalmol 2005 89:1; 74-80.*

exponentially, the long-term benefits of even a slight slowing of a rapidly progressive disease may result in significantly prolonged retention of visual function by delaying or preventing future visual loss. In less rapidly progressive disorders, early treatment has the potential to prevent visual loss altogether. Interestingly, TRT with MRT for diabetic retinopathy achieves permanent disease reversal in most cases with a single round of treatment (Luttrull et al 2006) (Figs. 14, 18, and 26). Intermediate in this spectrum appear to be AMD and OAG, for which periodic treatment every 3 to 4 months appears highly effective (although ARGA may eventually be found to benefit from even more frequent treatment) (Luttrull, Sinclair et al 2018, Luttrull et al 2020, Luttrull and Gray 2022). These time courses and periodicities of retreatment are informed by years of clinical experience and the results of long-term retinal and visual function testing and clinical monitoring of thousands of eyes. They are also consistent with what

we know about the pathophysiology of the disease processes, and the reset mechanism of retinal laser (Luttrull and Margolis 2016, Luttrull and Kent 2019). Thus, for the most common indications, MRT is best thought of as a process rather than as an event, to be applied with a dosing frequency reflecting the clinical setting and underlying disease process. This is another fundamental distinction of MRT from conventional RPC.

Key point: It helps to think of MRT like drug therapy.

I rob banks because that's where the money is.
—W. F. "Slick Willie" Sutton

Foveal treatment

Another major departure of MRT from the concepts and practices of the RPC era is routine treatment of the fovea (Luttrull and Dorin 2012, Luttrull and Sinclair 2014). When asked why he made a vocation of robbing banks, popular American entrepreneur and independent businessman William Francis Sutton replied, "Because that's where the money is." Why treat the fovea? Because that's where the vision is.

There has probably been no greater prohibition in ophthalmology than avoidance of the fovea with retinal laser treatment. Specifically, avoidance with RPC. This was due to the certainty of immediate treatment associated visual loss (Gitter 1989). Absent concern about treatment-associated visual loss, however, treatment of the fovea is eminently sensible for several reasons. First is that the safety required to offer and perform effective preventive treatment demands that there be no potential for inadvertent treatment-associated visual loss. Thus, ideal preventive treatment should not have the capacity for foveal harm. Second, the ability to treat the fovea safely, and thus the balance of the retina, is critical to unlocking the potential of MRT as homeotrophic therapy to slow and stop disease progression in CPRs, as LIRD worsens visual function and accelerates degeneration. This was demonstrated in the LEAD trial of nano second laser for dry AMD, which accelerated disease progression and visual loss in high-risk eyes (Guymer et al 2018). Third, and most obvious, is that the end goal of virtually every ophthalmic intervention is to preserve and maximize foveal function. The ability to treat and improve the fovea safely and effectively directly with laser, as do drug therapies, is thus a great therapeutic benefit denied to RPC and other damaging laser modes (Luttrull and Sinclair 2014) (Figs. 27-30).

As noted, visual loss from inadvertent treatment of the fovea was the most feared complication that could occur with PC (Gitter 1989, Morgan and Schatz 1989, Mainster 1999). This, and the other causes of RPC-associated visual loss, weighed heavily in the cost/benefit calculation for clinical use of RPC (Figs. 12 and 13). The inherent risks and adverse treatment effects of RPC dictated the indications for treatment. Thus, RPC was reserved for advanced disease, such as clinically significant DME (Early Treatment of Diabetic Retinopathy Study, ETDRS) and high-risk PDR (Diabetic Retinopathy Study Research Group, DRS) (Diabetic Retinopathy Study Research Group 1978, ETDRS 1985, Bandello et al 1993). To permit more effective early/preventive intervention and broadened treatment indications, treatment must be safe in the fovea. MRT makes this possible. The superiority of drugs over PC with regard to near-term visual acuity outcomes

demonstrated in virtually every clinical trial stem from two factors: first, drugs do not cause tissue damage that degrades visual function; and second, intravitreal drugs invariably treat the fovea directly, as well as the entire retina, maximizing the visual benefits of treatment. MRT shares this attribute with drugs, while eliciting a broader and longer-lasting restorative therapeutic response, without the risks or burden of drug therapy (Luttrull and Sinclair 2014).

As noted, MRT improves retinal function directly where it is applied. Nowhere is improved retinal function—and thus resistance to degeneration—more important than in the fovea. Second, it is important to consider both the mechanism of MRT action and the unique aspects of foveal anatomy. MRT works by initiating a catalytic chain-reaction of cascading events initiated by thermal activation of RPE HSPs. This cellular response is then amplified by confluent treatment of large areas of diseased retina to capture and recruit and functionally transform *en masse* as much dysfunctional retina as possible to maximize clinical effectiveness. Thus, RPE density, and the number of RPE cells directly exposed to treatment capable of a treatment response, is a key determinant of the treatment response. Nowhere is RPE density greater than in the central fovea, where it may be as high as 9,000 cells/mm^2, decreasing to 3,000 cells/mm^2 or less in the retinal periphery (Snodderly et al 2002). Third is the critical influence of the RPE on retinal function (Kolomyer and Zarbin 2014). In addition to maintaining the blood-ocular barrier and inhibiting subretinal neovascularization at its basal pole, photoreceptor function at its apical pole, and enhancing visual function by reducing reflections at the chorioscleral and outer retinal interfaces, the RPE has essential paracrine functions maintaining normal retinal function, retinal autoregulation, and retinal homeostasis via innumerable chemical mediators produced by, and responded to, the RPE. This tropic and regulatory role is greatest and most important in the fovea, reflected by its unmatched metabolic demand (Cohen et al 1965). Many RPE elaborated extracellular cytokines are diffusible and produced in sufficient quantities that they can be detected in the vitreous and anterior chamber (Nordgaard et al 2006, Midena et al 2020). This means they have the potential to influence all ocular structures to which they are exposed. Thus, inclusion of the macula is necessary to maximize the therapeutic clinical response to MRT

Summary of Survival Fits

The following plot shows the overall cumulative wet AMD conversion probabilities by group.

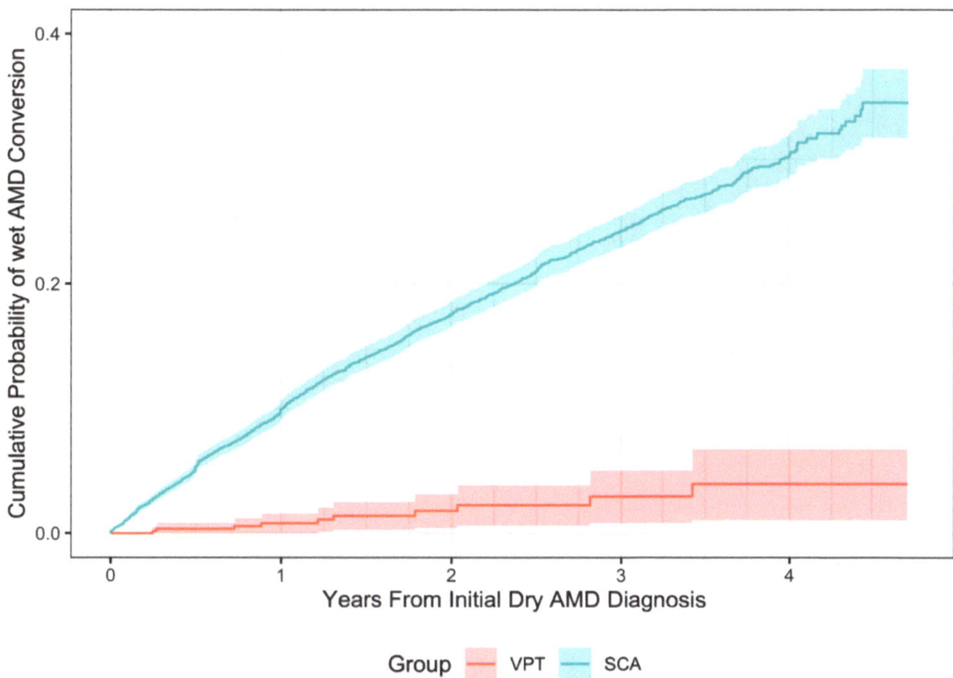

Fig. 27. Overall Kaplan-Meier cumulative wet AMD conversion probability by group. Shaded areas indicate 95% confidence intervals. Rate of neovascular conversion over 4.75 years in 9130 propensity scored eyes with bilateral dry AMD. Blue line, eyes receiving standard care alone (SCA) with AREDS supplements. Red line, eyes receiving SDM MRT as vision protection therapy (VPT) in addition to standard care. Hazard ratio 13.04. From: *Luttrull JK, Gray G. Real World Data Comparison of Standard Care vs SDM Laser Vision Protection Therapy for Prevention of Neovascular AMD. Clin Ophthalmol (2022) May, 16: 1555-1568.*

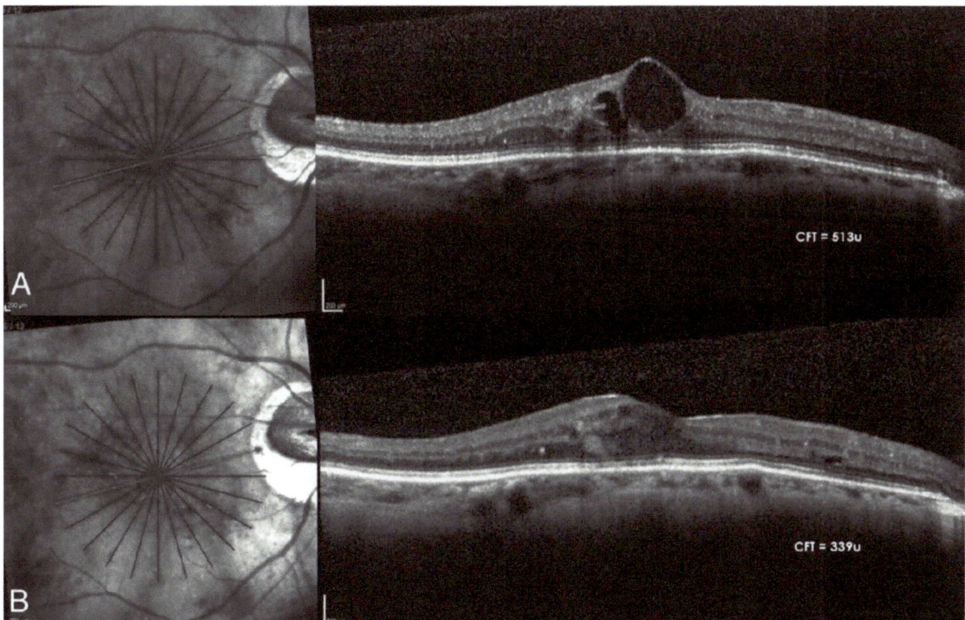

Fig. 28. Fovea-involving diabetic macular edema before (A) and 3 months after (B) TFSDM laser treatment. Preoperative visual acuity of 20/50. Visual acuity of 20/40 3 months postoperatively. (Fundus photographs on left depict SD-OCT scan positions and location of scans shown on right). From: *Luttrull JK, Sinclair SD. Safety of transfoveal subthreshold diode micropulse laser for intra-foveal diabetic macular edema in eyes with good visual acuity. Retina, May 2014 Oct; 34 (10): 2010-20.*

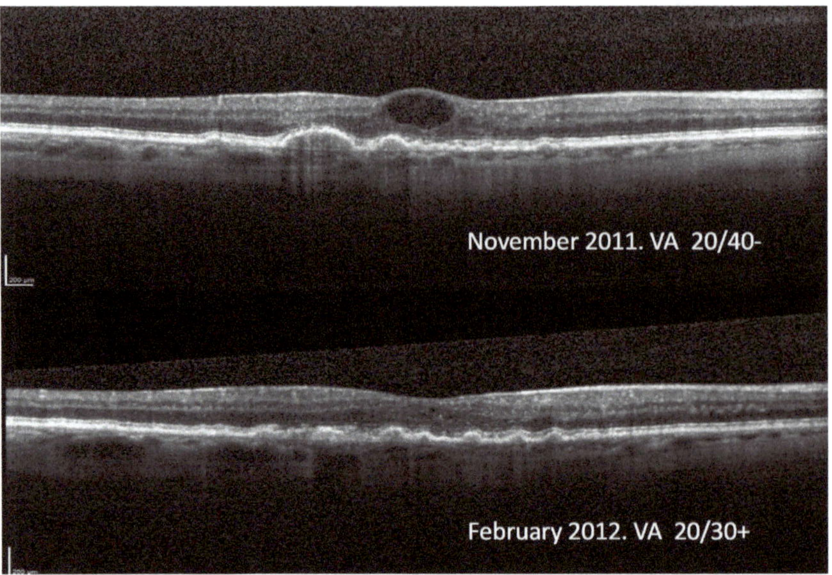

Fig. 29. Eye with intermediate AMD and DME with a central foveal cyst resistant to prior extrafoveal SDM laser,4 bevacizumab injections, and 7 ranibizumab injections. Due to the failure to respond, transfoveal SDM was performed. Top, before transfoveal panmacular SDM. Bottom, after. Note resolution of chronic foveal cyst following direct treatment of the fovea.

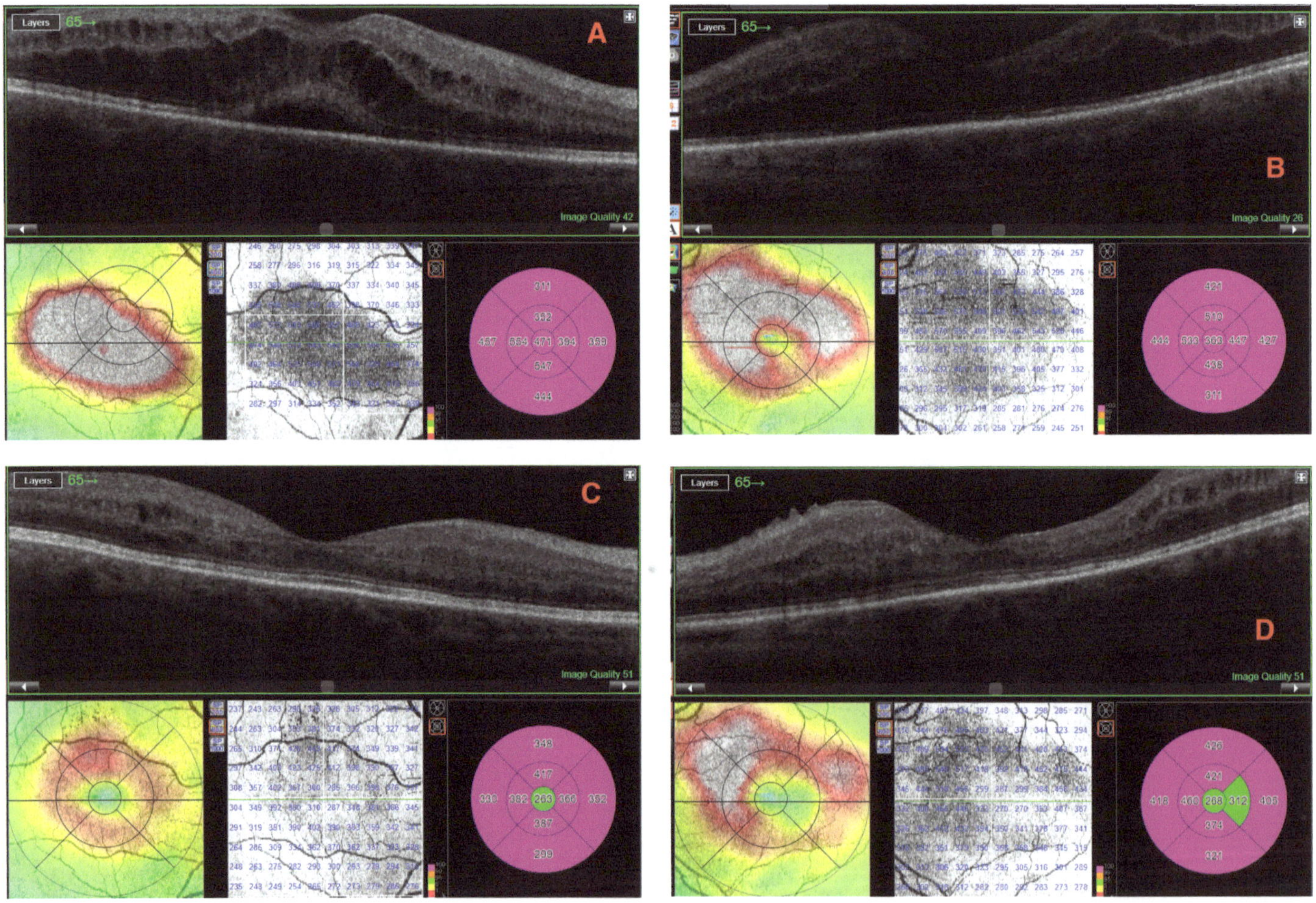

Fig. 30. OCT of 67 yo woman with Type I diabetes mellitus, severe NPDR, and severe DME unresponsive to two years of anti-VEGF therapy followed by intravitreal dexamethasone implants OU and membrane peeling OS. (A) right eye and (B) left eye before total retinal SDM MRT (TRT). VA 20/70 OD and 20/200 OS. (C) right eye and (D) left eye 12 months post TRT x 3 OU. Note reduction in DME OU and resolution of serous macular detachment OD. VA improved to 20/30 OD and 20/70 OS.

(Luttrull et al 2014, Luttrull, Samples et al 2018, Luttrull and Kent 2020).

Key point: Foveal treatment is not adventurism. It is good sense.

Combination therapy

Because the effects of MRT are to generically improve and normalize retinal function, promote repair, and reduce inflammation, MRT can be employed as monotherapy or in combination with any other intervention (Luttrull et al 2012, Luttrull 2020) (Figs. 20 and 26). Like any combination of therapies, three basic types of interaction may occur: inhibition, complementarity, or synergy. Applying different treatments in sequence also raises the issues of presentation order, temporal treatment intervals, and what effect(s) these may have on the desired outcome. This is because the first intervention alters the environment that will greet the second, and this alteration will also be reflected in the temporal distance from the first to the second intervention, and so on.

In inhibition, the combination of therapies may result in diminishing the effectiveness that would be achieved by either therapy alone. An example may be simultaneous use of MRT with anti-VEGF therapy (Luttrull et al 2012). If one thinks of MRT as a message to the retina to change its behavior for the better (more normal), and studies suggest that a complete MRT treatment response may require at least 3 weeks to manifest, what might be the effect of flooding the eye with a massive (pharmacologic) dose of anti-VEGF medication during that interval? (Luttrull et al 2012, Kern et al 2018). Might this be taken by the MRT-treated

RPE as a conflicting "never mind" message, attenuating the desired laser treatment response? Laboratory study suggests this may indeed be the case (Kern et al 2018). Concern over such a phenomenon informed the decision to delay rechallenge with anti-VEGF medication for at least a month after SDM treatment for drug tolerance in wet AMD, hoping to minimize the possibility that premature reintroduction of drug therapy might inhibit the development of MRT-induced tolerance reversal (Luttrull et al 2015). Complementary effects arise when combination of MRT with another intervention achieves results that are essentially additive. An example here may be MRT treatment of persistent macular thickening and visual loss following surgery for epiretinal membranes (Luttrull 2020). There is also the potential for combining MRT with another intervention to achieve results greater than the sum of their individual effects. Such synergy is more likely to arise if the two treatments are both effective, have different mechanisms of action, and do not compromise or inhibit one another. An example of such synergy is potentiation of photodynamic therapy with intravitreal triamcinolone acetate (TCA) (Luttrull and Spink 2007). TCA has no appreciable effect on age-related choroidal neovascularization (CNV) alone. However, co-administration of TCA with PDT for neovascular AMD prolongs the PDT effects, improving outcomes (Luttrull and Spink 2007). The greatest value of MRT remains, however, for MRT to preclude, replace, or reduce more invasive, short-acting, burdensome, expensive, and/or higher risk inventions such as RPC and intravitreal drug therapy.

Key point: MRT can be used with any other treatment to improve outcomes.

Section IV. Clinical Applications of Modern Retinal Laser Therapy

10. Diabetic Retinopathy

The past is not what it was.

—GK Chesterton

DME and the development of MRT

Before beginning a discussion of MRT for DME it is useful to recognize that there have been many large and well-done RCTs carried out over the years that provided the primary information regarding retinal laser treatment for DME to the ophthalmic community. In all of them, from the ETDRS to the Diabetic Retinopathy Clinical Research Network (DRCN), "retinal laser treatment" was RPC (ETDRS 1985, Glassman et al 2020). These studies of RPC for DME have established the treatment techniques, indications, and expectations for almost 50 years. What do these studies have to tell us about MRT?

Very little. We have clearly established that RPC is the most serious complication of retinal laser treatment, having no direct therapeutic effects while being the single cause of all the many risks, adverse effects, and limitations of retinal laser treatment. Thus, the results of studies on RPC for DME show us, at best, the worst-case scenario for the potential of retinal laser treatment for DME, with treatment effectiveness limited by low-density local and focal treatment and the inability to directly treat central swelling in the fovea; while at the same time destroying functional tissue and causing inflammation and retinal scarring, all detrimental to visual function and visual acuity. Unfortunately, the many subsequent studies on the path from conventional RPC to MRT provide only glimpses of the potential of retinal laser for DME.

The ETDRS found that high treatment intensity increased adverse treatment effects, while increased treatment density improved outcomes (ETDRS 1985). Thus were sown the seeds of MRT. Over time, treatment intensity decreased (Mainster 1999). However, presumed need for LIRD to achieve effective therapy persisted, and thus the SAEs of RPC, limiting treatment density, effectiveness, and visual results (Akduman and Olk 1999). Short-pulse CW and microsecond pulsed lasers came on the scene to be used to further reduce—but maintain—LIRD (Friberg and Venkatesh

1995, Moorman and Hamilton 1999, Roider et al 2000, Bandello et al 2001, Laursen et al 2004, Figueira et al 2009, Roider et al 2010, Casson et al 2012, Blumenkranz 2014, Park et al 2017, Hamada et al 2018). However, by reducing treatment intensity and maintaining low treatment density due to persistent LIRD these approaches were generally less effective than conventional RPC. While reducing treatment intensity did reduce the severity of laser SAEs somewhat, they remained, as did the risks of treatment. Thus, the move toward reduced treatment intensity while seeking to maintain the perceived necessity of LIRD was a change in style more than substance. Flames and racing stripes had been painted on the aged RPC jalopy (Fig. 31).

Key point: Studies of RPC tell us little about MRT

Low-intensity/high-density subthreshold diode microsecond pulsed laser for DME: 2000

The first report employing the modern retinal laser therapy paradigm of low-intensity/high density treatment described patients treated from 2000 to 2003 for DME (Luttrull et al 2005). In this retrospective study of 95 consecutive eyes of 69 patients followed for 3 to 29 months (mean 12.2), prior to availability of OCT and anti-VEGF medications, found the DME improved in 95% and completely resolved in 79% following SDM treatment. There were no adverse treatment effects, and no evidence of LIRD by clinical examination or intravenous fundus fluorescein angiography (FFA) in any eye (Figs. 5, 14, 26, and 27). VA was improved by three lines or more in 8.4%, unchanged in 76.8% and worsened by three or more lines in 14.7% of the patients. With availability of OCT, the time course of the treatment response to SDM was examined in 18 consecutive eyes of 14 patients, showing reduced macular thickening by 1 month, becoming statistically significant by 3 months (Luttrull and Spink 2007) (Fig. 36). Subsequently, 62 consecutive eyes of 42 patients followed a median 12 months following SDM treatment of DME evaluated

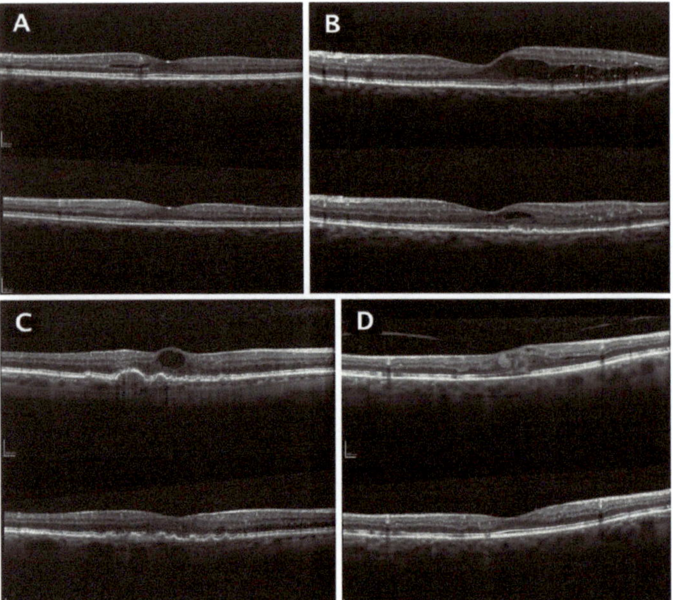

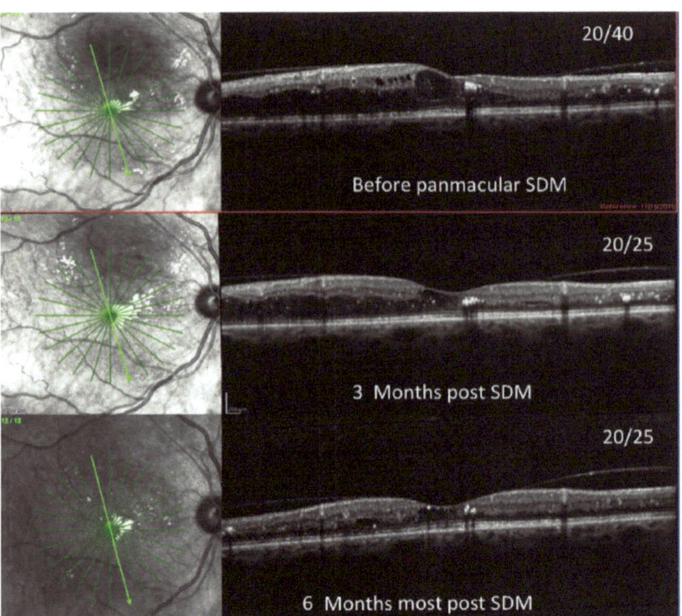

Fig. 31. OCTs of eyes with fovea-involving DME and VA > 20/40 before and after transfoveal SDM MRT. Despite mild macular thickening and good pre-treatment VAs, both macular thickening and VAs were significantly improved following treatment. No eye required intravitreal drug therapy. Types of FIDME in eyes with visual acuity of 20/40 or better treated with TFSDM in this study (In each pair, A-D, top of the frames represent preoperative SD-OCT and bottom of the frames represent postoperative SD-OCT). A. Intrafoveal cysts without retinal thickening. B. Intrafoveal thickening with minimal central foveal thickening. C. Isolated central foveal cyst. D. Diffuse macular thickening including the fovea. From: *Luttrull JK, Sinclair SD. Safety of transfoveal subthreshold diode micropulse laser for intra-foveal diabetic macular edema in eyes with good visual acuity. Retina, May 2014 Oct; 34 (10): 2010-20.*

Fig. 32. Optical coherence tomography before (top); 3 months after (middle); and 6 months after (bottom) panmacular SDM laser for center-involving diabetic macular edema. Note reduction in macular thickening and resolution of macular exudates without laser-induced retinal damage. Snellen visual acuity 20/40 before treatment and 20/25 after treatment. SDM, low-intensity/ high-density subthreshold diode micropulse laser. From: *Chhablani J, Roh YJ, Jobling AI, Fletcher EL, Lek JJ, Bansal P, Guymer R, Luttrull JK. Restorative retinal laser therapy: Present state and future directions. Surv. Ophthalmol 2018 May - Jun;63(3):307-328.*

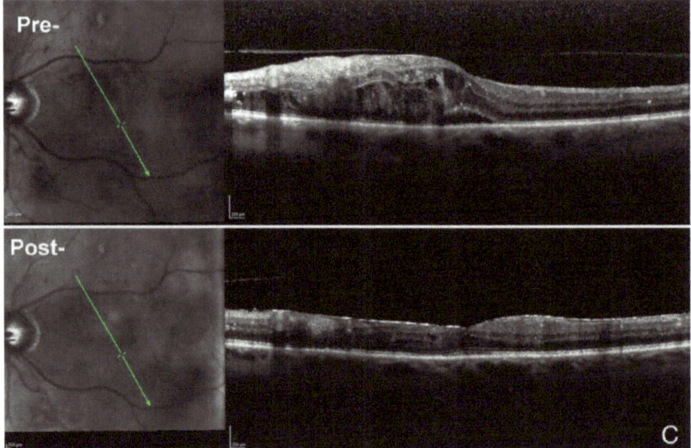

Fig. 33. Heidelberg Spectralis images of an eye treated for DME with extrafoveal SDM. This 66-year-old white man received 648 applications in a single session of macular SDM. Laser parameters: 131 retinal spot size, 0.93 Watt peak power, 5% DC, 500-Hz micropulse repetition rate, 0.3-second pulse (burst) duration. Visual acuity preoperatively was 20/80; 3 months postoperatively, it was 20/ 50. The images on the left were taken before treatment and those on the right 3 months after treatment. Note resolution of DME and the complete absence of laser-induced retinal injury postoperatively in all images. A. Autofluorescence fundus photographs (FAF). Arrows denote area of ME treated by SDM. B. Intravenous FFAs. C. Spectral-domain OCT before (top) and after (bottom) treatment. From: *Luttrull JK, Sramek C, Palanker D, Spink CJ, Musch DC. Long-term safety, high-resolution imaging, and tissue temperature modeling of subvisible diode micropulse photocoagulation for retinovascular macular edema. Retina 2012; 32 (2): 375-86.*

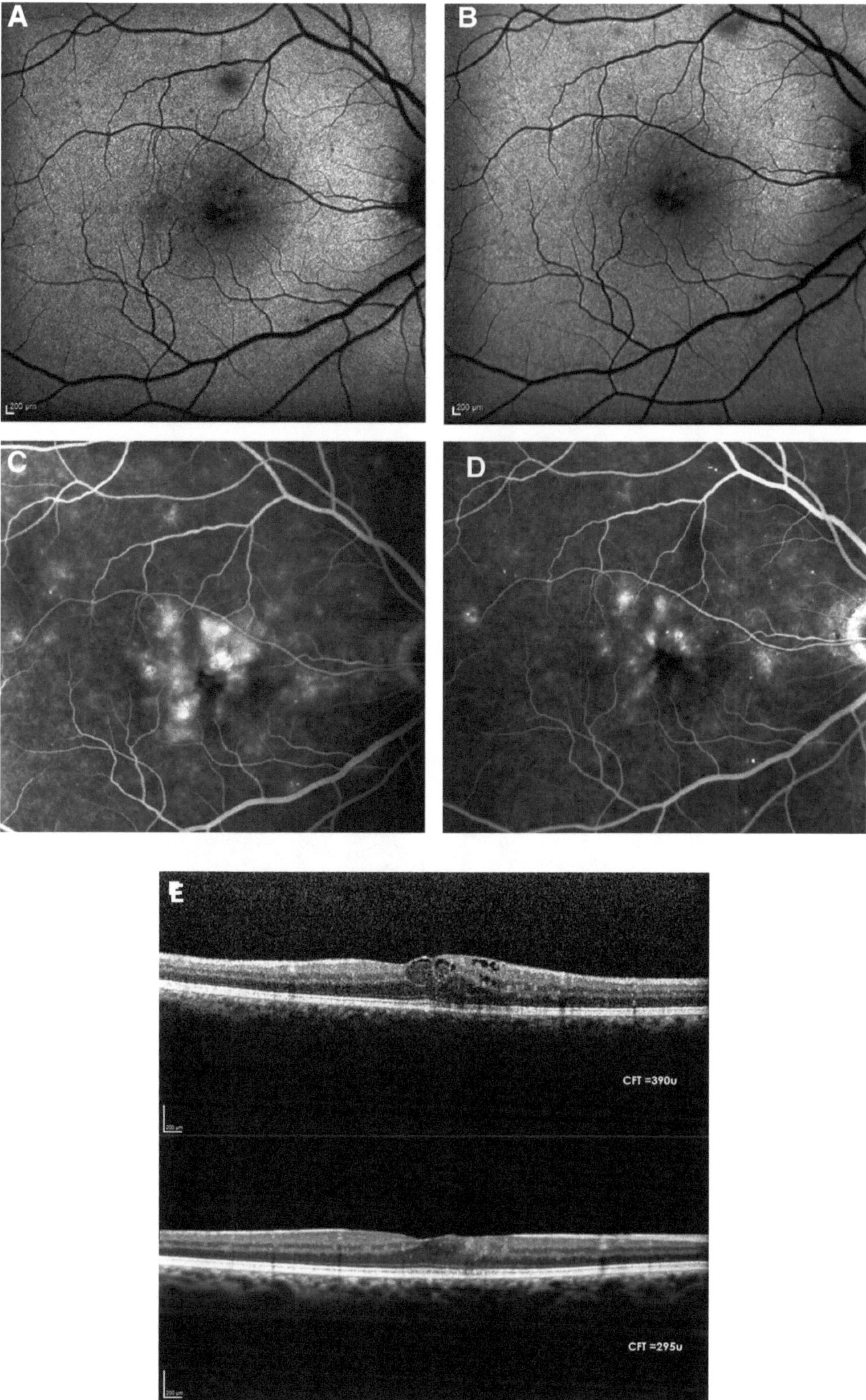

Fig. 34. Fundus autofluorescence photography of the right eye with FIDM and cystoid macular edema (CME) before (A) and after (B) TFSDM. Note the reduction in CME and absence of laser-induced retinal damage. Fundus fluorescein angiogram before (C) and after (D) TFSMD for FIDME. Note the reduced macular leakage and absence of laser-induced retinal damage. E. Spectral domain optical coherence tomography before (above) and after (below) TFSDM for FIDME. Note the reduced macular thickness and absence of laser-induced retinal damage. From: *Luttrull JK, Sinclair SD. Safety of transfoveal subthreshold diode micropulse laser for intra-foveal diabetic macular edema in eyes with good visual acuity. Retina, May 2014 Oct; 34 (10): 2010-20.*

Combination Therapy

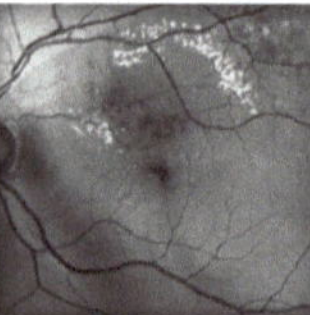

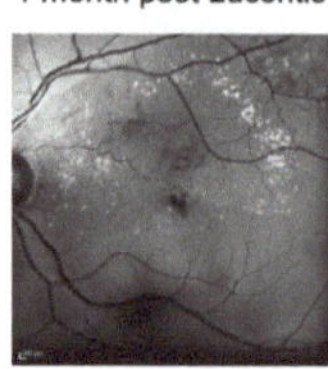

Pre-treatment
CFT 525 µm, VA 20/40

Avastin given

1 month post Avastin
CFT 275µm, VA 20/30

SDM Performed

4 months post MPLT
CRT 250 µm, VA 20/25

Red-free photo: BRVO
1 month post Lucentis

Red-free photo: BRVO
7 months post SDM

SDM for Lucentis nonresponse

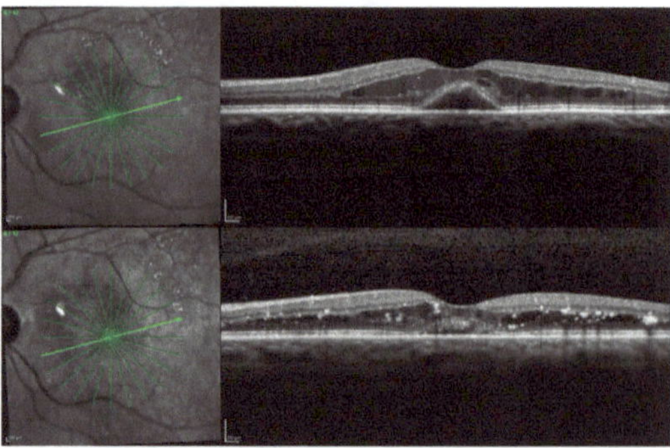

Top: SD-OCT 1 month post Lucentis. CFT 390 µm, VA 20/50-.
Unimproved. SDM performed.

Bottom: 7 months* post SDM. CFT 282 µm, VA 20/40+.
*Progressive improvement in ME from 6 weeks** post SDM by
SD-OCT.

Fig. 35. Examples of combination therapy with SDM MRT and anti-VEGF therapy for DME. (A) bevacizumab (B) ranibizumab.

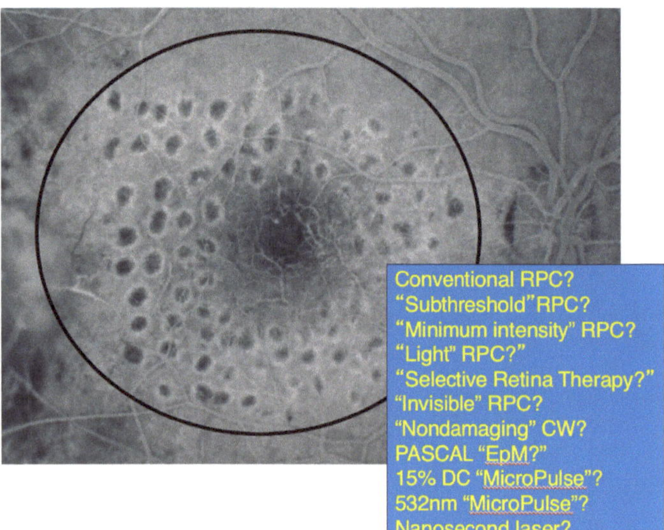

Subthreshold photocoagulation

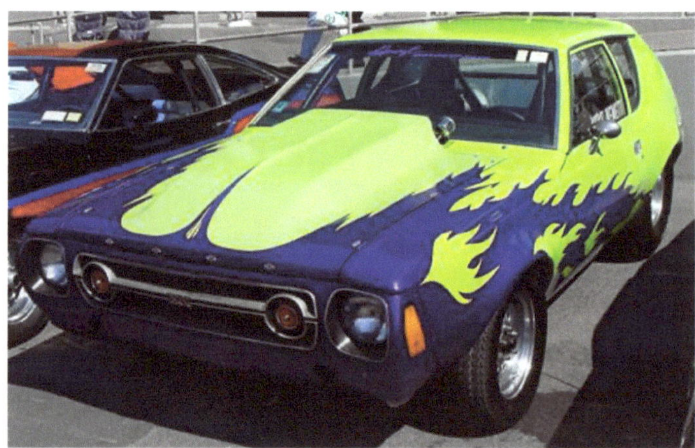

New? Different?

Fig. 36. (A) FFA illustrating the ambiguity of nomenclature used to evoke the impression of progress in the evolution of retinal laser treatment resulting from insistence on laser-induced retinal damage as the prerequisite for effective treatment. (B) Similar treatment of a popular automobile.

pre and post treatment by high resolution fundus autofluorescence photography and spectral-domain OCT (SD-OCT) found significant improvement in central (p=0.04) and maximum (p=0.0001) macular thickness following treatment, without LIRD (Luttrull et al 2012) (Table 5). Twenty four of these 62 eyes also received anti-VEGF therapy, usually due to worse initial visual acuities (p=0.0001). Final overall visual acuities were unchanged, and the addition of anti-VEGF therapy did not influence final visual or anatomic outcomes (Fig. 33). In none of these early studies was transfoveal treatment performed (Luttrull and Dorin 2012, Luttrull and Sinclair 2014) (Figs. 30-34). Subsequent reviews and meta-analyses of studies of various microsecond pulsed subthreshold laser approaches have confirmed these early reports, finding macular edema reduction on par with PC, but better visual results, including improved microperimetry (Vujosevic et al 2010, Chen et al 2016, Jorge et al 2018). The single trial comparing modified ETDRS PC to low-density subthreshold and high-density subthreshold treatment found clear superiority of the high-density/low-intensity approach for DME reduction, with visual results comparable to drug therapy (Lavinsky et al 2011).

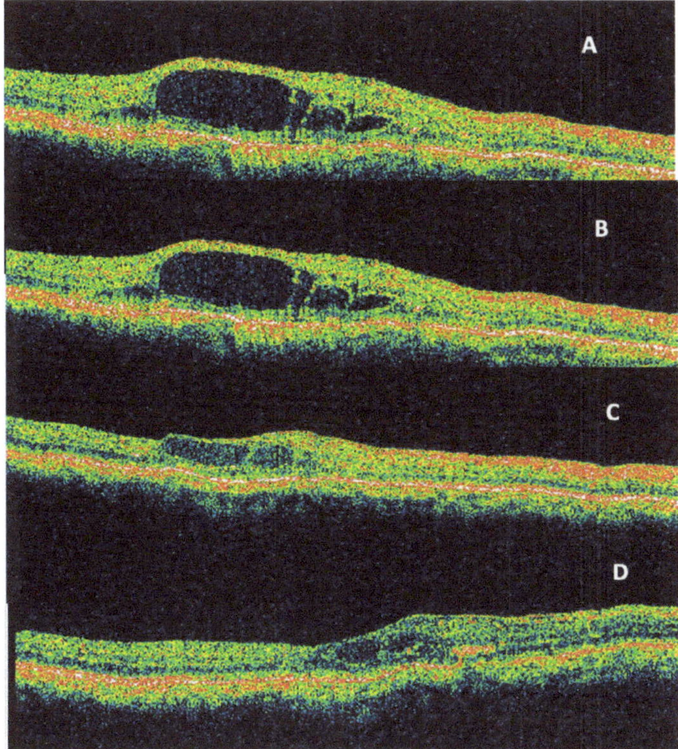

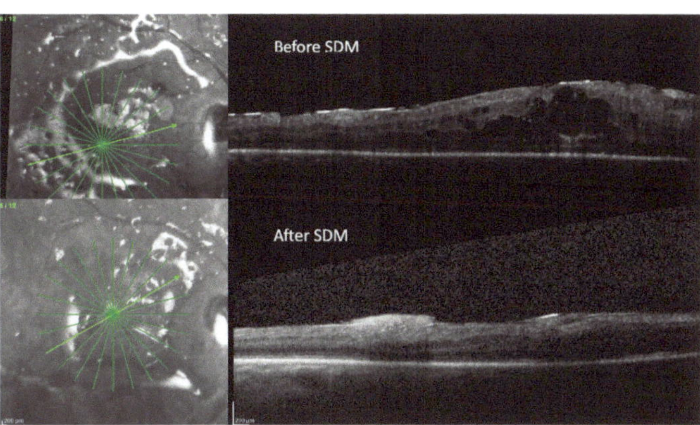

Fig. 39. OCTs of right eye (top) 6 months after vitrectomy and silicone oil for repair of recurrent diabetic traction retinal detachment with proliferative vitreoretinopathy. Note DME under silicone oil. (Bottom) Note resolution of DME 4 months after panmacular SDM MRT. VA 20/200 before and after.

Fig. 37. Example of time course of DME resolution following extrafoveal SDM 2004. (A) At presentation (B) one week post treatment (C) one month post treatment (D) 3 months post treatment.

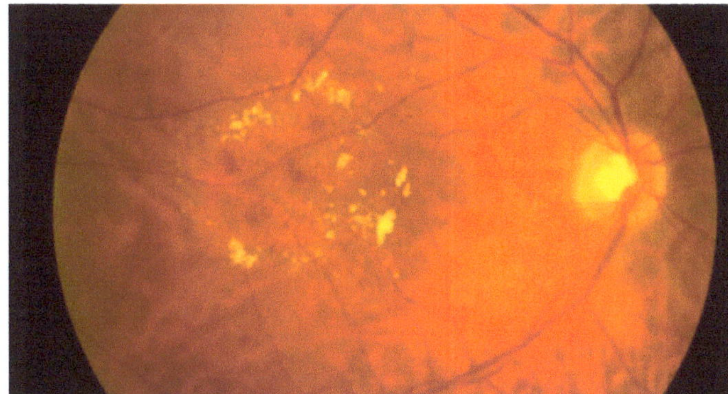

Fig. 38. Eye with clinically significant diabetic macular edema according to criteria of the Early Treatment of Diabetic Retinopathy Study. Contrary to the study terminology of "early", the anatomic derangements seen in this eye represents late, advanced disease, rather than early retinopathy.

Treatment of DME and the evolution of MRT "low-intensity" and "high-density" paradigm

The conceptual basis for the treatment of DME remains unchanged from the inception of SDM. However, both the "low-intensity" and "high-density" principles of MRT have evolved over the years, informed by clinical experience and an improved understanding of the mechanism of retinal laser action. This has led to the development of ever safer but still highly effective low-intensity MRT laser parameters by abandonment, after 20 years, of the previously widely preferred higher duty cycles for macular treatment, such as 15%, and adoption of high(er)-density treatment application. Hopefully, another 20 years will not pass before abandonment of visible wavelengths and titration (Figueira et al 2009, Chang and Luttrull 2020, Keunen et al 2020, Al-Barki et al 2021, Amoaku et al 2020, Chhablani et al 2022) (Figs. 4, 12, and 13) (Table 4). The definition of "high-density" has also evolved from the initial approach of confluent treatment of only the area of macular thickening indicated by contact lens examination in DME, to the current approach of total retinal treatment (TRT) for generalized retinopathies; and panmacular treatment for maculopathies (Luttrull et al 2005, 2008, Luttrull and Sinclair 2014, Luttrull 2018, Keunen et al 2020).

Early treatment

The more severe the condition, the more difficult it is to treat, the slower to improve, and the less complete the recovery. This is a reminder of the importance of early and preventive treatment when treatment is most effective and visual loss can be prevented. The ETDRS used ophthalmoscopically visible anatomic abnormalities to identify and define retinal pathology (ETDRS 1985). In the ETDRS, the anatomic changes that were identified as visually threatening and which responded to RPC described as *clinically significant (CS)* were recommended

Table 5. Clinical change within groups and overall for the subset treated with SDM for DME with pre- and postoperative HS SD-OCT information

Variables	All (*n* = 62 eyes; 48 subjects)			SDM + drug therapy (*n* = 24 eyes; 20 subjects)			SDM alone (*n* = 38 eyes; 28 subjects)		
	Mean (SD)	**Min, Max**	***P****	**Mean (SD)**	**Min, Max**	***P****	**Mean (SD)**	**Min, Max**	***P****
BCVA change	0.02 (2.04)	−7, 6	0.9505	−0.08 (3.03)	−7, 6	0.8942	0.08 (1.05)	−2, 3	0.6456
CFT change (*μ*m)	−25.0 (94.2)	−427, 340	0.0410	−42.7 (143.8)	−427, 340	0.1592	−13.8 (37.9)	−172, 49	0.0313
MMT change (*μ*m)	−49.1 (71.4)	−278, 71	<0.0001	−62.9 (94.9)	−278, 71	0.0035	−40.4 (51.2)	−209, 65	<0.0001

SDM, low-intensity/high-density SDM photocoagulation; BCVA, best-corrected visual acuity; visual acuity, 1 = 20/20, 2 = 20/25, 3 = 20/30, and so on.
*The t-test (all observations assumed to be independent).
From: Luttrull JK, Sramek C, Palanker D, Spink CJ, Musch DC. Long-term safety, high-resolution imaging, and tissue temperature modelling of subvisible diode micropulse photocoagulation for retinovascular macular edema. *Retina.* 2012;32(2):375-386.

for "early" RPC. In any other context, the findings of architectural tissue disruption and degeneration represented by CSDME would constitute advanced, if not end-stage disease, rather than "early" disease (Fig. 38). The designation of "early" for treatment of clinically significant DME primarily reflected the risks and adverse effects of RPC that recommended treatment be withheld until the development of advanced, visually threatening disease. Prevention of DME with RPC was not seriously considered due to the risks and SAEs. A major lesson learned from the ETDRS is the importance of early, preventative treatment before the development of anatomic damage occurs that is diagnosable by imaging and before the development of visual loss. Few eyes in the ETDRS that lost 20/20 vision regained it. Continuing to employ PC, the DRCR.net Protocol V trial reported little overall benefit from early treatment of eyes with center-involving DME and good VA. In this study, a significant percentage (16-19%) of eyes developed visual loss when treatment was deferred due to initially good VA (Glassman, Baker et al 2020). Absent adverse treatment effects, MRT allows such eyes to be treated promptly, safely, effectively, and repeatedly if necessary to maintain excellent vision and prevent visual loss (Luttrull and Sinclair 2014) (Figs. 31-34). The ability to treat early and directly in the fovea with MRT, when VA is excellent and DME most responsive to treatment, allows for more effective management and elimination of DME; and preservation, rather than attempted restoration, of excellent VA (Luttrull and Sinclair 2014) (Figs. 28, 30-34, 36). In the author's experience, early treatment with MRT has reduced the need for anti-VEGF in DME by 90% compared to the average U.S. retina specialist, requiring intravitreal drug therapy in less than 10% of eyes with DME, while preserving excellent VA. This is because SDM

MRT is effective, and because early treatment generally precludes progression to severe, chronic, intractable, and visually compromising DME requiring drug therapy (Luttrull et al 2005, Luttrull, Sramek et al 2012, Lai et al 2021) (JKL, unpublished data 2012-2021, Vestrum Health, Naperville, Ill, USA).

Key point: The ETDRS, relying on biomicroscopically visible anatomic signs, described late, not early treatment.

Preventive treatment and maintenance prophylaxis to prevent recurrent DME

It becomes quickly obvious to most as soon as they understand and begin to gain experience with MRT that the safety and effectiveness of MRT for DME will argue for use of MRT to prevent, and not just treat DME; and for use of MRT as maintenance prophylaxis after elimination of DME to prevent recurrence. Although the VA results of MRT are superior to RPC, nothing is more effective than prevention of visual loss in the first place. This is done by preventing the development of DME. Obvious candidates for preventive and prophylactic MRT are eyes without macular thickening, but with moderate to severe background retinopathy, especially if associated with diffuse microvascular leakage, macular microcystic changes or hyperreflective spots on OCT, and/or non-perfusion on FFA. As will be discussed again with respect to management of PDR and DR, FFA can be very useful in providing treatment endpoints in this context. By obtaining FFA prior to preventive treatment, and then 6-12 months later (sooner is often less informative) the activity of the microvascular disease can be easily visualized and appreciated, manifest by the degree of late leakage present (Figs. 5, 14, and 26). If the response is good, cessation of treatment is reasonable. If there is little response, treatment should be continued and FFA repeated until significant quiescence has been achieved. Once the leakage by FFA—an excellent indicator of disease activity—has been substantially reduced or eliminated, the risk of *de novo* or recurrent DME is generally low. In such eyes, as well as eyes in which DME has been eliminated but has the potential for recurrence, MRT allows periodic retreatment to suppress both occurrence and recurrence of DME.

Because treatment is simple, safe, and comfortable, MRT is well accepted by patients, unlike more painful, invasive, and burdensome treatments such as RPC and intravitreal drug injections (Wen et al 2017, Moore and Chao 2017, Chen et al 2018, Levine et al 2019, Maturi et al 2021). The safety of MRT also allows continuation of periodic treatments as long as needed until the eye is quiet and the DR has reversed and become minimal with little potential for new or recurrent DME. Once regressed, reworsening of DR is rare (Figs. 5, 14, and 26). The ability to treat preventively, therapeutically, prophylactically, as combination therapy when needed, and regularly, provides the doctor a range of management options with MRT not afforded by any other intervention to optimize clinical outcomes.

Those whose treatment armamentarium consists mainly of RPC and intravitreal drugs are generally unaccustomed to thinking preventatively and thus are not attuned to the opportunities for prevention that present themselves. According to Shah and associates, 14% of eyes with DME lost >10 letters and 55% had < 55 letters of VA despite intravitreal drug therapy for DME (Shah et al 2022). How to avoid?—By prevention. By fully incorporating MRT into DME management one becomes more keenly aware of the opportunities to intervene early and preventatively to reverse disease severity, prevent progression, and prevent visual loss. This is better medicine than waiting for things to first go bad, and then trying to repair the damage.

Key point: The safety of MRT allows preventive treatment. It is easier to keep good vision than to restore it.

MRT neuroprotective prophylaxis for post-DME macular damage

Another indication for panmacular MRT maintenance therapy are eyes with macular damage from chronic prior macular edema and/or severe retinopathy, and eyes RPC damage from prior conventional laser. Such eyes often exhibit diffuse macular thinning, microvascular abnormalities absent active DME, angiographic leakage and/or focal ischemia, and RPE damage from prior chronic DME or prior conventional RPC. Such eyes may continue to slowly worsen with time. Because MRT improves retinal function and thus stops or slows degeneration, there is an argument to be made for treating these eyes on a regular basis to maximize retinal and visual function and reduce the risks of visual loss from progressive degeneration. Such treatment may be especially useful in eyes with reduced VA but no DME, as MRT can improve and maintain improved visual function and VA in such eyes (Fig. 2, 11. 40). This is an application uniquely available to MRT as conventional RPC will clearly worsen such eyes, and drugs have nothing to offer in the absence of macular thickening.

MRT for DME: primary versus secondary treatment?

How should one decide whether to begin treatment with MRT or intravitreal drug therapy? Currently, there are two main approaches. The most popular is to be guided by OCT measured macular thickness, recommending drug injection if the macular thickness exceeds 400 um (Vujosevic et al 2013, Mansouri et al 2014, Othman et al 2014, Citirik 2019). After the macular thickness is reduced, MRT is begun to achieve complete and final elimination of the DME while minimizing the injection burden. An alternative, functionally guided approach, is informed by visual acuity rather than macular thickness (Luttrull 2017, Luttrull et al 2012). In this approach, for eyes with DME and VA of 20/50 or better, MRT is performed first. In such eyes, VA can generally be improved and DME eliminated without the need for drug therapy (Figs. 27 and 29). Because the benefits of anti-VEGF therapy are primarily early, with little if any advantage over laser in the long term, if injections are not needed initially in the management of DME it is likely they will never be needed (Luttrull et al 2012, Luttrull and Sinclair 2014, Frizziero, Calciati, Torresin et al 2021). For eyes with VA of 20/60 or worse, treatment can be initiated with anti-VEGF medication to hasten VA improvement and patient function, after which MRT is instituted to achieve long-term disease control and final resolution of DME, minimizing the need for further injections (Fig. 28, 30, 31). The advantages of such a reduction in injection frequency are a similar reduction in potential complications of injections, some of which, like endophthalmitis and glaucoma, are sight-threatening, avoidance of drug tolerance, and minimization of the treatment burden (Luttrull et al 2015).

It is always advisable, if not ethically required, to begin any treatment regimen with the simplest, safest, least burdensome, least expensive, and least invasive intervention that might be effective (Edelstein 1943). If a treatment fails to meet one or more of these criteria, it must be exceptional in the other criteria to compensate for the deficit. The author favors using VA to inform the initial treatment approach for DME, as it places the patient experience and functional capacity at the forefront of clinical decision making. Using macular thickness as the deciding factor assumes that rapid reduction, as results from anti-VEGF medication, is especially important. Anyone experienced with MPL (ideally sublethal to the RPE) for DME has noted that VA often improves significantly before macular thickness improves. Further, it is not that macular thicknesses greater than 400 um fail to respond to laser. Instead, it is simply that worse disease takes longer to resolve. However, resolve they will, given time and adequate patience, virtues forgotten in the era of fast-acting drugs (Luttrull and Spink 2007, Sivaprasad et al 2007, Luttrull et al 2012) (Figs. 26, 28-34, 37). While drug therapy is fast-acting, is it also short-lived with uncertain long-term benefits (Frizziero, Calcati, Torresin et al 2021) (Figs. 30, 32, 39). Studies of anti-VEGF therapy versus RPC for DME find RPC more effective at long-term reduction in DME, and that almost half of all eyes managed by regular long-term anti-VEGF injections still ultimately require RPC (Nguyen et al 2012, Brown et al 2013, Glassman et al 2020). It is speed of response where drugs excel compared to laser. Compared to RPC, drugs are also better at improving VA, particularly in the short-term. This is in part due to the loss of function and inflammation caused by RPC which often worsens VA early after treatment, and sometimes permanently (ETDRS 1991, Shimura et al 2009). Absent LIRD, the visual results of MRT are akin to drug therapy, but more durable. This is illustrated in an RCT of 164 eyes with DME randomized to aflibercept versus 577 nm MRT. In this study, drug injected eyes improved more quickly, but there was no difference between the groups at 2 years follow up (Frizziero, Calciati, Torresin et al 2021). By eliminating all adverse treatment effects—that tend to be detrimental to visual function, allowing early treatment prior to

visual loss, allowing foveal treatment, and producing long-lasting therapeutic effects, MRT offers the opportunity to optimize the management of DME while avoiding more invasive, intensive, burdensome and higher-risk intravitreal drug therapy. In the real world, given the option of an intravitreal injection versus MRT, the author has yet to encounter a patient preferring injection.

Key point: MRT is ideally suited as primary treatment for DME.

Adopt the pace of nature; her secret is patience.

—Emerson

Retreatment

Early in the use of SDM as MRT for DME, retreatment was performed as early as 6 weeks after initial treatment, hoping to hasten resolution of persistent swelling. With time, such frequent treatment was found to be unnecessary (Luttrull et al 2005, 2012). As noted, the first study of OCT of DME treated by MRT revealed that the time course of the treatment response was steady improvement becoming statistically significant by 3 months (Luttrull and Spink 2007) (Fig. 37). Clinical experience has shown that these posttreatment improvements may continue for several years following a single treatment session (Sivaprasad et al 2007). This phenomenon had been previously reported in eyes treated for retinal vein occlusion (Parodi et al 2006). During 3 years of posttreatment observation following sub-threshold microsecond laser applied focally and locally rather than in panmacular fashion, one study found recurrent DME was noted in 25% of eyes (Sivaprasad et al 2007). This emphasizes the fact that the great majority of eyes with DME achieve long-term resolution with a single laser treatment, even with suboptimal treatment according to current MRT criteria. Considering that the half-life of most enzymes in healthy cells is approximately 90 min, while in unhealthy cells it may fall to 18 min or less, the durable response to MRT in diabetic eyes reflects the fact that the reset effects of MRT extend far beyond initial intracellular protein repair to MRT normalization of transcription, translation, reduction in disease driving chronic inflammation, and therapeutic immunomodulation, all of which have been demonstrated experimentally and in patients. Recurrences of

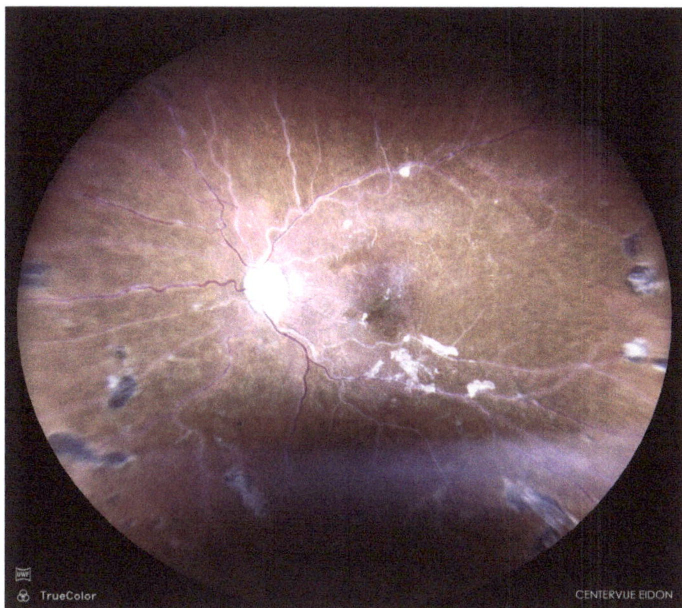

Fig. 40. Fundus photograph of left eye of 68 African American woman with Type 2 diabetes mellitus, following total retinal SDM (TRT) x 4 followed by pars plana vitrectomy for severe PDR and DME 2018. Preoperative VA 20/200, best postoperative VA 20/60. FFA demonstrated near total retinal ischemia and OCT diffuse macular atrophy. Note severe vascular attenuation and ghosting with diffuse retinal thinning. In such eyes, regular periodic panmacular SDM MRT (vision protection therapy, VPT) may help to maximize retinal and visual function to minimize the risks of further visual loss.

DME can usually be managed simply by repeat MRT. The evolution to total retinal (MRT) treatment (TRT) for DME/DR may help to reduce recurrent DME by reducing the overall level/severity of retinopathy and thus reducing inflammation and normalizing intravitreal balance of retinal cytokines, such as VEGF and pigment epithelial-derived factor (PEDF), in the vitreous (Fig. 41). Further study should be illuminating in this regard (Joussen et al 2004, Romero-Aroca et al 2016, Caballero et al 2017, Midena et al 2019, 2020, De Cillà et al 2019, Sinclair and Schwartz 2019, Chang and Luttrull 2020).

It is helpful to remember that eyes with DME can require many years of disease to deteriorate to that point, and that MRT elicits a physiologic, rather than pharmacologic response. Thus, time must be given for the response to MRT to develop, provided visual acuity is acceptable in the interim. It is difficult for practitioners steeped in the instant gratifications of drug response to exercise necessary patience in this regard. Experience has shown that it is best to give the MRT treatment response at least 3 to 4 months to allow treatment to become manifest before considering further treatment (Luttrull and Spink 2007) (Figs. 30, 32 33, 37). At that point, if the DME is improved,

one can continue observation, as continued improvement is likely. Evidence supporting retreatment of already improving DME at 3 to 4 months posttreatment is lacking (Luttrull and Spink 2007, Sivaprasad et al 2007, Luttrull et al 2012). It is interesting that Caballero, et al, found that the time course of initial response to SDM in an animal model required about 3 weeks to fully develop, capped off by recruitment of bone marrow immune cells to the retina of both eyes, even if only one eye was treated (Caballero et al 2017). Thus, despite the tendency for slowly progressive long-term improvement following MRT for DME, there may be an argument for retreating persistent DME after 3 to 4 months, once the near-term treatment reaction is complete, in hopes of renewing or reinvigorating the treatment response. Further study should reveal if such serial treatments are of benefit in DME.

Key point: The safety of MRT allows unlimited PRN retreatment

Posttreatment considerations

It is often most helpful to compare current findings with those at presentation, rather than the last visit, as this allows one to appreciate the overall progress more fully (Fig. 14, 34). If DME worsens, or fails to improve over consecutive 3 to 6 month visits, retreatment should be considered. Certain biomarkers for diabetic retinal inflammation, such as intraretinal hyperreflective spots, or foveal capillary plexus changes by OCT angiography (OCTA) may be helpful indicators of the direction of change, whether worsening or improving, as well. As indicators of disease severity, improvement in such findings may recommend continued observation (Vujosevic, Toma et al 2020, Vujosevic, Gatti et al 2020).

The presence of subretinal fluid in association with the DME is indicative of an exuberantly significant inflammatory component to the macular swelling, beyond the levels typically present in DR. Anti-VEGF medications are not anti-inflammatory, and thus tend to be of little benefit in this setting. However, as described earlier, MRT is anti-inflammatory, often allowing such eyes to be treated effectively to resolve both the DME and serous macular detachment without resorting to intravitreal steroids and their attendant concerns (Figs. 33, 33, 35).

Key point: MRT is anti-inflammatory. This is a good thing in treating DR and DME

Do you snore?

Long clinical experience indicates that worsening of DME/DR following MRT treatment is a very reliable indicator of poor or worsened systemic disease status. This might be a recent illness or hospitalization, uncontrolled systemic hypertension, poor glucose control, rapid glycemic tightening, or renal failure. However, by far most common (>95%) and consistent cause of worsening after initial MRT is undiagnosed and/or untreated obstructive sleep apnea (OSA) (Chiang et al 2021) (Figs. 41-43). While OSA typically affects obese patients, the nonobese can be affected as well. It is often helpful to ask the patient's spouse or partner if they snore, a common sign of OSA, as the patient (being asleep at the time) is usually unaware unless they have been told in the past. Occasionally one finds that the patient has been diagnosed previously but is noncompliant with treatment. In any case, the patient should be made aware that successful elimination of their DME, and/or arrest of their worsening DR, may not be possible until the aggravating issue, such as OSA, is effectively addressed. Once treated, rapid improvement (weeks to months) in the fundus findings including DME is generally observed. Patients often find treatment of OSA unpleasant and burdensome, so noncompliance is common and continued monitoring and encouragement is needed (Mehrtash et al 2019).

Key point: Lack of response or worsening after MRT is almost always due to untreated sleep apnea.

Combination therapy and comorbidities

No therapy is always, or never, effective. In those cases where MRT is ineffective, anti-VEGF or steroids may be helpful, just as MRT may be helpful when drugs are ineffective (Fig. 30, 35). Some eyes with DME fail to respond to any therapy. In such eyes, damage to the microvasculature renders it incapable of responding to regulatory factors, including exogenous anti-VEGF drugs and endogenous RPE-derived cytokines elicited by MRT. Such irreversible macular microvascular (and often eventual associated RPE) degeneration is best avoided by early treatment to prevent it from developing in the first place, as unresponsive DME is

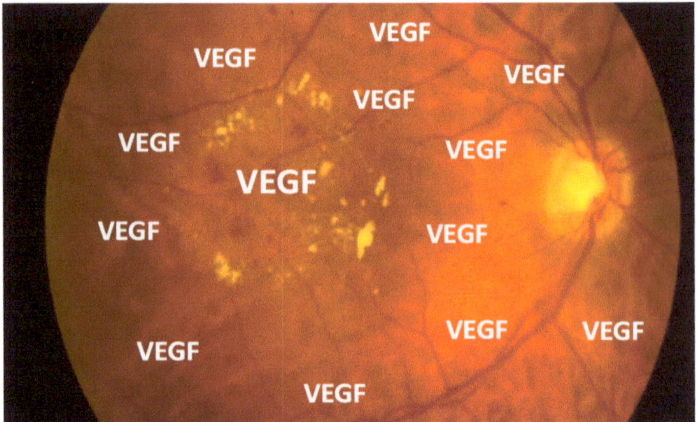

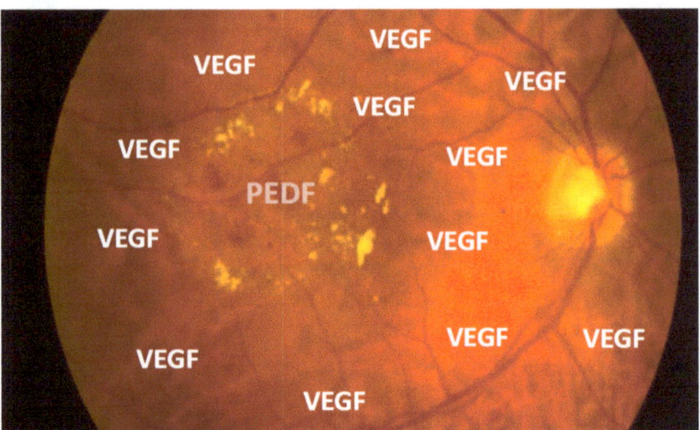

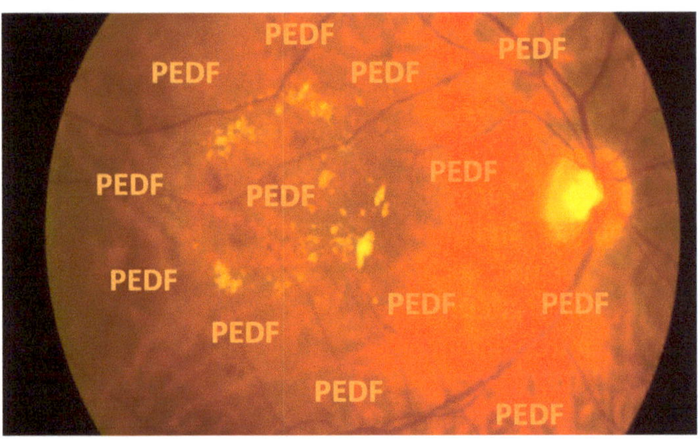

Fig. 41. Cartoon illustration of the strategy of total retinal treatment (TRT) with MRT for diabetic macular edema, and diabetic retinopathy in general. (A) eye with NPDR and DME with excessive VEGF production throughout the retina. (B) Focal / local treatment of the area of macular edema may reduce VEGF production and increase expression of pigment epithelial-derived factor (PEDF), but only locally. Vitreous levels of excessive VEGF due to widespread over expression would remain relatively unchanged and may interfere with elimination of the DME and foment disease progression. (C) TRT normalizes the VEGF / PEDF balance throughout the retina. This may aid elimination DME, reduce the chances of new or recurrent DME, reverse DR severity and reduce the risk of PDR. In this, TRT MRT acts little differently than an intra-vitreally injected drug, but more durably.

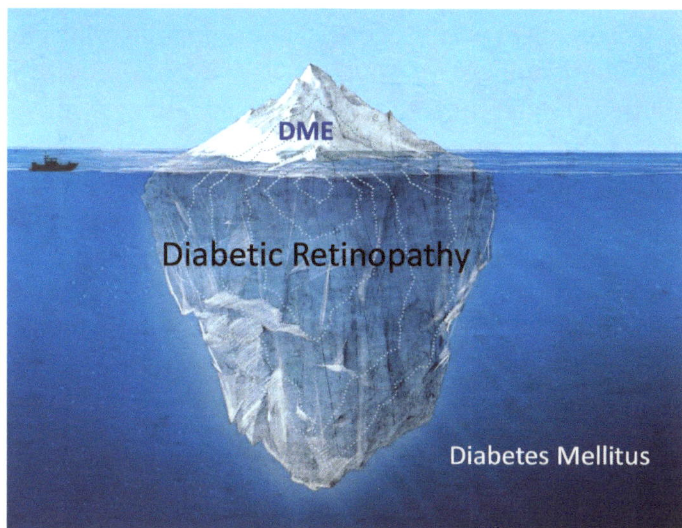

Fig. 42. DME can be thought of as the "tip of the iceberg" of diabetic retinopathy and thus chronic diabetes mellitus. In this context, focal and local treatment offends logic. Total retinal treatment with MRT more effectively addresses the entire retinopathy, much like intravitreal drug therapy.

virtually always the result of chronicity (Cicinelli et al 2017). In eyes with frank epiretinal membranes (ERM) or vitreomacular traction (VMT) MRT may improve VA enough to avoid the need for surgery, while postvitrectomy diabetic eyes may benefit from MRT in much the same way as nondiabetic eyes after membrane peeling (Luttrull 2020) (Fig. 39).

There have been a number of RCTs examining the effect of combining "subthreshold" laser with particularly anti-VEGF treatment for DME. Most find that addition of laser reduces the number of injections required to manage the DME. Unfortunately, these studies are difficult to interpret as they employed different treatment protocols and most either do not describe the laser parameters or techniques or employed different laser modes altogether. As such, relatively uniform anti-VEGF therapy is compared to highly nonuniform and often surgeon-specific macular laser. Thus, it is reasonable to conclude that these studies, none fully incorporating MRT treatment principles, underestimate the potential benefits of laser therapy (Othman 2014, Frizziero, Calcati, Torresin 2021, Tatsumi et al 2022). In the author's experience, early treatment and application of MRT principles to macular laser results in successful laser monotherapy in over 90% of eyes with DME (Fig. 31-33, 43 and 44).

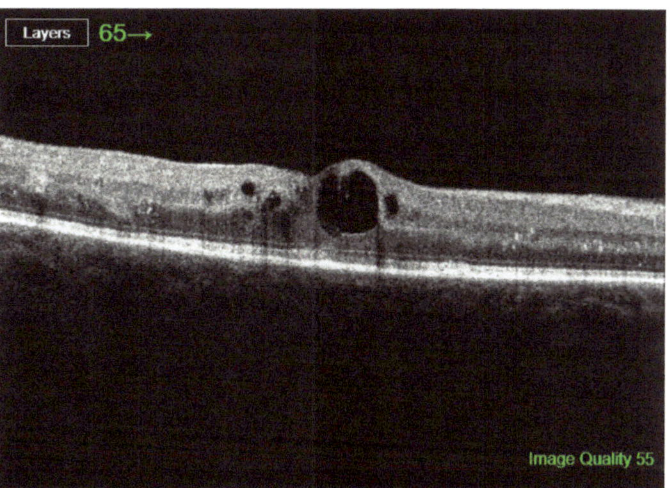

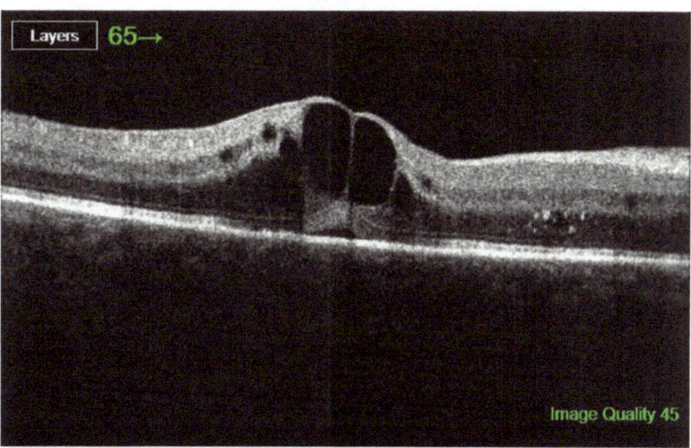

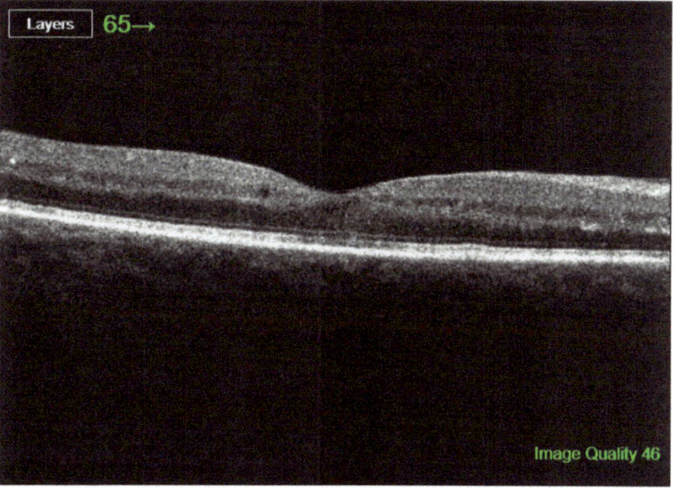

Fig. 43. 69 yo woman with type 2 diabetes mellitus and PDR with (A) DME by OCT in her right eye. VA 20/30. Panmacular SDM performed. (B) 4 months later, VA has worsened to 20/50- with increased DME. Worsening of DR or DME after MRT is virtually always due to untreated or undiagnosed sleep apnea. Unless this is addressed, response to any treatment, including drug therapy, may be limited. Obstructive sleep apnea (OSA) diagnosed following recommended sleep study. Treatment was instituted. Panmacular and peripheral retinal SDM performed (total retinal treatment, TRT). (C) 4 months later, VA 20/25 with DME resolved.

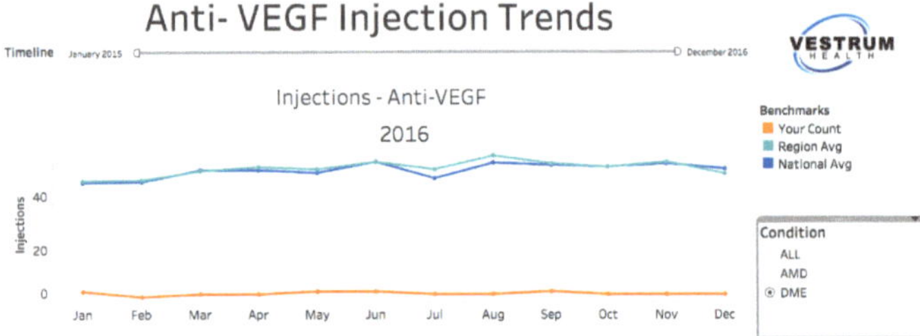

Fig. 44. Monthly anti-VEGF injection rates for diabetic macular edema for the year 2016, from Vestrum Health, Inc, Naperville, Illinois. Top lines, U.S. national and western U.S. per physician averages reflecting use of anti-VEGF drugs as first line treatment for DME. Bottom line, the author's practice employing SDM MRT as first line treatment for DME. Note that these rates indicate very few eyes managed by primary SDM MRT require intravitreal drugs.

Key point: Early treatment with MRT can virtually eliminate the need for intravitreal injections for DME.

Proliferative diabetic retinopathy (PDR)

History of MRT for PDR

The first and still largest report of subthreshold laser/ MRT for PDR described 99 consecutive eyes of 63 patients with DR ranging from severe nonproliferative (SNPDR) to severe PDR treated with peripheral retinal SDM, between 2000 and 2003, followed a median of 1 year (Luttrull et al 2008, 2009). Illustrating the principle that you cannot learn anything new if you do not do anything different, several notable findings arose from this first study of retina-sparing peripheral (pan) retinal laser treatment. First, it was that progression of retinopathy severity was noted in only 4 of 99 eyes posttreatment despite total absence of LIRD clinically, or by FFA. Three were from the 35 eyes treated for SNPDR. As 50% of eyes with SNPDR are expected to advance to PDR within 1 year absent treatment, the finding of only 8.5% progression from SNPDR to PDR was highly significant (p>0.001). Another notable finding was that only few eyes went on to require vitrectomy. Despite four eyes presenting with iris neovascularization, none progressed to neovascular glaucoma. Of the 14% of eyes undergoing surgery following panretinal SDM, the indications were nonclearing vitreous hemorrhage in half, and macular pucker in the other half. Thus, the risk of requiring vitrectomy after panretinal SDM appeared to compare favorably with conventional PRP. Despite many eyes presenting with severe PDR, no eye with at least 12 months follow-up developed neovascular glaucoma after peripheral retinal SDM. Finally, and most interestingly, the clinical course following panretinal SDM was found to be quite different from that following conventional PC. In the absence of LIRD there was no posttreatment inflammation. In the absence of inflam-

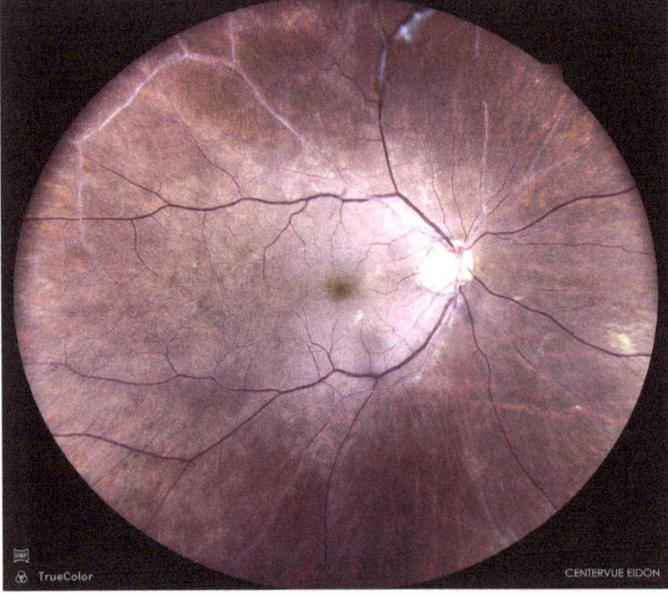

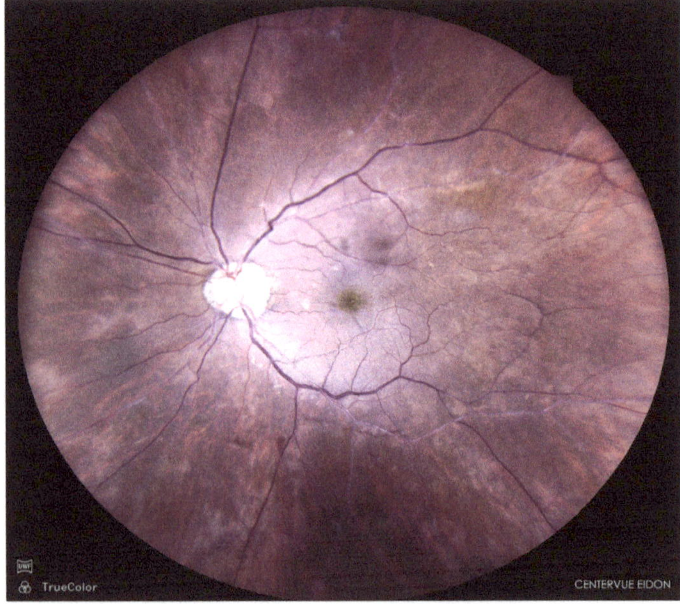

Fig. 45. Fundus photographs dated July 2022 of 74 Asian male with Type 1 diabetes. The patient presented July 2016 with active proliferative diabetic retinopathy and DME in both eyes, and a vitreous hemorrhage in the left eye. Presenting VAs were 20/30 OD and 20/70 OS. Starting in 2016, total retinal SDM performed once each year until 2020. VA 20/30 OU July 2022. Note marked peripheral retinal vascular attenuation with resolution of DME and PDR without pre-retinal fibrosis and absence of laser-induced retinal damage.

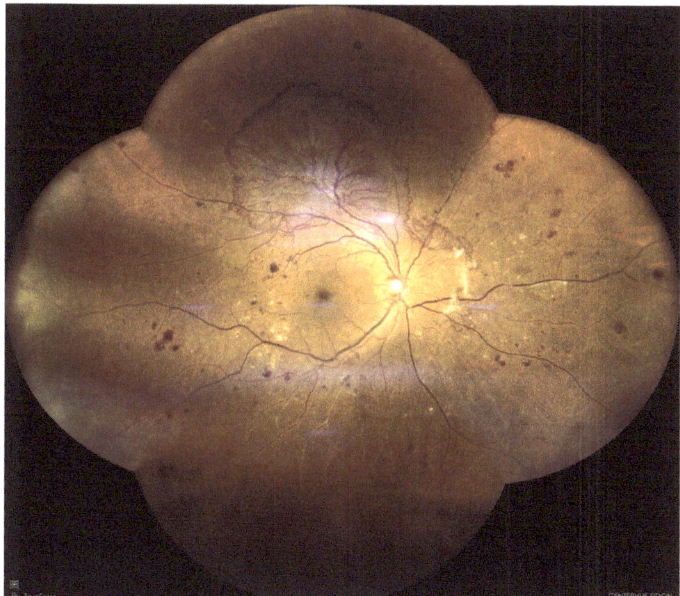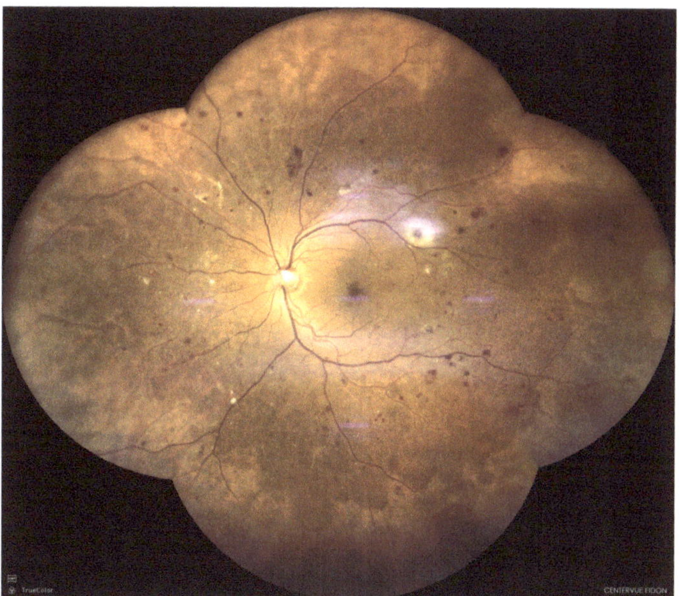

Fig. 46. Fundus photographs August 2022 of 54 yo Hispanic woman with Type 1 diabetes mellitus s/p total retinal SDM MRT OU x 5 since 2018 for severe PDR with near-complete circumferential retinal ischemia and DME OU. VA 20/30 OU. Note resolution of disc and retinal neo-vascularization and DME in the left eye without evidence of pre-retinal fibrosis or traction. Of note is the right eye. The DME has resolved and there is a very large frond of persistent retinal neovascularization superiorly; regressed, stable, and non-progressive since TRT was begun in 2018. Note the absence of fibrosis, contraction, or elevation despite the size of the neovascular frond. Note arterialization of the marginal vessels with peripheral shunt formation, and resolution of fine vascular structure within the frond. These are reliable signs of NV arrest and regression indicating that no further or re-progression will occur. Absent fibrosis and contraction, involutional and regressed neovascularization following TRT in PDR behave benignly, without reprogression, new NV, significant vitreous hemorrhage, or traction retinal detachment. As a rule, areas of arrested and regressed NV continue to stain on FFA indefinitely, and do in both eyes of this patient.

mation, DME was not caused or worsened. Of special note was the near absence of neovascular fibrosis or contraction following panretinal SDM MRT. Instead, neovascularization regressed, angiographic leakage diminished, and the neovascularization (NV) showed decreased vascularity with arterialization and shunt formation at the distal margins of the NV (Figs. 45-55). Once arrested and involuted, the NV did not reprolif-erate. It was noted in that report that these attributes of panretinal SDM suggest that it may be especially well-suited to eyes with the most severe and active disease, to quieten the eye and arrest proliferation without precipitating vitreous hemorrhage and/or retinal detachment. Over 20 years of clinical experience with panretinal SDM MRT has confirmed these early lessons.

VEGF in reserve

Laser-untreated eyes, or eyes long since their last anti-VEGF injection, may have high vitreous concentra-tions of VEGF (Wakabyashi et al 2012). In such eyes, the vitreous acts as a VEGF reservoir in which biologically active concentrations of VEGF may persist for 6 weeks or

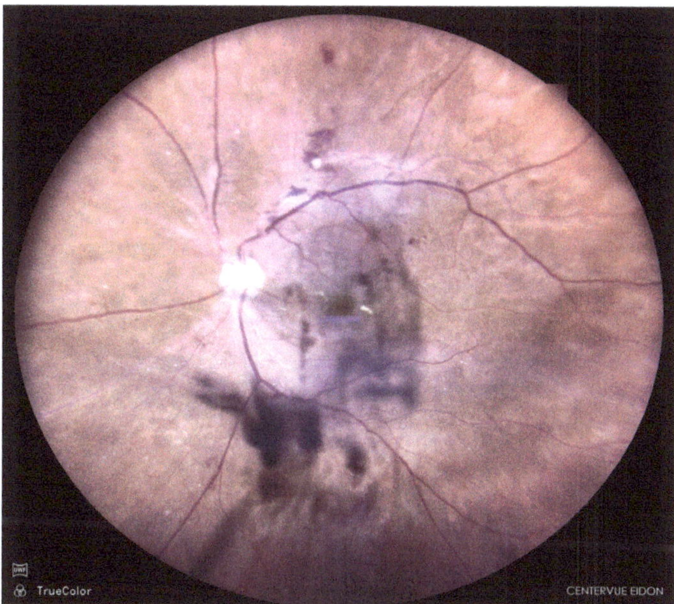

Fig. 47. Fundus photograph of left eye of 63 yo Hispanic male with Type 2 diabetes mellitus. The patient presented with a dense vitreous hemorrhage precluding visualization of most of the retina, despite relatively good chart acuity of 20/80. Peripheral retinal SDM MRT was begun as permitted by visualization over 3 months, aided by the lack of absorption of 810nm laser by blood. The vitreous hemorrhage resolved with improvement in VA to 20/30. Note residual central vitreous hemorrhage (expected to continue to clear) and regressed and involutional neovascularization without contraction and with minimal pre retinal fibrosis following SDM MRT TRT.

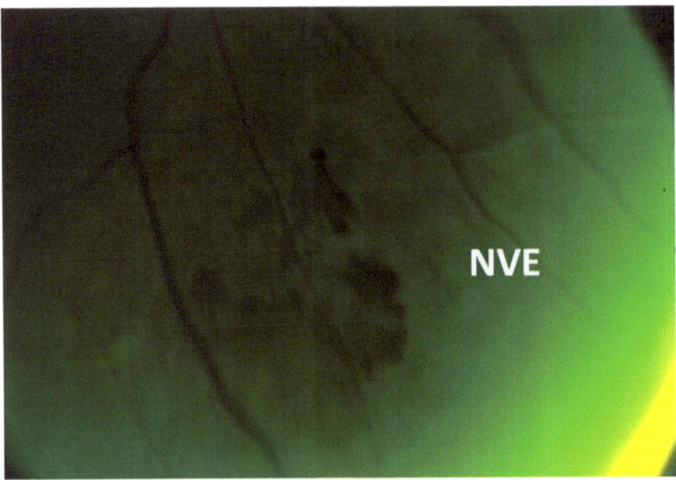

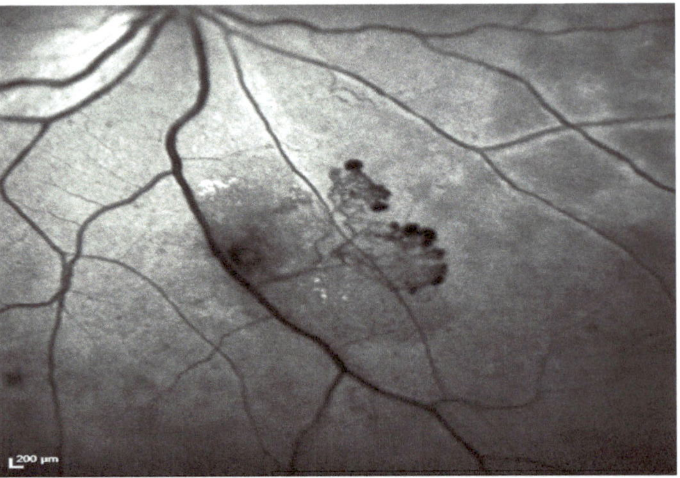

Fig. 48. Fundus photograph of a frond of diabetic retinal neovascularization (A) before and (B) 16 years after total retinal SDM MRT. Note lack of progression and absence of fibrosis and contraction and LIRD. Note decreased microvascularity with distal shunt formation.

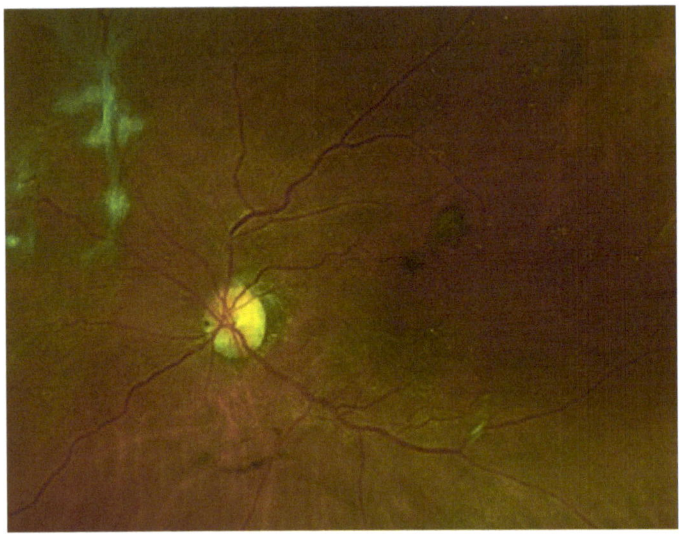

Fig. 49. Fundus photograph of left eye 1 year following total retinal SDM MRT for PDR with multifocal retinal neovascularization and vitreous hemorrhage. Note small foci of minimal avascular preretinal fibrosis without contraction following regression of the NV.

more even after VEGF production is markedly reduced by MRT. The author has seen one case (in 22 years) where both eyes of a patient with highly ischemic but early PDR progressed rapidly over 2 months following total retinal MRT, presumably due to the influence of a preexisting high vitreous concentration of VEGF (Edington et al 2017).

PDR and DME: one disease, or two?

While the clinical manifestations of chronic diabetes mellitus are different in the peripheral retina (NV) compared to the macula (DME), the underlying disease process is the same. Therefore, it makes sense that the treatments should be the same as well (Fig. 56). While this seems obvious, it is remarkable that in recent years many have become comfortable with subthreshold/retina sparing treatments for DME but continue to believe in the need for retinal ablation with RPC for PDR. The psychology that underlies this belief seems to be that PDR is more serious, and thus requires more serious treatment (retinal ablation). This reflects both a lack of understanding of the mechanism of laser action, and lack of experience with peripheral retinal MRT such as SDM for management of PDR. How could one entrust a clearly visible and threatening clinical problem (PDR) to an invisible (and apparently thus ineffectual) treatment, seems to be the sentiment. Curiously, the invisibility and retina sparing properties of anti-VEGF therapy do not elicit the same concern. Thus, such thinking belies the fact than many practitioners continue to associate visible retinal destruction by RPC with the efficacy of laser treatment (Figs. 1, 2, and 11). This is an emotional, not rational connection. Insistence on a conventional 1980s approach to PRP is easily the single most intransigent area of thinking regarding laser treatment held by clinicians at the time of this writing. It is difficult to change 50 years of thinking. However, as previously noted, the advent and implementation of SDM treatment for both PDR and DME were simultaneous, reflected the same reasoning and understanding that the disease process of DME and PDR are the same,

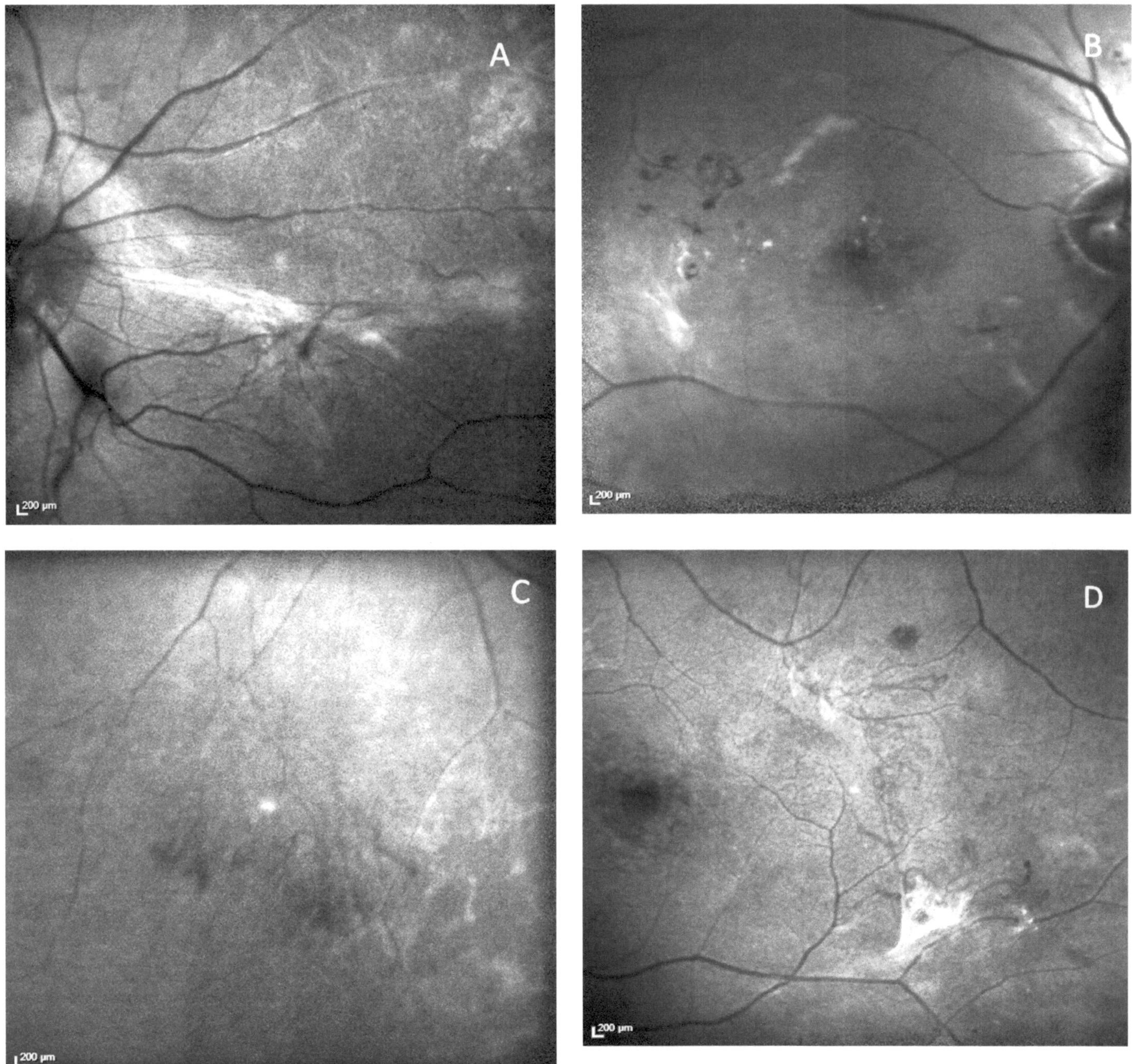

Fig. 50. Red-free fundus photographs of patient 20 years post total retinal SDM MRT (TRT) for florid proliferative diabetic retinopathy and diffuse macular edema in both eyes, presenting VA of 20/25 OU. Despite severity of retinopathy and DME, in the 20 years of follow up the VA never fell below 20/30 and no injections or surgery were required at any point post TRT. Note involution of widespread multifocal NVE and NVD with without contraction, and minimal fibrosis.

and thus the same techniques were applied for both (Luttrull et al 2005, 2008).

MRT, inflammation, and disease progression

Both MRT and drug therapy differ from conventional PRP in the absence of proinflammatory LIRD.

However, unlike either PC or anti-VEGF therapy, MRT is anti-inflammatory (Karu 1989, Luttrull and Kent 2019). Chronic inflammation is a key component to all chronic progressive retinopathies, including diabetic retinopathy (Joussen et al 2014, Romero-Aroca et al 2016, Sinclair and Schwartz 2019, Pillar et al 2020, Sinclair and Luttrull 2022). Reduced chronic inflamma-

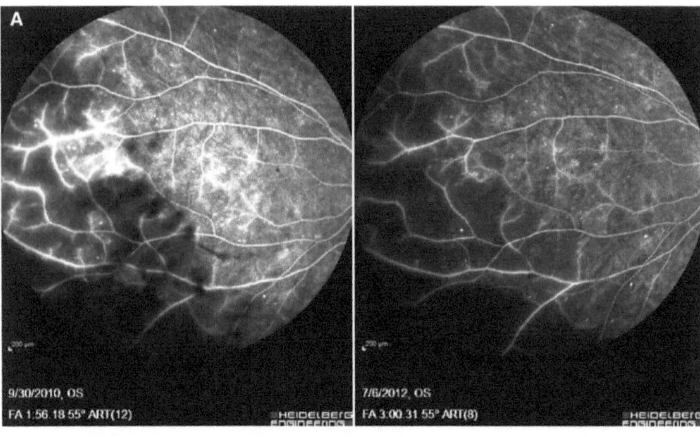

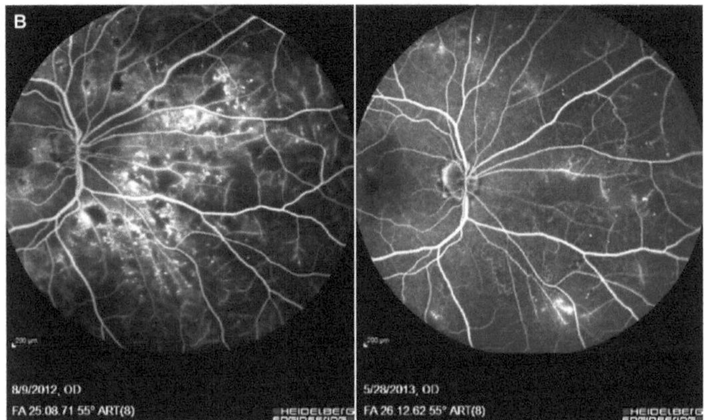

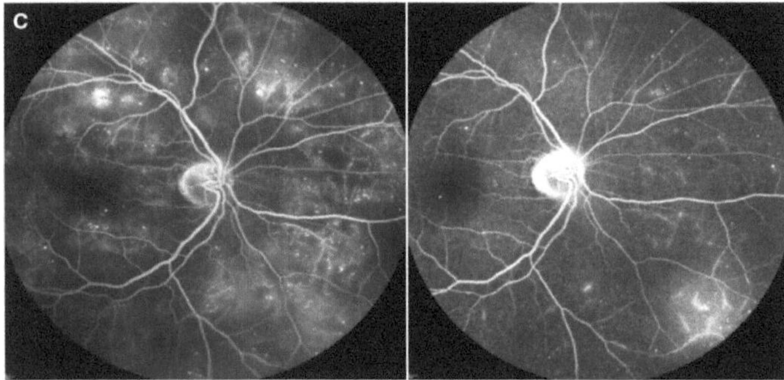

Fig. 51. Intravenous fundus fluorescein angiograms (FFA) of diabetic retinopathy (DR) following total retinal SDM laser (TRT, panmacular and panretinal) in three patients (a), (b) and (c). No VEGF inhibitors, steroids, or other medical treatment for DR was used. Left photo, before treatment; right photo after treatment. Note reduction in macro and microvascular leakage along with reversal/ diminution of retinopathy severity in each case From: *Luttrull JK, Kent D. Laser therapy to prevent choroidal neovascularization. Choroidal Neovascularization. Chhablanni J, Ed. Springer Verlag. July 2020. DOI: 10.1007/978-981-15-2213-0_30*

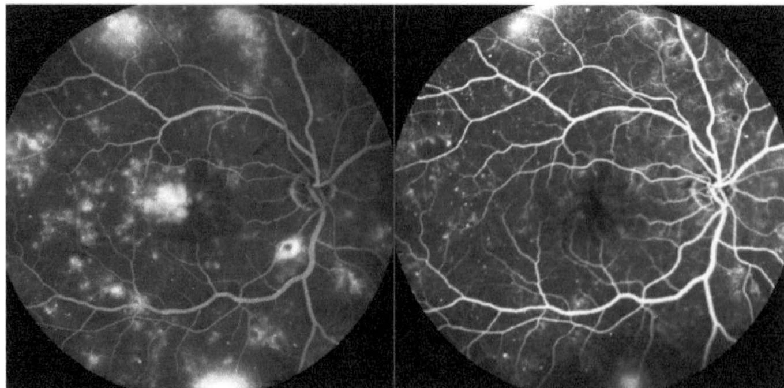

Fig. 52. Ten-minute post injection intravenous fundus fluorescein angiographs of eye with proliferative diabetic retinopathy before (left) and 3 years after (right) a single treatment session of panretinal SDM laser. Note regression of neovascularization inferiorly, with decreased leakage of dye and reversal of background retinopathy severity. From: *Chhablani J, Roh YJ, Jobling AI, Fletcher EL, Lek JJ, Bansal P, Guymer R, Luttrull JK. Restorative retinal laser therapy: Present state and future directions. Surv. Ophthalmol 2018 May - Jun;63(3):307-328.*

of PC, the visual benefits of drug therapy, with the added benefit of long-term reduction in disease-driving chronic inflammation, clearly demonstrated by FFA before and after treatment (Figs. 5, 14, 26, and 45-55).

Most people see what they expect.

—John Steinbeck

A landscape of preserved retina: a needle in a haystack is lost. A needle on a shiny table is easily seen

It is important at this juncture to recognize that one's expectations of the treatment response go a long way in determining the "success" or "failure" of any treatment. Patience and a new perspective are needed to allow a treatment response to develop following MRT for complications of DR. Besides the immediate, if short-lived, gratifications of anti-VEGF therapy, the picture of an intact, normal-appearing and functional retina following MRT is disconcerting if one is accustomed to a landscape of obliterated and scarred peripheral retina after conventional PRP. (Figs. 1-3, 11, 45-50) First, one may feel as if one has not done anything and is negligent about the destroyed retina. Second, after MRT regressed, the involutional and inactive NV could still be easily seen, particularly by FFA. On FFA, regressed NV will continue to stain, although leakage is diminished because the NV is regressed and no longer proliferative (Figs. 45-55). This may continue indefinitely, or eventually resolve altogether. Such persistent staining of NV may cause one to think treatment has failed. This

tion following MRT reduces disease severity and the impetus to progression. While drug therapy has been found to be as effective as retinal photoablation for PDR without the inherent SAEs of PC, discontinuation of drug therapy suppression usually results in disease reactivation and reprogression (Luttrull et al 2006, Maturi et al 2021). Instead, total retinal MRT offers the durability

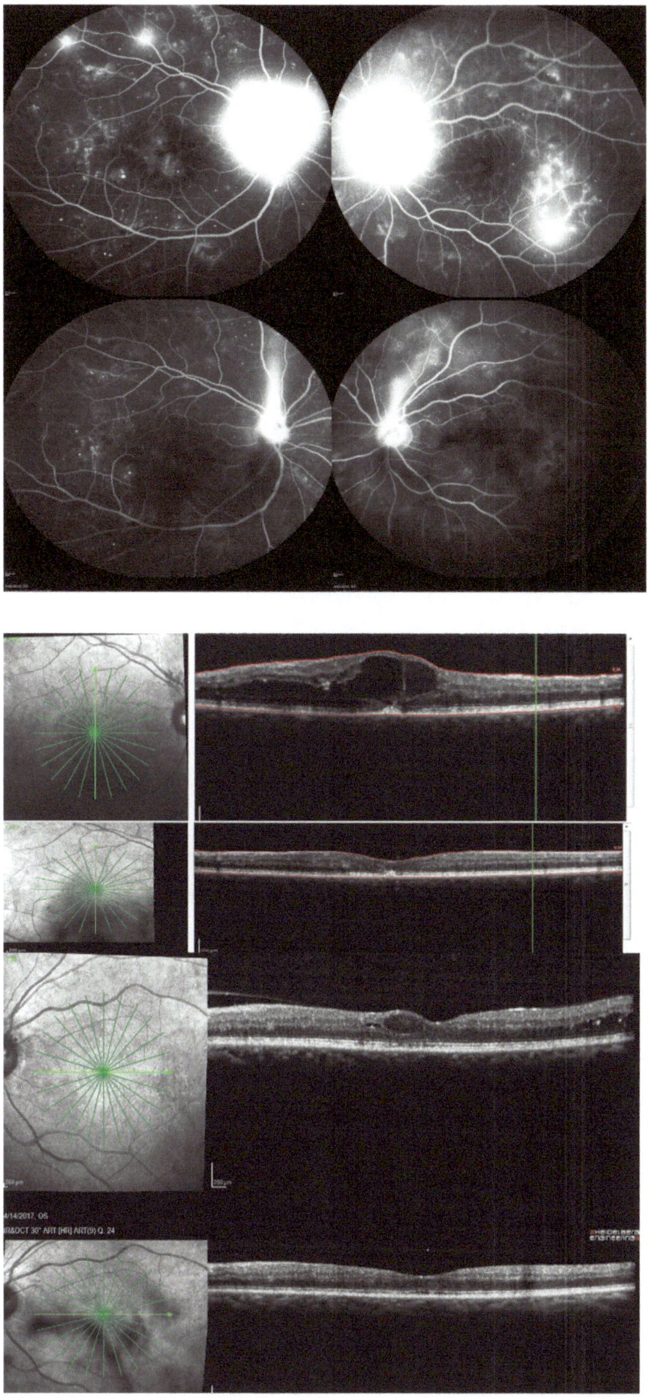

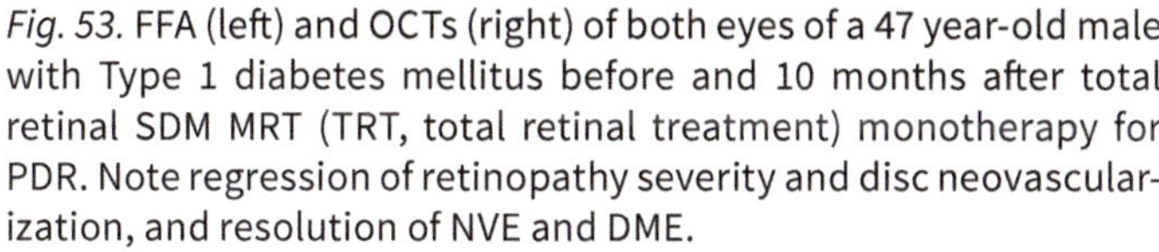

Fig. 53. FFA (left) and OCTs (right) of both eyes of a 47 year-old male with Type 1 diabetes mellitus before and 10 months after total retinal SDM MRT (TRT, total retinal treatment) monotherapy for PDR. Note regression of retinopathy severity and disc neovascularization, and resolution of NVE and DME.

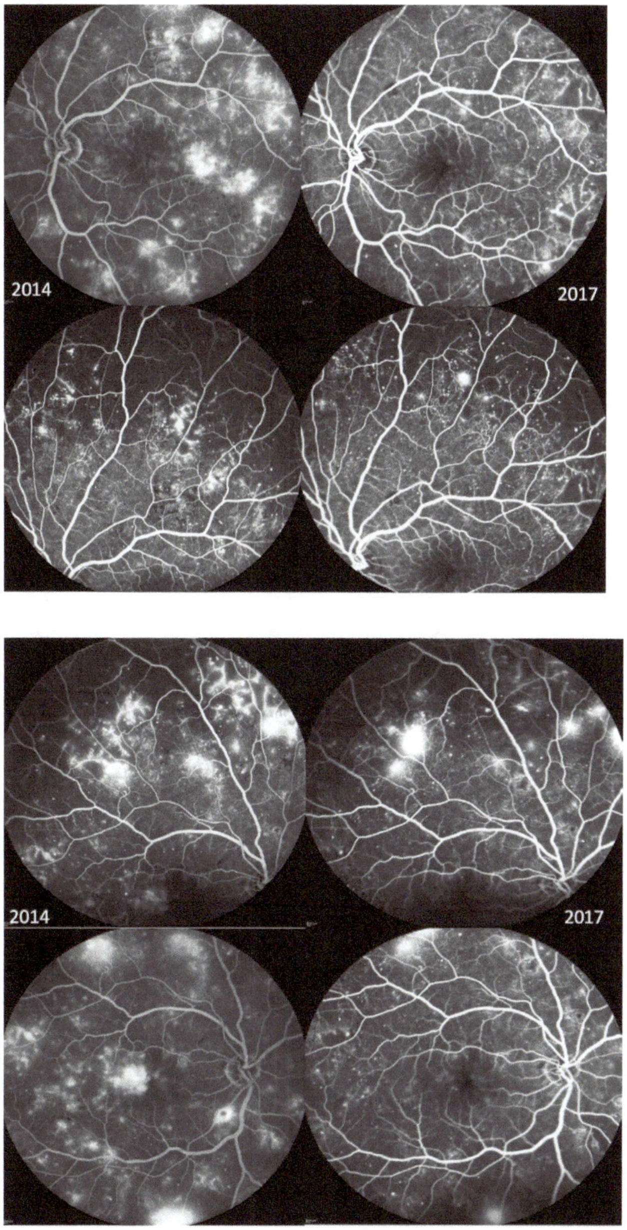

Fig. 54. FFA of patient with PDR given a single session of SDM MRT TRT in 2014 and subsequently lost to follow up until 2017. Note durable reversal of retinopathy severity with regression and involution of retinal neovascularization in both eyes.

is because such persistence of regressed NV and angiographic leakage, also typical following conventional PRP, are simply difficult to see against the backdrop of scarred retina. If one sees this against the backdrop of normal appearing retina after MRT, one may feel one has not done anything, or enough, to rid the eye of the NV. If one should see exactly the same regressed and persistently leaking NV against the background of heavily scarred retina post RPC, one feels one has done all that could be reasonably expected to address the problem. Thus, the pathology is not retinal, it is psychological. For such reasons, only one subsequent study has been done looking at retina-sparing laser for PDR since the initial report in 2006 (Luttrull et al 2006,

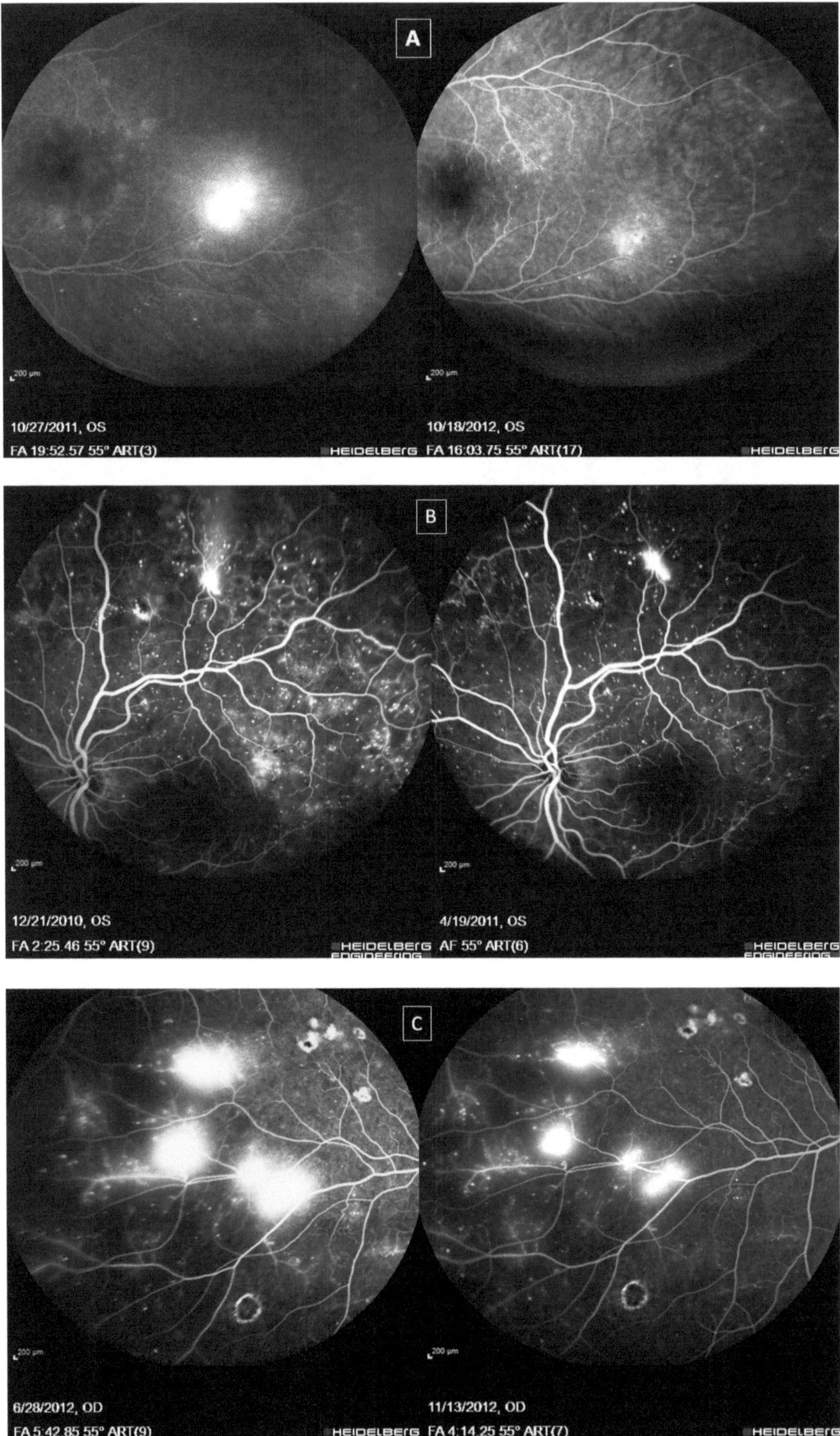

Fig. 55. Examples of regression of PDR following SDM MRT TRT. Note persistent staining of involutional neovascularization (A-C). Example of the same in an eye treated by conventional PRP RPC. (D)

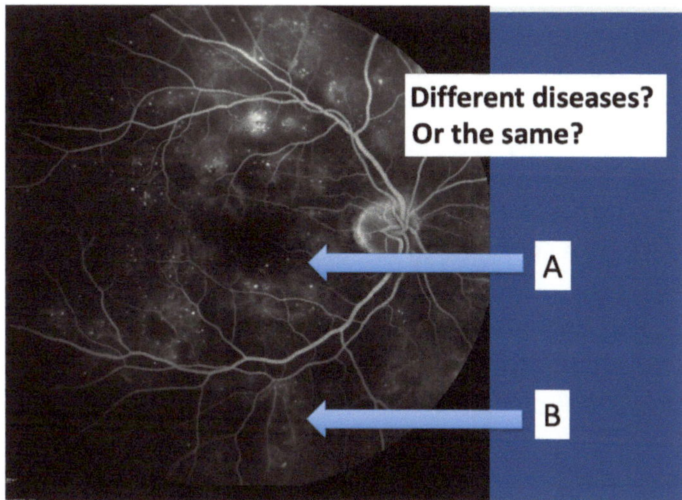

Fig. 56. While the manifestations of DR may be different in different parts of the eye (DME vs NV), the underlying disease, and thus primary treatment options, are the same. This fact challenges the still remarkably wide-spread idea that retina-sparing treatment in the macula is reasonable, but retinal photoablation by convention-al RPR is still necessary outside the macula.

Jhingan et al 2018). While this study found benefit from both short-pulse CW and microsecond pulsed laser PRP, both arms employed insufficient treatment leading to unimpressive results.

More study of MRT for peripheral retinal treatment of PDR is sorely needed, considering the morbidities—visual loss, visual field loss, photophobia, nyctalopia, loss of driving privileges, sleep disturbance, to name only some of the long-term SAEs—associated with conventional PRP; and the treatment burden, tolerance rate, and recurrences with reprogression following discontinuation or loss to follow-up associated with intravitreal drug therapy (Gross et al 2015). Who will fund such studies? The author has actually personally contacted Novartis, Genentech, and Regeron to access their interest in sponsoring retinal laser studies. They declined. As the cost of a major RCT typically exceeds the market capitalization of most ophthalmic laser companies, the prospects for such studies do not appear bright. Regardless, in light of retina and vision sparing alternatives, jus-tification for the continued intentional wholesale destruction of the retina with conventional RPC for PRP rests entirely on those who continue to do it (Edelstein 1943). Appeals to tradition, convention, and custom no longer seem tenable.

Key point: It is difficult if not impossible to justify continuation of conventional PRP when effective reti-na-sparing treatments are available

Posttreatment monitoring and retreatment

Intravenous fundus fluorescein angiography (FFA) is especially useful in the management of DR, because more than static OCT angiography (OCTA), FFA is a dynamic functional test. The degree of micro and mac-rovascular leakage on FFA in DR is a very useful indicator of disease activity and accompanying inflammation. Thus, it is helpful to obtain a pretreatment wide-field FFA of any eye to receive peripheral or total retinal MRT to establish a baseline of disease activity. By repeating the FFA no sooner than 4 to 6 months post treatment, one can gain an easy appreciation of the treatment response. In the vast majority of eyes, posttreatment FFAs demonstrate diminished leakage throughout the fundus consistent with reversal of clinical retinopathy severity, and often reperfusion of areas of retinal ischemia (Luttrull et al 2006, Luttrull and Sinclair 2014). A decrease in the number of the microaneu-rysms in both retinal capillary plexuses, and especially in the deep capillary plexus following MRT in DME can be documented and monitored by OCT angiography (Vujosevic, Gatti et al 2020, Vujosevic, Toma et al 2020).

Once there is regression of retinopathy severity following MRT and involution of NV it is unclear if additional or continued treatment is of any benefit, as continued improvement is the rule, and reprogression or de novo NV after retinopathy reversal is rare. However, due to the safety and ease of treatment, an occasional retreatment may benefit one's peace of mind, if nothing else. That said, it is the author's habit to repeat total retinal SDM MRT 2 to 3 times in the first 2 years of treatment of SNPDR and PDR, even if there is complete resolution of the absence of DME and clinical and angio-graphic reversal of retinopathy severity. This may be simply the doctor treating himself. However, the ease and safety of treatment makes such occasional "insurance" or "booster" retreatment reasonable and preferrable to any worry. Future study will show whether this is actually necessary or beneficial (Figs. 5, 14, 26, and 45-55).

Key point: While the author has found SDM MRT highly clinically effective for PDR for over 20 years, more studies are needed to gain wider acceptance.

A durable response

There is much more to be learned from the half-life of treatment effects of MRT in various disorders. By virtue of the etiologically agnostic "reset" mechanism of action, it is expected that the effects of MRT will wear off at some point, due to the continuing influence of the primary stressor of the underlying disease process, and the fact that most MRT elicited effects are time-limited. While protein misfolding is the currency of cellular dysfunction, the "menu" of especially affected proteins, and thus compromised cellular processes, is unique to each disease. As noted, the half-life of typical enzymes prior to misfolding and failure in even normal cells is short, and much shorter in sick cells (Chang and Luttrull 2020). Despite this, improvements in retinal and visual function following SDM MRT tend to return to baseline in retinitis pigmentosa (RP) in about 3 months, and in AMD around 6 to 9 months. Because MRT elicited clinical improvements far exceed the half-life of repaired intracellular proteins, it is clear that HSP 70-mediated protein repair is just the first and initiator of many other and longer-lasting restorative changes triggered by treatment (Karu 1989, Kregel 2002, Hattenbach et al 2005, Flaxel et al 2007, Beckham 2008, Sramek et al 2011, Inagaki et al 2015, Lavinsky et al 2016, Luttrull and Margolis 2016, Caballero et al 2017, Kern et al 2018, Midena et al 2019, Luttrull 2018, De Cillà et al 2019, Luttrull and Kent 2019).

This makes particularly interesting the case of DR, in that the great majority of eyes demonstrate durable and essentially permanent reversal of retinopathy severity following only one or two sessions of MRT (Luttrull et al 2006) (Figs. 46-50). This is clearly seen in the permanent reductions in micro and macro vascular leakage and permanent involutional response of diabetic neovascularization following MRT (Karu 1989, Kregel 2002, Richter et al 2010, Stetler et al 2010) (Figs. 5, 11, 14, 25, and 44-53). Exactly why the effect of MRT on DR is so durable compared to other CPRs is unclear, but the retina appears to become insensitive or tolerant to the continuing metabolic abnormalities constituting diabetes mellitus. Acquired tolerance to drugs is, as a rule, a permanent condition (except for the unique ability of SDM MRT to reverse anti-VEGF drug tolerance in wet AMD) (Luttrull et al 2015). There is no reason MRT should not be also able to induce "tolerance" to the abnormal metabolic milieu of diabetes in eyes with diabetic retinopathy, as a part of functional normalization. There is no one path to tolerance. However, it is clear that MRT very likely causes epigenetic changes in exposed cells that could easily account for such long-term if not permanently induced changes (Dayeh et al 2016). The key here is whether MRT reverses or induces tolerance, the direction of the reset effect is always toward normalized function. Thus, unlike the current approach to treatment of PDR that depends on long-term administration of short-acting drug therapy, SDM MRT for PDR can either prevent or minimize the need for intravitreal injections, and the associated treatment burden in all but a few eyes (Gross et al 2015, ASRS 2021) (JKL, unpublished data 2012-2021, Vestrum Heath, Naperville, Ill) (Fig. 44).

Key point: The durability of disease regression following MRT for DR suggests laser-induced "tolerance" of retina to diabetes mellitus.

Nonproliferative diabetic retinopathy

Prevention

The safety and effectiveness of MRT creates the unique opportunity for the most effective application of any therapy—preventive treatment. As noted many times previously, it is axiomatic that earlier treatment is more effective, and preventive treatment is most effective. It is further axiomatic that any treatment that is effective therapy is also preventative if given early. Of all currently available therapeutic modes, only MRT is sufficiently safe for general preventive use.

When to start?

The characteristic response to MRT is durable reversal of retinopathy severity without reprogression (Luttrull et al 2006) (Figs. 5, 14, and 26). Therefore, early treatment, especially prior to the development of DME or significant DR, can effectively preclude diabetic vision loss in most eyes. But how early is best? In principle, the earlier the better (Hawkes 2019). Diabetic retinal neuronal dysfunction precedes clinical retinopathy (Sinclair and Schwartz 2019, Pillar et al 2020, Sinclair and Luttrull 2022). Thus, there is an argument, based on the safety of MRT, for treatment even before evidence of clinical DR appears, to try to prevent clinical DR altogether. Again, FFA is a particularly useful indicator of the success of such a strategy, by showing reversal of retinopathy severity after treatment. Of all indications for MRT in diabetics, early preventive treatment is arguably the most important, as (a) there are many more patients at risk for vision loss than with sight-threatening complications of disease at any point in time; and (b) the only way to guarantee excellent visual acuity in diabetic eyes is to prevent vision loss in the first place (Flaxman et al 2017). No treatment is effective absent compliance. The safety of MRT not only permits preventive treatment, but importantly also makes it acceptable to patients because treatment is quick, long-lasting, safe, painless and without adverse treatment effects, thus fundamentally unlike long-term frequent intravitreal injections that have been advocated by some for the same purpose (Gross et al 2015).

Key point: Total retinal treatment with MRT is a safe, durable, and highly effective disease reversing strategy for prevention and therapy for all stages of diabetic retinopathy.

11. Modern Retinal Laser Therapy for Age-Related Macular Degeneration

Dry AMD

Prevention of neovascular conversion: laser NOT for drusen

Neovascular conversion is the most important cause of visual loss from AMD. Prevention of neovascular conversion is thus the highest priority in the clinical management of AMD. MRT appears to be the most effective measure toward this end.

Early experience with SDM as MRT showed that SDM did not cause short-term drusen reduction, which, at that time, was the presumed prerequisite for improving dry AMD and preventing neovascular conversion (Luttrull and Kent 2020) (Fig. 57). Thus, there was initially no expectation that MRT would be beneficial for AMD. However, elucidation of the mechanism of action of retinal laser treatment made it clear that MRT might indeed be therapeutic for AMD by improving retinal health and function in the absence of drusen reduction (Luttrull et al 2015, Luttrull and Margolis 2016, Luttrull and Kent 2020). This expectation was based on the principle that achieving, and then maintaining, improvement in retinal function is the minimum requirement for slowing disease progression and reducing the long-term risks of visual loss in any CPR. The hypothesis, integral to reset theory, was explored clinically in two ways.

The first, and most novel hypothesis to arise from the reset theory of laser action, was that MRT should reverse tolerance to anti-VEGF medications in wet AMD. This was subsequently confirmed in a small clinical study (Luttrull et al 2015). The power of the reset theory was thus demonstrated not only by the ability to predict this novel treatment application; but also, by the fact that it remains the only example of reversal of drug tolerance known in medicine (Fig. 57-59).

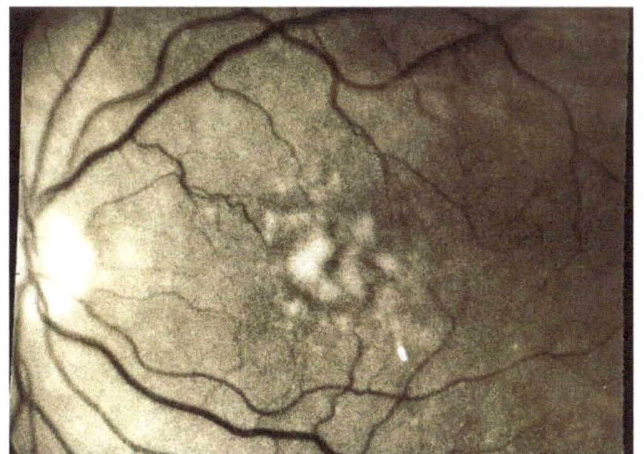

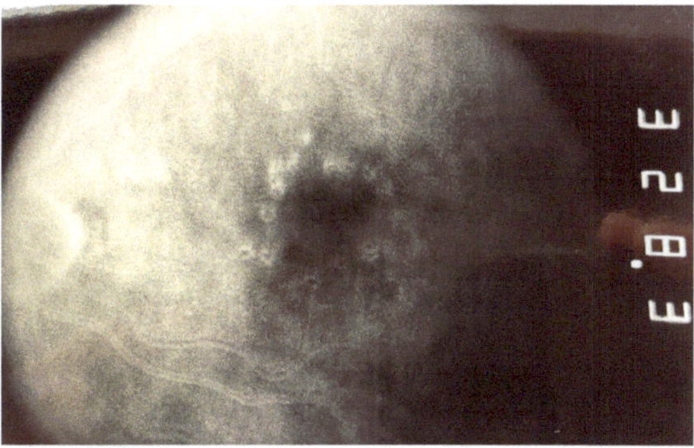

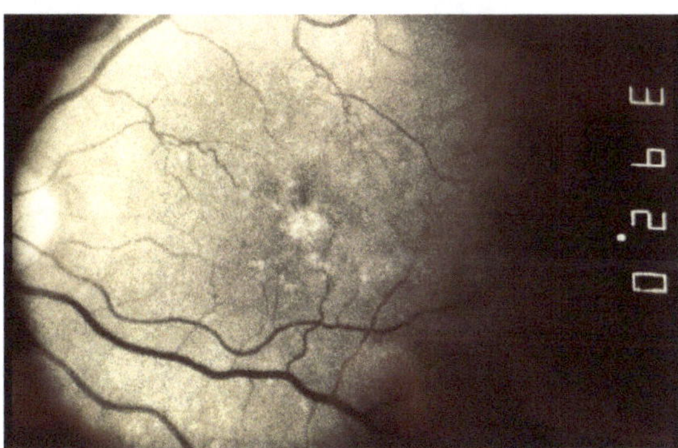

Fig. 57. Fundus photograph of eye with (A) subfoveal soft drusen prior to conventional CW "subthreshold" grid laser treatment to try to eliminate the drusen, circa 1990. (B) Poor quality post treatment FFA showing ring of photocoagulation scars after treatment. (C) Fundus photo showing resolution of drusen following RPC. Because the effectiveness of laser treatment to provoke resolution of drusen parallels the degree of photocoagulative damage to the retina, any benefit achieved by drusen reduction is more than offset by an increased likelihood of choroidal neovascularization arising in the laser-damaged retina.

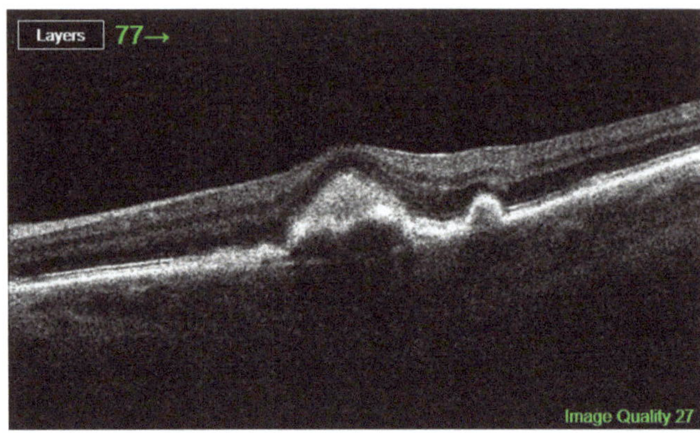

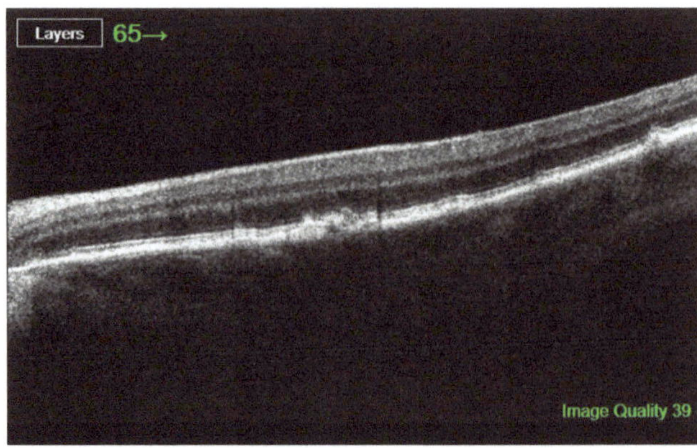

Fig. 58. OCT of left eye of 78 yo patient with intermediate AMD who began SDM MRT VPT in 2017. OCT (Left) shows subfoveal high-density material with underlying serous pigment epithelial detachment first noted January 2019. VA 20/30. This lesion remained unchanged while ongoing SDM MRT vision protection therapy until it resolved May 2022 (Right). Note resolution of PED and subretinal high-density material without the development of geographic atrophy. VA remained 20/30.

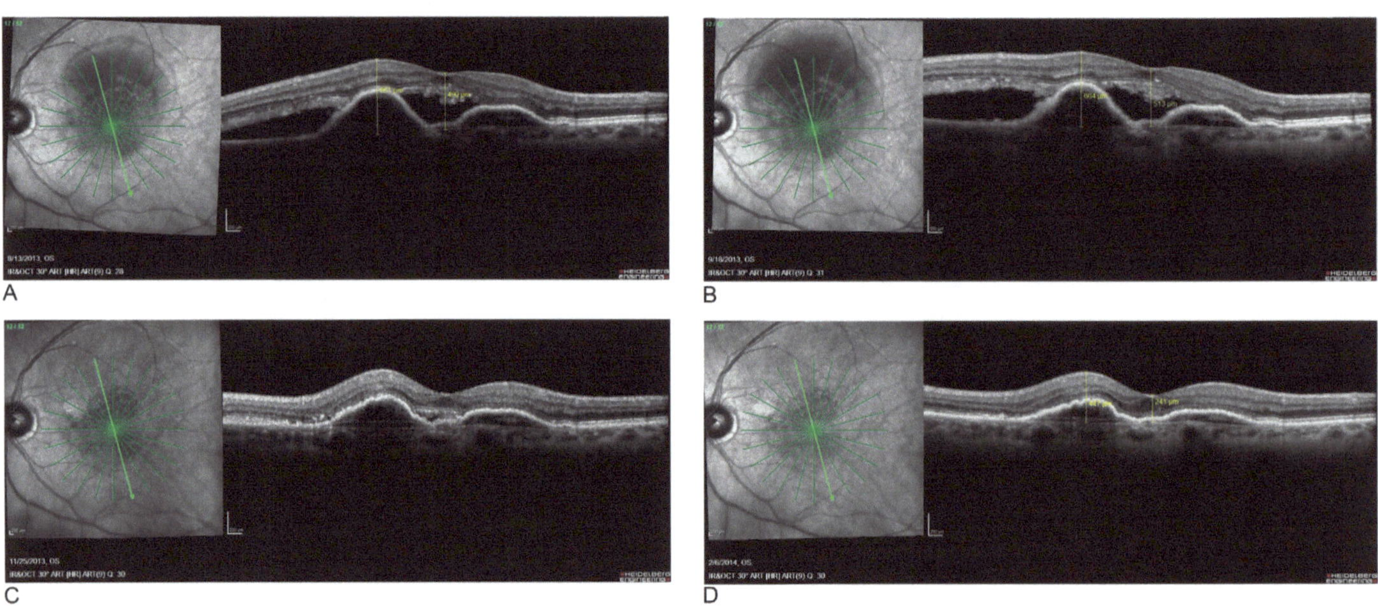

Fig. 59. Spectral-domain optical coherence tomography series demonstrating the resolution of macular fluid after SDM reversal of tolerance to anti-VEGF medication in NAMD. Treatment before SDM included injections of intravitreal bevacizumab x 8, then ranibizumab x 7, and finally aflibercept x 9. A. Left eye 1 month before SDM treatment. Multifocal serous PEDs and subretinal fluid unresponsive to anti-VEGF medications were noted. Aflibercept injection repeated. B. One month later, persistence of subretinal fluid despite continued aflibercept treatment. Anti-VEGF medication tolerance diagnosed, and SDM treatment was performed. C. Two months after SDM treatment and 1 month after rechallenge with aflibercept. Reduction in subretinal fluid and decreased height of PEDs were noted. D. Four months after SDM treatment and 3 months after reinstitution of monthly intravitreal aflibercept. Further reduction in macular thickness with complete resolution of subretinal fluid and a "dry" treatment response designation were noted. From: *Luttrull JK, Chang DB, Margolis BWL, Dorin G, Luttrull DK. Laser re-sensitization of medically unresponsive neovascular age-related macular degeneration: Efficacy and implications. Retina 2015 Jun; 35(6): 1184-1194.*

Clinical monitoring treatment of diabetic retinopathy is fairly straightforward because the clinical response to treatment is generally well demonstrated by retinal imaging. Monitoring the effects of treatment on dry AMD, in the absence of drusen resolution or other acute or short-term laser-induced morphologic change, presents a different challenge, as there is nothing visibly indicative of improved retinal function. Thus, currently available imaging modes are not helpful. Even if one were to improve retinal function in dry AMD by MRT enough to prevent later progression to wet AMD, how would one know without treating large numbers of eyes and waiting many years to observe the result? Only physiologic testing to confirm an initial treatment response, and then monitoring that response over time, could indicate if maintained improvement in retinal function had been achieved and with it the hope of an improved long-term prognosis (Luttrull and Margolis 2016, Luttrull and Kent 2020).

A second confirmation of reset theory in AMD was, as discussed previously, use of pattern electrophysiology (PERG) and various visual function tests to detect and monitor MRT treatment effects. Highly significant improvements in retinal function in dry AMD and various IRDs were documented following SDM MRT (Luttrull and Margolis 2016). Because PERG measures full-thickness retinal function and not just the photoreceptor layer, it is useful even in retinitis pigmentosa (RP) where there is often no measurable photoreceptor function by electroretinography (ERG). Further, PERG unexpectedly confirmed the reset hypothesis of MRT as a nonspecific trigger of disease-specific repair, by identifying characteristic disease-specific PERG improvement signatures following SDM (Luttrull 2018, Luttrull, Samples et al 2018, Luttrull and Kent 2019).

Visual function improvement following MRT was also found to be significant by all measures, including visual acuity, contrast visual acuity, microperimetry, and MVFT, reflecting the underlying improvement in retinal function (Luttrull and Margolis 2016, Luttrull and Kent 2019). Like PERG, mesopic visual function, contrast acuity, and dark adaptometry are early predictors of AMD (Puell et al 2012, Lains et al 2021) (Figs. 16, 17-23) (Table 6). By improving these traditional predictors of disease progression and visual loss, MRT would be expected to slow down disease progression and reduce the risks of vision loss (Luttrull et al 2015, Luttrull and Margolis 2016, Luttrull, Sinclair et al 2018, Luttrull et al 2020, Luttrull and Gray 2022).

All-comers study of incidence of neovascular conversion following MRT in dry AMD

The first study of wet AMD prevention by MRT as vision protection therapy

It is not enough to improve retinal function. The improvements must be maintained, either via long-lasting treatment or regular periodic treatment. Clinical studies found that not only could retinal function be improved in AMD by MRT, but that these improvements could also be renewed and maintained by periodic retreatment indefinitely, as predicted by reset theory (Luttrull and Kent 2019). In 2017, a first study was undertaken in an attempt to ascertain the effect of regular periodic SDM MRT (what we now call *vision protection therapy*) on the incidence of neovascular conversion in eyes with dry AMD.

Table 6. Summary of calculated difference (post- minus pretreatment) for ORP (Omnifield Resolution Perimetry) mesopic visual function testing (*in open angle glaucoma*)

Variable	Mean (SD)	Median (IQR)	p-value
BA 6°, LogMAR	−0.17 (0.34)	−0.11 (−0.30, 0.00)	<0.0001
GMA, LogMAR	−0.15 (0.31)	−0.10 (−0.24, 0.02)	0.003
Visual area (N_{miss} = 3)	70.5 (92.7)	51 (16, 122)	<0.0001

The mean and median differences for the covariates of interest are shown. Each row shows the difference (post- minus pretreatment) in BA 6°, GMA, or visual angle (for only those eyes with improvable pretreatment visual area and not equal to 400°). In order to test whether the mean difference is different from zero, linear mixed models predicting the measure were performed using an indicator for time as a covariate, adjusting for left or right eye, and including a random patient intercept. The p-values are those associated with the time (pre- vs. post-) regression coefficient. A significant p-value indicates that the mean difference is significantly different from zero. All measures are significantly different pre- versus posttreatment. This method accounts for intereye correlation. BA6: best logMAR visual acuity within 6° of fixation. GMA: global macular logMAR visual acuity. N_{miss}: number of missing values. SD: standard deviation. IQR: interquartile range.

From: Luttrull JK, Samples JR, Kent D, Lum BJ. Panmacular subthreshold diode micropulse laser (SDM) as neuroprotective therapy in primary open-angle glaucoma. In: Samples JR, Knepper PA, eds. *Glaucoma Research 2018-2020*. Kugler Publications; 2018:281-294

The electronic medical record (EMR) of the author's vitreoretinal practice was searched to identify all active patients with the diagnosis of dry AMD in at least one eye, to determine the effect of SDM MRT on neovascular conversion. As a retrospective review, inclusion of eyes in the EMR, an "all-comers" approach, was employed to minimize selection bias. Study revealed that SDM was offered to 373/392 (95%) patients with dry AMD and elected by 363/373 (97%) between 2008 through 2017 (most eyes beginning treatment after 2014). SDM MRT was performed on average every 3 to 4 months in treated eyes. Follow-up was available for 354/363 patients (547 eyes, 98%) (range 6-108 mos., avg. 22). The study population constituted one of the highest risk populations for neovascular conversion of any yet reported. CNV risk factors included advanced age (median 84 years, 67% > 80 years); high incidence of reticular pseudodrusen (214 eyes, 39%); high Age-Related Eye Disease Study (AREDS) risk categories (78% category 3 and 4); and high incidence of fellow eye CNV (128 eyes, 23%). New CNV developed in 9/547 eyes (1.6%, annualized rate 0.87%). Visual acuity was unchanged (AREDS 2001). There were no adverse treatment effects (Tables 7-10).

Table 7. Descriptive statistics by new CNV events for patient-level and eye-level covariates

Variable	Value	CNVM		
		No	**Yes**	**Total**
Patients, N (%)		345 (97.5)	9 (2.5)	354
Sex	Female	201 (56.7)	6 (66.7)	207 (58.5)
	Male	144 (40.6)	3 (33.3)	147 (41.5)
Age		82.6 (9.0)	81.0 (6.1)	82.5 (8.9)
Age	<80	115 (33.3)	4 (44.4)	119 (34)
	80 +	230 (66.7)	5 (55.6)	235 (66)
Hypertension	No	142 (41.3)	7 (77.8)	149 (42.0)
	Yes	202 (58.7)	2 (22.2)	205 (58.0)
Smoker	No	325 (94.2)	9 (100.0)	334 (94.4)
	Yes	20 (5.8)	0 (0.0)	20 (5.6)
All eyes, N (%)		538 (98.4)	9 (1.6)	547
Eye	OS	270 (50.2)	5 (55.6)	275 (50.3)
	OD	268 (49.8)	4 (44.4)	272 (49.7)
Follow-up time, months		21.7 (11.8)	15.4 (8.8)	21.6 (11.8)
Pre-SDM LogMAR		0.4 (0.3)	0.2 (0.2)	0.4 (0.3)
Post-SDM LogMAR		0.4 (0.4)	0.2 (0.1)	0.4 (0.4)
SDM treatments	1	100 (18.6)	0 (0.0)	100 (18.3)
	2	149 (27.7)	4 (44.4)	153 (28.0)
	3	145 (27.0)	4 (44.4)	149 (27.2)
	4	115 (21.4)	1 (11.1)	116 (21.2)
	5	25 (4.6)	0 (0.0)	25 (4.6)
	6	4 (0.7)	0 (0.0)	4 (0.7)
AREDS class	1	9 (1.7)	0 (0.0)	9 (1.6)
	2	107 (19.9)	0 (0.0)	107 (19.6)
	3	278 (51.7)	7 (77.3)	284 (51.9)
	4	145 (27.0)	2 (22.2)	147 (26.9)
Reticular pseudodrusen	No	332 (61.7)	1 (11.1)	333 (60.9)
	Yes	206 (38.3)	8 (88.9)	214 (39.1)
Fellow eye AREDS class	1	9 (1.7)	0 (0.0)	9 (1.6)
	2	86 (16.0)	0 (0.0)	86 (15.8)
	3	224 (41.7)	3 (33.3)	227 (41.6)
	4	218 (40.6)	6 (66.7)	224 (41.0)
Fellow eye pre-SDM CNVM	No	415 (77.1)	4 (44.4)	419 (76.6)
	Yes	123 (22.9)	5 (55.6)	128 (23.4)

Significance testing was not performed due to the very low number of events. N = number. CNV = choroidal neovascularization. SDM = panmacular low-intensity/high-density subthreshold diode micropulse laser. AREDS = age-related eye disease study. AMD = age-related macular degeneration. VA = visual acuity. From *Luttrull JK, Sinclair SH, Elmann S, Glaser BM. Low incidence of choroidal neovascularization following subthreshold diode micropulse laser (SDM) for high-risk AMD. PLoS One. 2018;13(8):e0202097. doi:10.1371/journal.pone.0202097*

Table 8. Age-specific rates of progression using two different age groupings

Age	Number of progressions	Person-eye months	Rate (per 1,000 person-eye months)
All	9	11,799	0.763
55–69	0	1,018	0.000
70–79	4	2,884	1.387
80–89	5	5,345	0.935
90 +	0	2,552	0.000
55–79	4	3,902	1.025
80 +	5	7,897	0.633

There are no progressions in the youngest or oldest eyes. The second grouping shows that the rate of progression is higher for those under 80 compared to those 80 or over. In this study, the incidence rate ratio is 1.619 comparing those younger than 80 to those 80 or older. From: *Luttrull JK, Sinclair SH, Elmann S, Glaser BM. Low incidence of choroidal neovascularization following subthreshold diode micropulse laser (SDM) for high-risk AMD. PLoS One. 2018;13(8):e0202097. doi:10.1371/ journal.pone.0202097*

Table 9. Univariate Cox regression models that estimate the effect of covariates on the hazard of progression

Covariate		HR (95% CI)	*p*-value
Sex:	Female	1.78 (0.48, 6.64)	0.39
	Male	REF	
Age		0.98 (0.94, 1.02)	0.24
Pre-SDM LogMAR		0.06 (0.00, 1.91)	0.11
HTN		0.21 (0.04, 0.98)	0.048
RPD		14.62 (1.82, 117.65)	0.01
Fellow eye pre-SDM CNVM		3.64 (0.98, 13.59)	0.054

A sandwich estimator to obtain robust standard errors was used in order to counteract possible inter-eye correlation. There were too few new CNV events to permit analysis by AREDS category. Systemic hypertension, reticular pseudo-rusen, and fellow-eye CNV all predisposed to development of a new CNV. From: *Luttrull JK, Sinclair SH, Elmann S, Glaser BM. Low incidence of choroidal neovascularization following subthreshold diode micropulse laser (SDM) for high-risk AMD. PLoS One. 2018;13(8):e0202097. doi:10.1371/ journal. pone.0202097*

Table 10. Characteristics of treated eyes with dry AMD developing choroidal neovascularization following SDM

Patient	Age	Sex	AREDS class treated eye	AREDS class fellow eye	CNV fellow eye	VA	HBP	Smoke	RPD	No. SDM	Mos. to new CNV
1	87	M	3	4	+	20/30				3	17
2	83	F	3	4	+	20/25	+		+	1	2
3	88	F	3	4	+	20/40			+	1	4
4	73	M	3	3		20/25			+	2	24
5	73	M	4	4	+	20/60			+	2	9
6	82	F	3	3		20/25			+	2	15
7	77	F	3	4	+	20/30			+	2	28
8	82	F	3	3		20/30			+	2	14
9	89	M	4	4		20/60	+		+	4	25
Avg.	82		3.2	3.7	5/9	20/36	2/9	0/9	8/9	2	15

Avg. = average. M = male. F = female. AREDS = age-related eye disease study. CNV = choroidal neovascularization. VA = Snellen visual acuity. HBP = high blood pressure. RPD = reticular pseudo drusen. No. = number. Mos. = months. From *Luttrull JK, Sinclair SH, Elmann S, Glaser BM. Low incidence of choroidal neovascularization following subthreshold diode micropulse laser (SDM) for high-risk AMD. PLoS One. 2018;13(8):e0202097. doi:10.1371/ journal.pone.0202097*

Compared to the AREDS (avg. age 69 years), SDM treated study eyes (avg. age 84 years) had an 83% reduction in the expected annual rate of neovascular conversion. However, using the results of the Beaver Dam and Reykjavik studies to correct for the age disparity between the all-comers study and the AREDS, estimated a 95% to 98% per year lower than expected incidence in neovascular conversion in the SDM treated study group (Klein et al 2002, Jonasson et al 2011, Luttrull et al 2018). While this all-comers study is retrospective and limited, the robust nature of these results suggested that regular periodic SDM MRT is highly effective at reducing the risk of neovascular conversion in eyes with dry AMD, even those with high risk factors for conversion.

Key point: MRT improvements in retinal function appear to be accurate surrogate indicators of long-term risk reduction in AMD

Prevention of neovascular AMD: real world comparison of standard care versus vision protection therapy

The second study of prevention of wet AMD by MRT as vision protection therapy
The results of the Luttrull, Sinclair et al (2018) all-comers study were tested further in a second, larger real-world data (RWD) study employing a different study population, different time window, and different method of analysis, using propensity scoring to compare the rate of neovascular conversion in patients with bilateral dry AMD receiving vision protection therapy (regular periodic panmacular SDM MRT maintenance therapy Q 3 to 4 months) versus standard care with AREDS vitamin supplements alone (standard care alone, SCA) (Rosenbaum and Rubin 1983, Greenhouse 2009, Jupiter 2017, Luttrull and Gray 2022).

Propensity scoring is a statistical method of matching existing populations to achieve high quality data comparisons by randomizing patients retrospectively according to the criteria of interest, analogous to a "reverse" RCT (Jupiter 2017). In this RWD study, all data was obtained from Vestrum Health, Inc (Naperville, Ill, USA) a publicly available database of patient unidentified data aggregated from the electronic medical records from over 300 retina practices in the United States, including one employing vision protection therapy (VPT) (regular periodic SDM maintenance therapy) for dry AMD. The study period was 4.75-year time window, from January 4, 2016, through September 20, 2020.

392,250 eyes coded for dry AMD were identified. Filters for inclusions (diagnosis of dry AMD and age of 50 years or more) and exclusions (prior injections, wet AMD in fellow eye, diabetes mellitus, retinal vein occlusion, and other confounding diagnoses and indications for anti-VEGF injection, prior macular photocoagulation) were applied by Vestrum, and patients matched for risk factors including age, sex, systemic hypertension, smoking, and AREDS vitamin use. Because a patient encounter is a prerequisite for identification and documentation of a conversion event, patients were also matched for encounter frequency as an additional risk factor. Data included both ICD-9 and -10 codes, precluding stratification of dry AMD severity. As age is the principal risk factor for the presence and severity of AMD, propensity score

matching for age and all other identifiable conversion risk factors, as well as the large number of study eyes, was expected to balance AMD severity equally between the study groups. VPT was routinely performed by only one practice in the Vestrum database, simplifying comparison between VPT and SCA. However, all data for both groups was harvested from the Vestrum database in the same manner with the same inclusions and exclusions, except for the difference of VPT in that group. Consequently, not all eyes in the VPT group were treated, as treatment was not offered for early, low-risk dry AMD. These eyes were kept in the VPT group to balance it demographically with the SCA group, which also included early, low-risk eyes, to avoid skewing of conversion risk in favor of the SCA group. Because AREDS vitamins are not indicated for early, low-risk AMD, use of AREDS vitamin use between the groups (64.4% in the VPT group, and 56.8% in the SCA group) is an indicator of the proportion of low-risk versus intermediate to advanced dry AMD eyes in both groups. Based on AREDS vitamin use, the proportion of early, low-risk AMD eyes may have been slightly higher in the SCA group. For the SCA group, the date of study entry was the date of first diagnosis of dry AMD, and for the VPT group, the date of initial SDM treatment (Figs. 27, 60, 61).

Propensity score matching was then performed by biostatistician Gerry Gray, PhD, using the R "Matchit" package (in the publication Supplemental data). Using the resulting propensity scores, all VPT cohort eyes were nearest-neighbor matched with standard care alone (SCA) cohort eyes in a 1/10 ratio (VPT/SCA) to create the analysis data set. This resulted in 9,130 eyes for study (830 VPT, 8300 SCA) (Rosenbaum and Rubin 1983, Greenhouse 2009, Austin 2011, Jupiter 2017). Subjects were then divided into five strata based on propensity scores, and standard stratified analyses were applied. Propensity scoring analysis showed excellent matching for each population quintile (Fig. 60). To minimize the risk of false positives, two-factor confirmation of neovascular conversion was used, including both a change in coding from dry to neovascular AMD, and simultaneous initiation of anti-VEGF therapy. Comparison of the propensity-score matched study groups using a stratified Cox proportional hazards model found a markedly lower rate of neovascular conversion in the VPT group compared to the SCA group (hazard ratio 13.04; 95% bootstrap CI (5.5, 18.5]. The cumulative probability of neovascular conversion in the VPT group was approximately 4% after 4 years from dry AMD

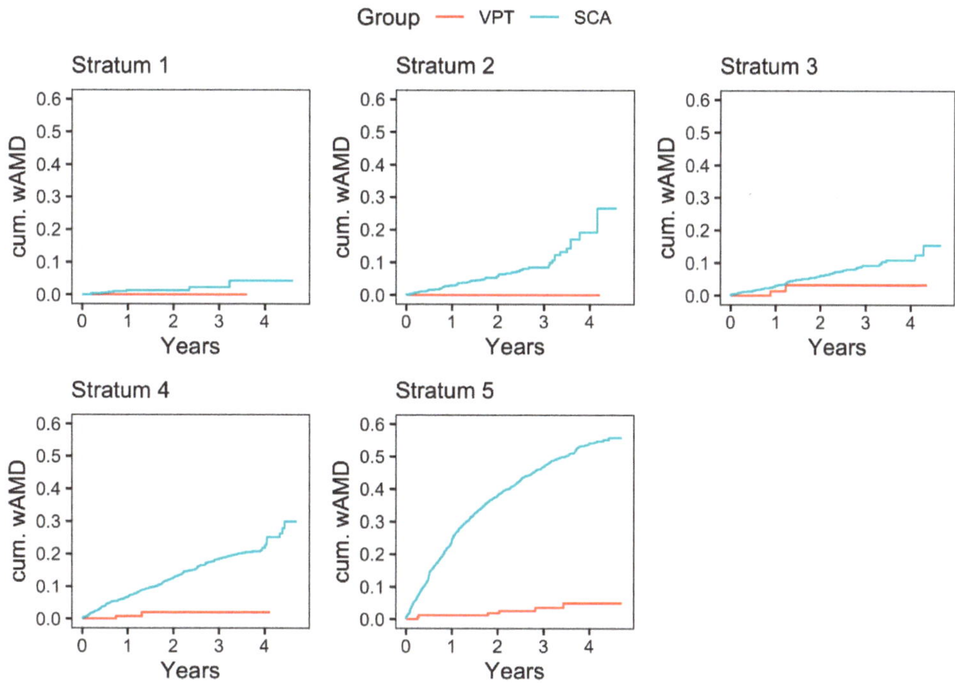

Fig 60. Kaplan-Meier survival plots by propensity score strata. Note that for each quintile, eyes receiving panmacular SDM in a program of vision protection therapy (VPT, red line) suffered significantly fewer conversion events from dry to wet AMD compared to eyes managed standard care with AREDS vitamins alone (SCA, blue line). *From: Luttrull JK, Gray G. Real World Data Comparison of Standard Care vs SDM Laser Vision Protection Therapy for Prevention of Neovascular AMD. Clin Ophthalmol (2022) May, 16: 1555-1568.*

diagnosis, compared to approximately 31% in the SCA group (Fig. 27). All statistical diagnostics indicated that the Cox model provided an acceptable fit. Reflecting the consistency of MRT data, the results of this large RWD (avg age 78) were thus nearly identical to the previously published all-comers study (avg age 84), finding a 93% to 98% annual reduction in the rate of neovascular conversion compared to standard care with AREDs vitamins alone, with the greatest advantage afforded to the highest risk (older) patients, as reset theory would predict (Luttrull et al 2018, Luttrull and Grey 2021).

In the same propensity scored RWD study, chart VA showed gradual improvement in the VPT group, compared to progressive worsening of VA in the AREDS only group (Fig. 61). These studies support the hypothesis that improving and maintaining improved retinal function in AMD is a useful surrogate indicator for reduced long-term risks of visual loss (Luttrull and Margolis 2016, Luttrull et al 2018).

According to Diaz et al, as many as 18% of eyes with high-risk dry AMD may harbor occult neovascularization detectable by OCT angiography. Within 12 months, as many as 21% of these will become active, requiring anti-VEGF therapy (Diaz et al 2018). The annual neovascular conversion rate on the order of 1%

in eyes with high-risk dry AMD after SDM MRT suggests treatment is also effective at suppressing clinical activity in most eyes with preexudative subclinical macular neovascularization.

Vision protection therapy for prevention of neovascular AMD

Report No. 3
The findings of the retrospective cohort study and the subsequent RWD study finding regular periodic SDM (vision protection therapy) markedly reduced neovascular conversion in AMD was then examined in a third study, also using the same Vestrum RWD (Luttrull and Bhavan 2022, Luttrull and Gray 2023). Because the first RWD study of VPT included ICD-9 codes for AMD, AMD severity stratification was unavailable and could not be matched by propensity scoring. To address this deficiency, a second RWD study was performed using the same data source, inclusions, exclusions (with the addition of macular telangiectasis), and statistical methods, but this time restricting the data to include only the time during which ICD-10 coding data was available, January 2017 through June 2022. From an eligible population of 424,324 eyes with AMD, eyes were

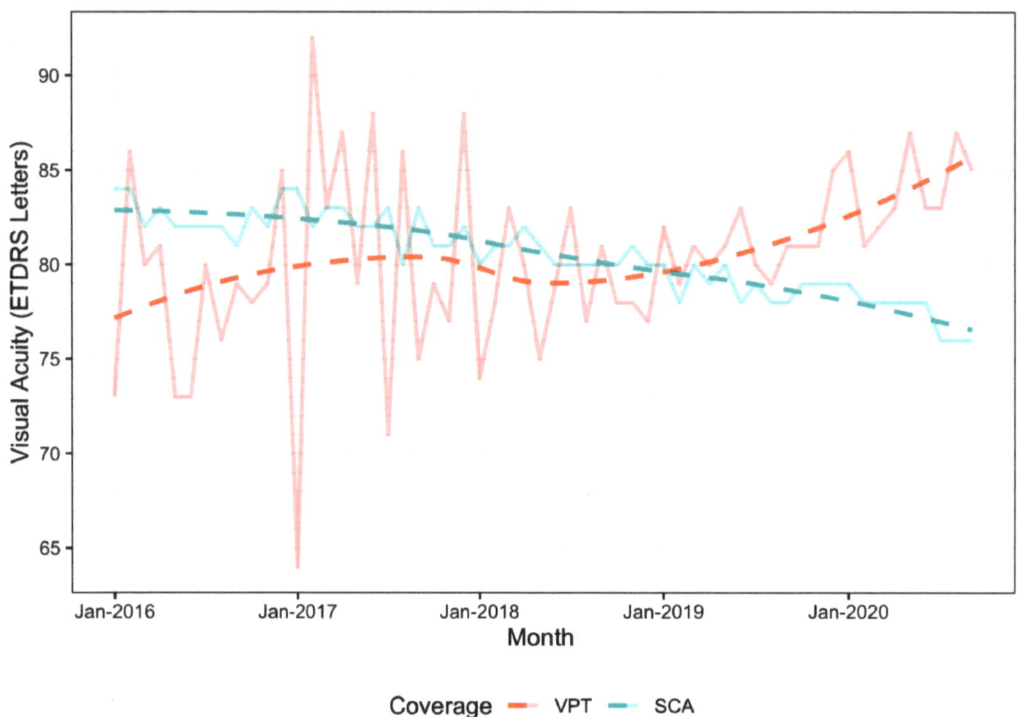

Fig. 61. Visual Acuity by month, SCA, VPT Groups, with loess smooths, comparing 9130 propensity scored eyes with bilateral dry AMD over 4.75 years, comparing average VA of eyes receiving standard care alone (SCA, blue line) to eyes receiving SDM MRT as vision protection therapy (VPT, red line) in addition to standard care. Note trend for progressive VA loss in standard care eyes compared to trend for improved VA in VPT MRT eyes. *From: Luttrull JK, Gray G. Real World Data Comparison of Standard Care vs SDM Laser Vision Protection Therapy for Prevention of Neovascular AMD. Clin Ophthalmol (2022) May, 16: 1555-1568.*

filtered and then matched by propensity scoring, and then matched for comparison in a 1/10 ratio of 675 VPT managed eyes and 6,750 conventionally managed eyes without VPT ("standard care alone," or SCA) for all risk factors. In this study, because eyes managed by SCA are examined infrequently, two analyses of these groups were performed, one with and one without matching the number of clinical encounters.

When matched for encounter frequency (10.4 office visits for the VPT group and 10.5 for the SCA group) incidence of neovascular conversion was 2.27% for the VPT group and 16.1% for the SCA group (hazard ratio 8.3) (Figs. 62 and 63). When not matched for encounter frequency, reflecting the actual clinical observation intensity of the SCA group for patients with dry AMD in the community of 7.9 encounters over the 5.5 year study window, the documented conversion rate in the SCA group fell from 11.1% (HR 7.5). In both analyses, eyes with the highest risk factors for conversion benefited most from VPT, the opposite of the LEAD trial of nanosecond laser, which accelerated degeneration and visual loss. The only significant risk factor for neovascular conversion not specifically accounted for

in this study was the presence of reticular pseudodrusen (RPD), because images were not available. However, RPD are highly correlated with age and AMD severity, which were matched between the groups (Luttrull et al 2018). Thus, because the VPT and SCA were matched for all risk conversion factors available in the database, this 33% drop in documented neovascular conversions in the SCA group resulted from the decrease in encounter frequency alone. When the encounter frequency was balanced between the VPT and SCA groups (to 10.5 and 10.4 encounters, respectively), the 33% increase in encounter frequency from 7.9 to 10.4 for the SCA group resulted in a 45% increase in recognized and documented neovascular conversions. This suggests that standard of care for dry AMD as currently implemented fails to recognize many, if not most, cases of neovascular conversion because of the infrequency of patient examinations. The outcome of the eyes in the SCA with undocumented conversions cannot be determined from this study. However, they would either go undiagnosed and untreated, or have received delayed treatment, compared to the VPT group, who are examined more often and thus diagnosed earlier. Human nature being

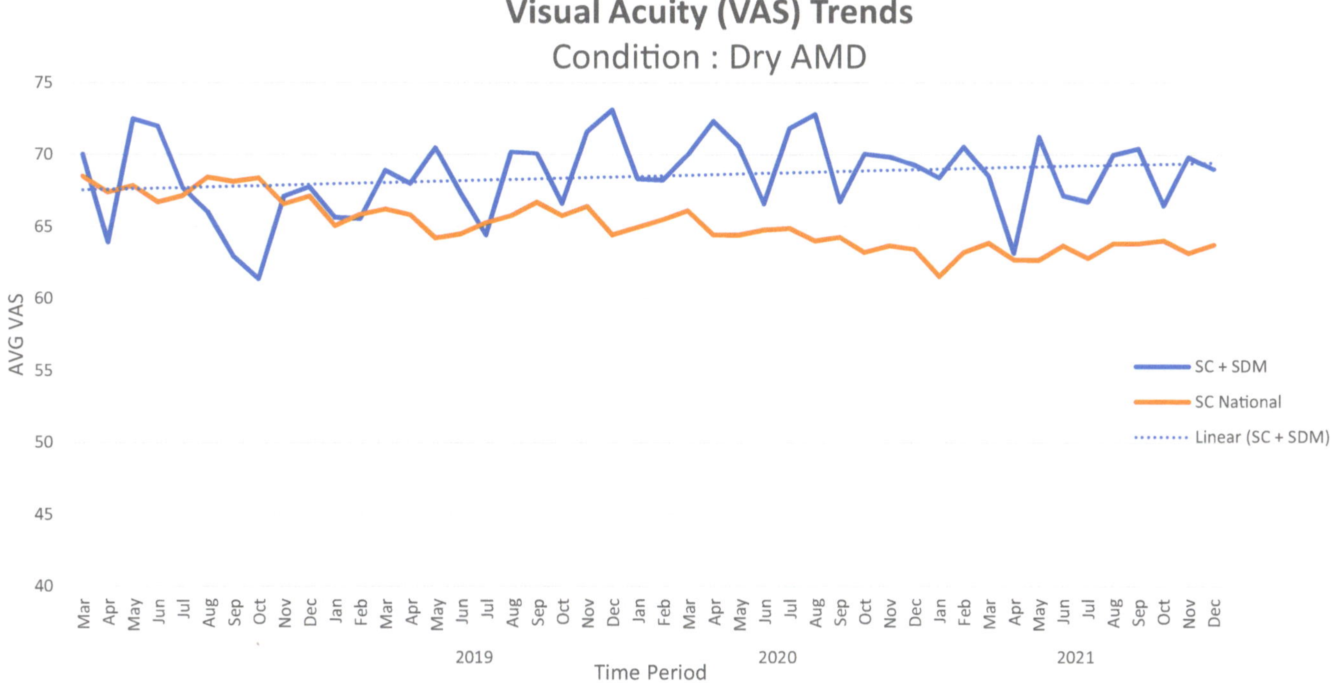

Fig. 62. Bar graphs showing risk factors for neovascular conversion in eyes with dry AMD in propensity scored RWD study including ICD-10 code matching of dry AMD subtypes. Distribution of risk factors in study population on left, raw data prior to matching by propensity scoring; right after matching by propensity scoring. Note balance of risk factors in the control, standard care alone group, with the group treated by the addition of vision protection therapy.

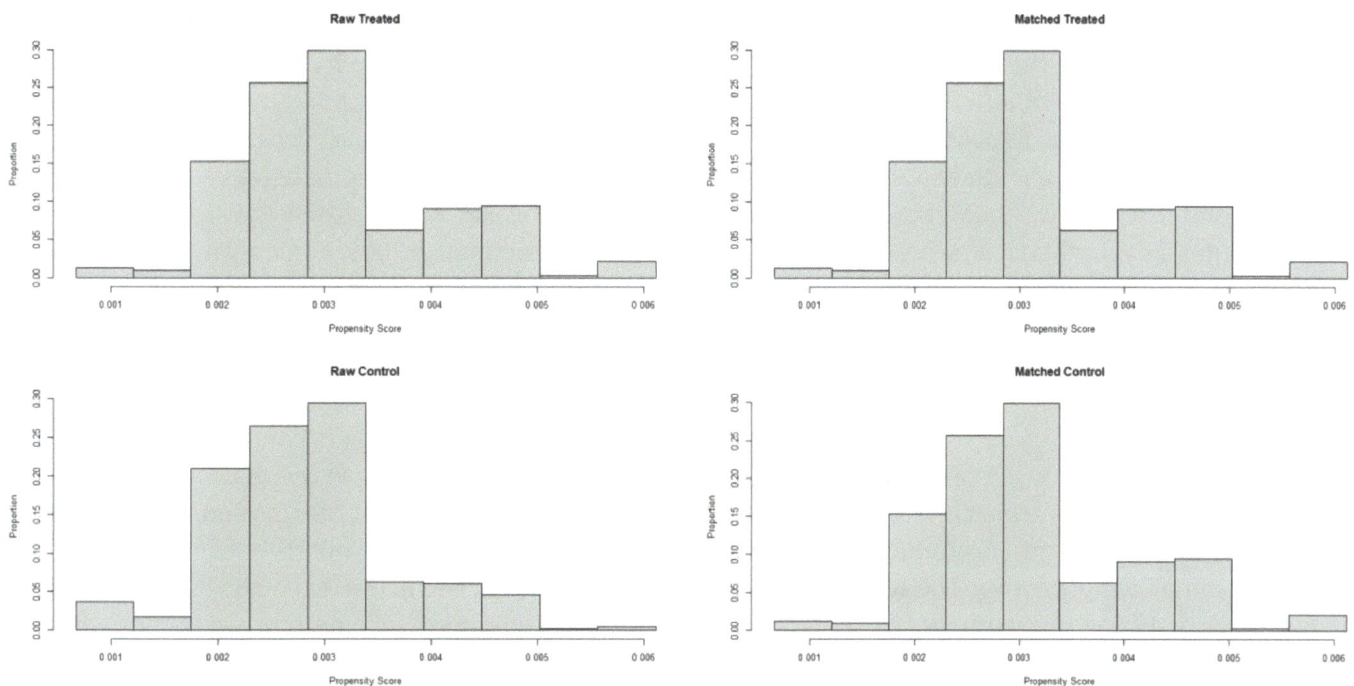

Fig. 63. Long-term visual acuities (VAS) in eyes with dry AMD from propensity scored eyes matched for major neovascular AMD risk factors including ICD-10 dry AMD severities. Blue line (SDM+SC) = Vision Protection Therapy (VPT) group. Red line (SCA) = Standard care alone group. Dotted lines depict trends with loess smoothes. As in the prior study without ICD1-10 codes, VA appears to favor the VPT group, in this case at all times in the study window.

what it is, when doctors have little to offer they tend not to be as deeply engaged. Thus, the current approach to the management of dry AMD can reasonably be described as little more than, "Take these pills (AREDS supplements) and call me when you lose your vision." This is problematic, as experience is clear that most patients with wet AMD are diagnosed incidentally rather than presenting for evaluation with new symptoms. This is because many older patients either do not notice the visual changes occurring with early wet AMD, when treatment is most effective; or they simply accept visual loss as normal with age and do not seek attention. Thus, only frequent examination can detect neovascular conversion in a timely fashion. Indeed, an entire industry has developed around this fact, producing a plethora of monitoring and diagnostic devices designed to detect neovascular conversion at home. Both lack of treatment and delayed treatment for neovascular AMD worsen the long-term visual prognosis (Ciulla et al 2018, 2019). Thus, not only do VPT managed eyes appear to have a markedly lower risk of neovascular conversion, but if conversion occurs in VPT patients, they are more likely to be diagnosed and treated in a timely fashion, improving their long-term visual prognosis compared to the current standard of care in which dry AMD patients are examined very infrequently.

It is noteworthy that these three studies of the effect of MRT VPT all show that VPT markedly reduces the incidence and risk of neovascular conversion in AMD. This is despite different study methods, different inclusions and exclusions, different time windows, and different study patients and controls. Only the treatment (VPT) and study endpoint (neovascular conversion) were constant. This leaves little room to doubt the reliability of these findings.

"This is not an RCT"

"This is not an RCT!" is a remarkably common first comment of many peer-reviewers in response to a study that is described in the title, introduction, methods, and discussion as retrospective. The tone is generally triumphant, suggesting the reviewer has seen through the authors' ruse and has presciently discovered the hidden fatal flaw in the study. The implication is that, because the study is not an RCT, it is without meaning or merit.

Obviously, such a view is problematic in general, and with regard to MRT in particular, as thus far the best evidence for the effectiveness of MRT in AMD is RWD.

RWD—retrospective data—is very often summarily dismissed as "not an RCT." The implication, of course, is that any RWD study is uninformative and less meaningful than any RCT.

The ability to do significant RWD studies is relatively new and rapidly improving, paralleling the development of the internet and large databases and our ability to mine and analyze vast amounts of data. With time, finely detailed RWD of all types will be available on masses of subjects over entire lifetimes, and then generations. This will allow studies based on RWD whose power could not even be approximated by an RCT. Thus, RWD studies will be increasingly important with time and may well replace RCTs for most purposes. With application of statistical methods such as propensity scoring to match RWD study populations to a degree comparable to an RCT, meaningful and useful data can be obtained, made more powerful by the large numbers and lengthy time frames available to RWD. Statistical methods like quintile analyses allow biases to be identified and minimized (Austin 2011, Jupiter 2017, Kim and Schneeweiss 2019). Further, the low cost of RWD analyses makes such analyses available to virtually anyone, not just entities with commercial interests and vast financial resources. The weaknesses of RWD studies are essentially the same as RCTs—garbage in, garbage out. The results are only as meaningful as the quality of the data and analysis. In 2014, a Cochrane collaborative systematic review found no significant difference between RCTs and RWD studies if the RWD studies were large and demonstrated robust results, such as the RWD studies of VPT MRT for AMD (Greenhouse 2009, Anglemyer et al 2014, Lundh et al 2017, Kim and Schneeweiss 2019). When there is a difference between RCT and RWD studies, the results of a given intervention are typically better in the RCT than in real-world implementation (Ciulla et al 2018, 2019). This is because of the highly controlled idealized environments of RCTs lacking in the real world. In fact, one can reasonably argue that the main enemy of the RCT is RWD. This is because the positive results of most RCTs are seldom matched in the real world, while the adverse effects of treatment become more apparent with time and application. The RCT is the best-case scenario. RWD is the reality check. This suggests the results of the RWD studies of VPT for wet AMD prevention would be confirmed, and likely found even more robust, in any subsequent RCT (Greenhouse 2009, Austin 2011, Anglemyer et al 2014, Lundh et al 2017, Ciulla et al 2018, 2019, Kim and Schneeweiss 2019, Enríquez et al 2021).

For this reason, RWD has historically been used to verify RCT results, rather than the obverse. As an example, emergency approval of the first COVID vaccines was granted based on RCT data. Full approval required RWD. While additional research is always desirable and will certainly be done, there is little reason to doubt the reliability of the large propensity scored RWD studies showing a substantial benefit from VPT in dry AMD (Anglemyer et al 2014, Kim and Schneeweiss 2019).

Key point: The effectiveness of MRT for prevention of neovascular AMD is robust, unprecedented, reliable, and predicted by reset theory.

MRT for geographic atrophy

Since all models are wrong the scientist cannot obtain a "correct" one by excessive elaboration. On the contrary; following William of Occam he should seek an economical description of natural phenomena. Just as the ability to devise simple but evocative models is the signature of the great scientist, so overelaboration and overparameter-ization is often the mark of mediocrity.

—George E. P. Box

The effect of regular periodic panmacular SDM MRT on the progression of age-related geographic atrophy (ARGA) was examined by looking at the rate of radial linear ARGA progression in eyes with GA reported as part of the 2018 neovascular conversion study cohort (Luttrull , Sinclair et al 2018).

A brief digression

If one could slow the progression of GA, how would one know? Originally, GA expansion was measured as a function of increased area over time, until it was realized that area progression was strongly influenced by initial lesion size. In response, the square root of the area was used to eliminate the confounding variable of initial lesion size. Despite this, determination of lesion area was curiously still employed to derive the square root. Determination of lesion area was done by manual tracing of the lesion margins, or a wide range of automated and semiautomated processes, often proprietary, specific to the operator—typically an academic image reading center (Uji et al 2010). All methods of area determina-tion are inherently very complex as the margins of GA

appear different depending on the imaging method, are often indistinct, and thus uncertain and subject to subjective interpretation. We know from Occam and his predecessors that complexity introduces the opportunity for error and that the inaccuracy introduced by accumulated errors reduces accuracy exponen-tially (Baker 2010). Complexity, while it confers the impression of superiority, technical sophistication, and nuance, is thus to be avoided rather than embraced. In fact, there is no evidence that any of the current models for determination of GA expansion based on area deter-mination are objectively correct. All are approximations (Uji et al 2010). So, why not use a simpler one?

When one takes the square root of the area, what is one left with? Radius. Why not measure it? As demon-strated in Figure 64, finding of the radius of GA lesions is straightforward and fairly easily done. To determine the radius, one simply determines the lesion diameter and divides by 2. Fewer data points and vastly increased simplicity is the reason for the reduction in potential for error and increased likelihood of reproducibility. A meta-analysis of GA measurement studies found that, absent treatment, the radial linear progression velocity of GA in any given eye is constant in all directions over time, independent of size and location (Shen et al 2016). This means that all that is needed to measure the rate of GA expansion is to measure the diameter of the lesion in exactly the same meridian over time. Proletarian, to be sure, but not for that reason illegitimate, and as it is a simpler method, it is to be preferred.

MRT slows GA in AMD

Employing this method (Luttrull et al 2018). 77 eyes of 49 consecutive patients were identified, average age 86 years, followed an avg. of 2.5 years prior to MRT treatment (controls), and 2.2 years after initiation of regular panmacular SDM MRT every 3 to 4 months. ARGA lesion measurements were masked for treatment versus control for the purpose of diameter measurements by a nontreating physician. The rate of linear radial progression was found to decrease 47% per year on average following initiation of regular periodic panmacular SDM MRT (Fig. 64). Although not statistically significant due to the small sample size, posttreatment annual progression of ARGA lesions <1 mm in diameter was reduced twice as much (>80% per year) compared to lesions >1 mm diameter (Fig. 65). This suggests that, as one might expect, early treatment of ARGA, when disease is less severe (*i.e.,*

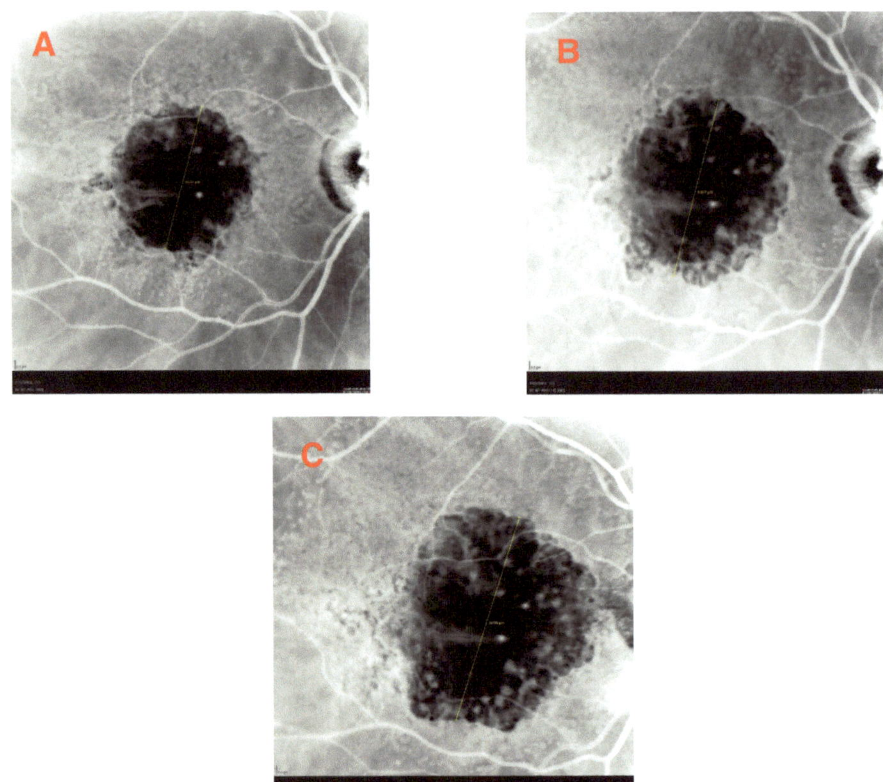

Fig. 64. Infrared autofluorescence fundus photograph of age-related geographic atrophy at presentation (A), at the time of initial panmacular SDM treatment 51 months later (B), and at the last visit 43 months following initiation of panmacular SDM treatment (C). *From: Luttrull JK, Sinclair SH, Elmann S, Chang DB, Kent D. Slowed progression of age-related geographic atrophy following subthreshold laser. Clin Ophthalmol (2020) Oct 1;14:2983-2993. doi:10.2147/OPTH.S268322. eCollection 2020*

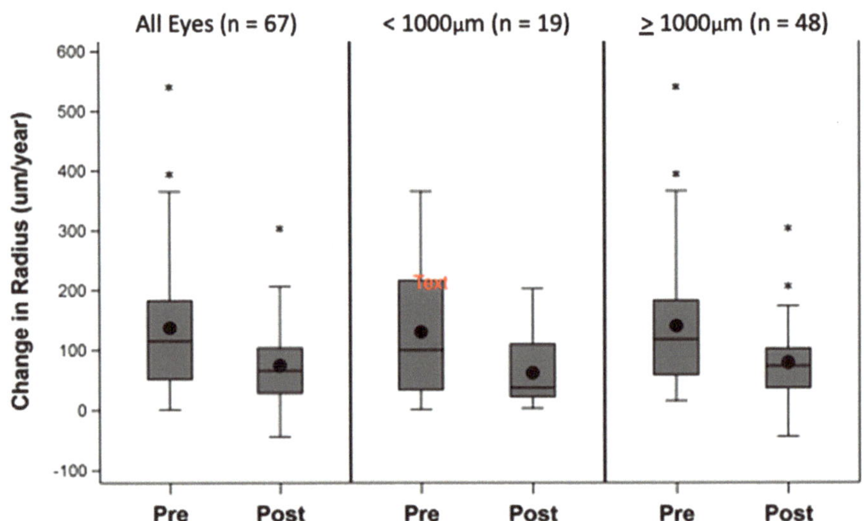

Fig. 65. Boxplots showing the distribution of change in radius, pre and post treatment. Plots are stratified by samples of all eyes (n=67), eyes with initial diameter <1000um (n=19) and eyes with initial diameter >1000um (n=48). Boxplots display the mean (black dot), median (line within the box), interquartile range (IQR) including the 25th percentile (bottom of the box) and the 75th percentile (top of the box), observations within 1.5 times the IQR (upper and lower fences) and outliers (asterisks, observations outside 1.5 times the IQR). For each comparison panmacular SDM laser significantly reduced the annual rate of linear radial progression of geographic atrophy (p<0.0001, linear regression analysis). A linear mixed model accounting for inter-eye correlation was performed to test the potential difference between eyes with smaller (< 1000um) vs larger (>1000um) initial lesion diameters. Initial lesion size did not significantly affect rates of progression either before or after SDM treatment (pretreatment continuous measure (p=0.919), dichotomized scale (p=0.824); post treatment continuous measure (p=0.408), dichotomized scale (0=0.269). From: *Luttrull JK, Sinclair SH, Elmann S, Chang DB, Kent D. Slowed progression of age-related geographic atrophy following subthreshold laser. Clin Ophthalmol (2020) Oct 1;14:2983-2993. doi:10.2147/OPTH.S268322. eCollection 2020*

smaller lesions) and more amenable to treatment, may be most effective. As usual, these MRT treatment benefits were achieved without adverse treatment effects (Fig. 31) (Luttrull et al 2018). These results are in marked contrast to inherently damaging retinal laser modes such as selective retinal therapy (SRT) and nanosecond laser, both of which have been shown to accelerate and worsen ARGA progression and visual loss in similar high-risk eyes (Roider et al 2000, Guymer et al 2018). Unlike damaging laser modes, MRT has been shown in every application to benefit the worst—thus highest risk—eyes the most. It will be important to confirm these MRT findings in further study, and to see if more frequent treatment might slow GA progression even more.

Key point: SDM MRT as vision protection therapy can significantly and safely slow progression of geographic atrophy in AMD

Geographic atrophy: where to treat, and why

By definition, panmacular treatment entails confluent treatment of the entire area of ARGA, because it is normally encompassed by the posterior vascular arcades. In more severely affected eyes, the area of ARGA may take up the majority of the panmacular area, and sometimes even extend outside it. Retinal function testing has shown that eyes with ARGA have measurable retinal function within the areas of ARGA that improves in response to MRT (Luttrull and Margolis 2016). This indicates that there is residual retina within the areas of ARGA that is bioactive, and that this activity is modifiable (normalizable) by MRT. Further, linear regression analysis showed that the most dysfunctional eyes, such as those with largest areas of GA, demonstrated the greatest degree of improvement following MRT, as reset theory would predict (Luttrull and Margolis 2016, Luttrull et al 2020).

Laser scar expansion as a model for GA

Prior theories of PC scar expansion proposed that initially sublethal thermal affects at the margins of PC lesions lead to slowly progressive death of this affected retina at the PC spot margins, causing the atrophic chorioretinal scar to expand radially with time (Schatz et al 1991, Mainster 1999). We now know, however, that the thermally affected but not killed retina at the margins of PC burns are instead vitalized, not de-vitalized, through RPE HSP activation. In

addition, expansion of PC scars with time often eventually exceeds the radius of the heated, but not immediately killed, lesion margins (Morgan and Schatz 1989). (Figs. 2, 8, 11) This expansion of PC scars cannot be explained by thermal effects at the margin of the PC lesion. Depending on the clinical setting, PC scar expansion may also progress through areas of otherwise normal retina. These three observations suggest that the impetus for PC scar expansion does not come from the margins of the atrophic lesion, or the retina outside the lesion, but from within the lesion itself. Thus, any treatment intended to slow progression of PC scars, and by extension ARGA, must necessarily target the GA directly, rather than the surrounding retina. Slowing of ARGA progression following panmacular SDM MRT suggests that dysfunction of residual retina surviving within ARGA, measurable by PERG, is the modifiable source of a factor or factors responsible for driving progression of lesion growth (Luttrull and Margolis 2016). This factor, or factors, appears to cause progressive failure at the proximate margins of the atrophy, and is thus highly locally acting. This also suggests that loss of RPE-derived trophic factors is the cause of choriocapillaris atrophy, rather than choriocapillaris atrophy being the cause of RPE failure, as the choriocapillaris is not a significant source of cytokines or other such modifiable chemical factors, and the congruity of choriocapillaris atrophy is with the overlying RPE atrophy, rather than the obverse of RPE atrophy mirroring choroidal vascular lobular structure (Kolomyer and Zarbin 2014). Normalization of this residual retinal function within the area of ARGA by MRT, and therefore homeotrophic alteration of the factor(s) driving ARGA progression, appears to account for slowing of ARGA progression following panmacular SDM as VPT. Although not yet studied, in the absence of other available treatment, based on the findings in ARGA it seems reasonable to consider panmacular MRT to try to slow expansion of fovea-threatening PC scars in the same way (Figs. 11 and 21).

Pigment epithelial detachment (PED)

It has been noted that MRT has no notable effect on morphology, such as drusen, in the short term. This reflects the absence of LIRD and inflammation. As has been discussed extensively elsewhere, because drusen reduction is generally associated with a worse prognosis and increased risk of neovascularization, this is a good thing (Luttrull and Kent 2019). The same can be said for PEDs. Long clinical experience indicates that MRT rarely results in short-term resolution of PEDs. As PED resolution typically results in acute visual loss due to the development of ARGA, this is also a good thing. For the same reasons, MRT does not cause RPE rips in eyes with PED. Treatment of eyes with PEDs, as with eyes with drusen, is directed at maximizing and preserving the health and function of the overlying macular RPE to maximize visual function, slow progression of RPE atrophy, and minimize the risk of neovascularization. If this is successful and the PED resolves prior to the development of secondary pigment atrophy, visual loss may be avoided or minimized (Fig. 58). It may also be noteworthy that, in long experience, de novo development of a PED following initiation of MRT vision protection therapy, has been observed very rarely, if at all. Might this be another salutary effect of MRT in AMD? Further study will tell.

Early treatment is best. What is early?

The vision protection therapy (VPT) program of regular periodic panmacular SDM appears to markedly reduce the risk of neovascular conversion and thus visual loss in dry AMD, particularly for eyes with high-risk findings in at least one eye (Luttrull et al 2018, 2020, Luttrull and Gray 2021). Eyes with early AMD have little risk of neovascular conversion and visual loss. Should the logic of early treatment be extended to them? In favor is to note that high-risk dry AMD must begin somewhere, and this is low-risk AMD. By slowing progression of the most aggressive form of dry AMD, ARGA, MRT appears to be the only treatment to safely slow AMD progression (Luttrull et al 2020). Might treatment of early AMD be of benefit to prevent or delay high-risk AMD? As we await a prospective trial, a simple evidence-based testing approach can offer guidance and aid decision making in this regard.

As noted, abnormal electrophysiology, MVFT and dark adaptation (DA) precede the development of clinical disease in most if not all CPRs, including AMD, and have been shown to predict future progression and the risk of future visual loss (Arden et al 1982, Riggs 1986, Banitt et al 2013, Katz et al 2010, Lahav et al 2011, Feigl et al 2011, Puell et al 2012, Jackson et al 2014, Gutstein et al 2015, Stringham et al 2015, Luttrull and Margolis 2016, Luttrull and Kent 2019, Hirji et al 2021). Clinically, MVFT and DA are the simplest to perform and interpret. Recently, the author has found automated perimetry using the macular threshold 10-2

and "M-Top" programs of the Octopus 600 perimeter to be very useful as well, and generally even easier and quicker for patients (Haag-Streit AG, Koniz Switzerland) (Fig. 72). In eyes where it is unclear whether or not to begin treatment, such testing can be obtained to determine if visual function is normal or abnormal. If abnormal, MRT can be formed as a provocative test. An improved result after treatment (usually tested 1 to 4 weeks post treatment) indicates the presence of a significant dysfunction correctable by treatment. As this correction represents temporary reversal of the disease process, this suggests that maintenance treatment should be considered to slow progression and reduce the long-term risks of visual loss (Figs. 17-23, and 71-72).

MRT for neovascular "Wet" AMD

Reversal of anti-VEGF drug tolerance

As noted earlier, understanding the mechanism of retinal laser action as a physiologic reset phenomenon suggested that MRT should reverse tolerance to the anti-VEGF medications used for treatment of AMD. This first test of the reset theory was also in many ways the most severe and novel, as reversal of drug tolerance was previously unknown in medicine. Reversal of anti-VEGF drug tolerance was subsequently demonstrated as predicted by reset theory in a small clinical study of 13 consecutive eyes chronically unresponsive to all available anti-VEGF drugs (Luttrull et al 2015). Panmacular SDM MRT was performed one month following the last ineffective anti-VEGF injection (aflibercept) and the eyes were rechallenged with aflibercept one month later. 12/13 eyes responded with resolution of exudation (Fig. 59). This was the first and still only demonstration of reversal of drug tolerance report in medicine, in any setting. Drug tolerance may occur by any number of mechanisms. Thus, the mechanism whereby MRT reverses drug tolerance to anti-VEGF drugs is unknown, and may actually be due to different effects in different eyes. Recent studies on reset-like phenomenon suggest that MRT may induce or reverse epigenetic changes in tolerant eyes (Zhang et al 2020, Ramaiah et al 2021).

Essential to the validation of any theory not only its ability to explain prior observations—such as how

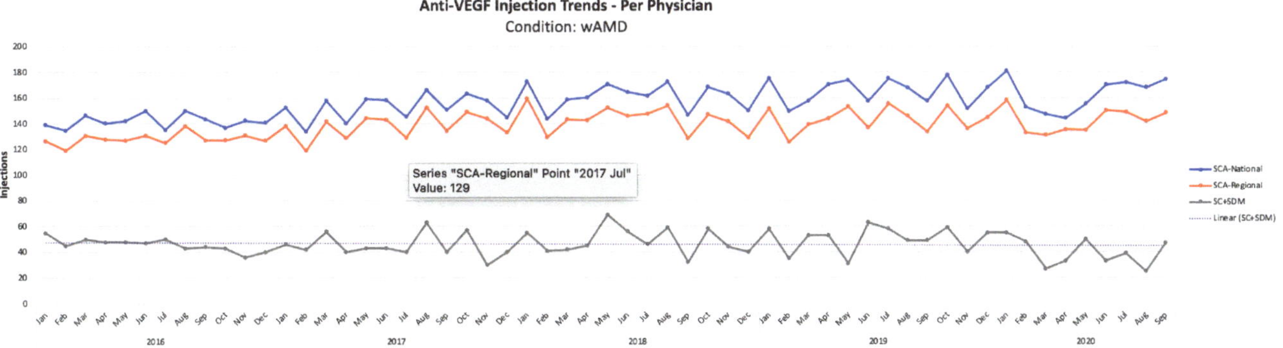

Fig. 66. Anti-VEGF injection frequency in eyes with neovascular AMD managed with standard care with injections alone ("SCA" group, n=72,243 eyes, top lines, regional and national) compared to eyes managed standard care and the addition of regular periodic SDM MRT ("SC+SDM", n=195 eyes). Final average monthly injections for national SCA group was 0.73 injections / eye / month, compared to 0.27 / eye / month for SC+SDM eyes. Injections per physician SCA group avg 163/month, SC+SDM group 63/month. Note the average 69% per eye lower in injection frequency in the SDM MRT (SC-SDM) group. The low injection per physician rate in the SC+SDM group reflects the cumulative effects of both the low injection frequency per eye due to SDM-elicited extension anti-VEGF drug effectiveness; as well as a low number of eyes with dry AMD converting to wet AMD in the SC+SDM VPT group.

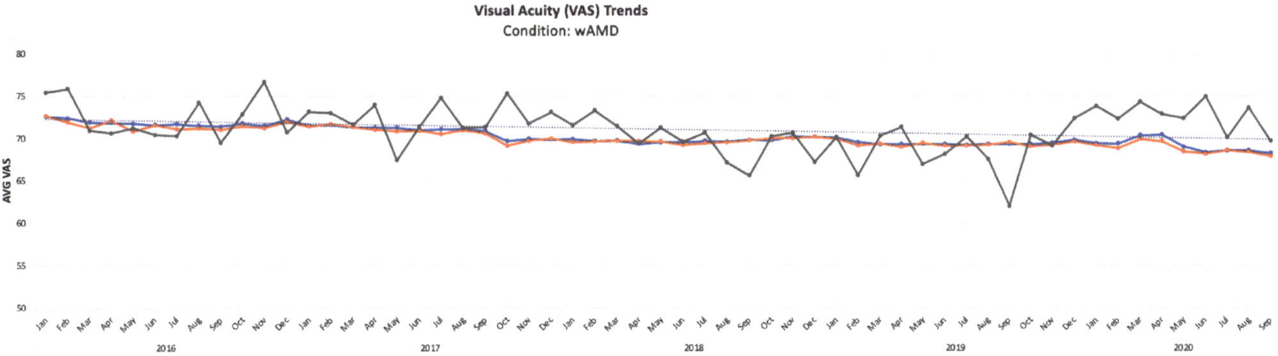

Fig. 67. VA averages for in eyes with neovascular AMD managed with injections alone (top lines, national and regional US averages) compared to eyes managed with regular periodic SDM MRT VPT (SC-SDM). Note that despite average 69% per eye reduction in injection frequency in SDM group over the 4.75 year study window, VAs are the same.

retinal laser might improve disparate diseases such as CSR and DR—but also is its ability to predict new and previously unknown phenomena (Fazlollah 1994). The success of reset theory to predict reversal of drug tolerance was the first of many novel predictions subsequently confirmed (Luttrull et al 2015, Luttrull and Margolis 2016, Luttrull 2018, Luttrull, Samples et al 2018, Luttrull, Sinclair et al 2018, Luttrull et al 2020, Luttrull and Gray 2021). Long clinical experience finds, not unexpectedly, that MRT reversal of anti-VEGF drug tolerance in AMD is generally temporary, ususally lasting 3 to 9 months, before recurring. As reset theory also predicts, retreatment is effective at reversing recurrent drug tolerance as often as subsequently necessary in most eyes.

Reduction of the anti-VEGF injection burden

Because the clinical response to long-term anti-VEGF drugs tends to diminish with time, representing a state of partial or incomplete tolerance, the ability to reverse complete anti-VEGF tolerance in wet AMD suggested that regular periodic SDM MRT in eyes receiving anti-VEGF injections for wet AMD should improve drug effectiveness by preventing or minimizing partial as well as complete tolerance. If so, this would improve the effectiveness of drug therapy, prolonging the treatment effect. The longer the treatment effect, the fewer injections that would be required to maintain a dry macula (Luttrull et al 2015). This effect was also confirmed in the Vestrum retina database RWD AMD study. As predicted by reset theory, eyes with wet AMD receiving SDM MRT every 3 to 4 months along with anti-VEGF drugs required an average of 69% fewer anti-VEGF injections per eye, compared to eyes receiving injections alone. Despite significantly fewer injections, the average VA results were the same as the non-SDM managed eyes (Luttrull and Gray 2021) (Figs. 66, 67).

Inhibition of anti-VEGF injection-associated geographic atrophy

Ultimately, visual acuity in most eyes with wet AMD is limited by subretinal fibrosis, ARGA or most often, both (Toth et al 2019, Okeagu et al 2021). A recent meta-analysis found a linear correlation between the number and frequency of anti-VEGF injections and the development and progression of ARGA in wet AMD (Eshtiaghi et al 2021). Whether the tendency of eyes with wet AMD to develop geographic atrophy is due to, or aggravated by, anti-VEGF medications; or simply reflects disease activity and severity is unclear. However, because MRT can slow progression of ARGA in dry AMD, the addition of regular periodic panmacular SDM MRT as vision protection therapy to anti-VEGF therapy may also help reduce ARGA-associated vision loss in wet AMD (Luttrull, Sinclair et al 2018).

Summary: MRT for AMD

MRT is thus the first retinal treatment to safely and significantly slow progression of ARGA, markedly reduce the risk of neovascular conversion and thus vision loss in dry AMD, improve long-term VA in dry AMD, and significantly reduce the frequency of anti-VEGF injections and thus the treatment risks and treatment burden in wet AMD.

Key point: Uniquely, MRT can help all types and stages of AMD

12. Open-Angle Glaucoma and Modern Retinal Laser Therapy

Neuroprotection, neuroenhancement and neuroregeneration and MRT

One of the most interesting and compelling applications of MRT is treatment of OAG. A fundamental precept of reset theory is that the effect of MRT is retinotrophic, thus neurotrophic and neuroprotective. Dropping the IOP (intraocular pressure) significantly in OAG can be thought of as neuroprotective. In 2005, Ventura and Porciatti reported improved PERGs in eyes with OAG following IOP reduction, indicating improved retinal ganglion cell function (Ventura and Porciatti 2005). The neuroprotective effect of MRT in OAG was thus suggested by the effects of MRT on the PERG and mesopic visual function in dry AMD, which showed baseline abnormalities like those demonstrated by previous investigators in OAG, that then improved following SDM MRT (Ventura and Porciatti 2005, Ventura et al 2012, Luttrull and Margolis 2016). As approximately 95% of the optic nerve arises in the macula, any treatment hoping to modify the course of OAG via neuroprotection must necessarily target and improve macular function. Clinical application has confirmed the reset theory prediction of neuroprotective effects in OAG, and, once again, the hypothesis of disease-specific repair. After MRT for OAG, significant improvements in optic nerve function by electrophysiology, VA, and mesopic VA and visual fields following panmacular SDM MRT are noted, representing neuroenhancement via rescue and revitalization of previously nonfunctional, nonrecordable preapoptotic cells (Tables 7 and 8) (Johnson et al 2022). As we will see in the following pages, the effects of MRT may extend beyond neuroprotection and neuroenhancement to actual neuroregeneration (Levin et al 2017, Johnson et al 2020). Disease-specific repair is reflected in the electrophysiologic response of OAG to MRT, which is characteristically different from that seen in AMD and IRDs, manifest by significant increases in VER and PERG signal amplitudes, rather than improvements in signal latencies as seen in other retinopathies, such as AMD and the IRDs. It is difficult to imagine how better to define neuroprotection in the eye other than by the range of improvements elicited by MRT in the CRPs, including OAG (Luttrull, Samples et al 2018, Luttrull and Kent 2019) (Figs. 16, 19, 20, 22, 68, and 69).

Discovering the unexpected is more important than confirming the known.

—George E. P. Box

ROAG: The retinopathy of open angle glaucoma

Reflecting on the above, one of the most remarkable discoveries attributable to MRT is the discovery that there is a previously undetected retinopathy at the heart of OAG. The most robust electrophysiologic response to MRT in OAG is improvement in optic nerve function measured by VER signal amplitudes (Fig. 16, Table 12). MRT is the only measure known thus far to improve the VER in any setting, clinical or otherwise (Luttrull, Samples et al 2018). It is notable that following MRT in eyes with both AMD and OAG, it is the OAG PERG response that predominates over the AMD response, showing the greater improvements in signal amplitudes (characteristic of OAG) compared to improvements in signal latencies (characteristic of AMD and IRDs) (Luttrull, Samples et al 2018). Thus, the results of selective treatment of the RPE in OAG reveal the presence of a hitherto unrecognized retinopathy in OAG, or ROAG (retinopathy of open-angle glaucoma), characterized by a hyponeurotropism correctable by MRT. This is a novel statement. How can it be made?

(1) SDM has no effect on normal tissue. (2) The only effect of SDM is to improve the function of dysfunctional tissue. (3) SDM treats only the RPE. (4) Following treatment of only the RPE by SDM, visual function, ganglion cell (by PERG) and optic nerve function (by VER) improve. (5) This improvement indicates an RPE/retinal dysfunction in OAG. (6) The RPE acts at distance by chemical mediators. (7) Therefore, the improve-

ments in ganglion cell and optic nerve function indicate a chemical (cytokine) hyponeurotropism of retinal origin in OAG (ROAG) that is modifiable and responsive to SDM MRT.

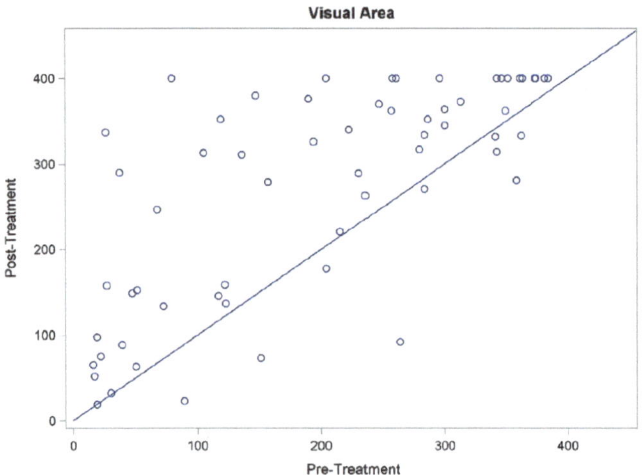

Fig. 68. Scatter graph of Omnifield resolution (mesopic) perimetry visual area (VA) before and after SDM treatment (for open angle glaucoma). Note significant improvements in recordable visual areas following SDM treatment (BA6 and GMA also showed similar levels of improvement following SDM). From: *Luttrull JK, Samples JR, Kent D, Lum BJ: Panmacular subthreshold diode micropulse laser (SDM) as neuroprotective therapy in primary open-angle glaucoma. Glaucoma Research 2018-2020, pp. 281-294 Edited by: John R. Samples and Paul A. Knepper © 2018 Kugler Publications, Amsterdam, The Netherlands*

Thus, OAG appears to be a panocular disease. Recognition of this association, evident in the response of OAG to MRT, improves our understanding of OAG, presenting new opportunities for more effective management and prevention of visual loss. Identification of a previously unrecognized ROAG may explain why glaucomatous optic neuropathy and visual loss continues to progress in the majority of OAG patients despite IOP lowering. It will be important and interesting to find out if long-term mitigation of ROAG by MRT neuroprotection and neuroenhancement can reduce visual loss from OAG as it does in AMD and DR.

Improved nerve fiber layer (NFL) and ganglion cell complex layer (GCC) thickness trends following MRT vision protection therapy (VPT) in eyes with OAG and AMD. Evidence of neuroregeneration?

Normal aging is associated with progressive thinning of the retina, including steady thinning of the NFL and GCC. Because no one gets younger, these measures only worsen with time and do not improve. This loss of tissue thickness has been attributed to loss of retinal ganglion cells and supportive neural and glial elements with age. Superimposition of disease, such as a CPR like AMD or OAG, increases the rate of thinning. Thickening of these layers with time in normal aging or disease has

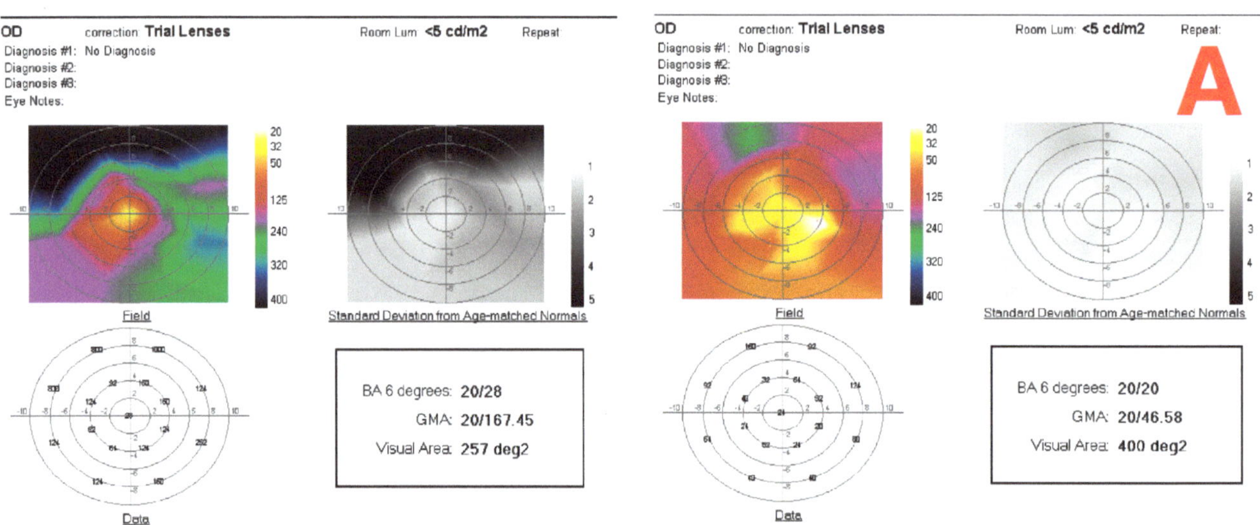

Fig. 69. Omnifield resolution (mesopic) perimetry findings for patients with primary open angle glaucoma and glaucomatous optic neuropathy. Each row A-C represents a different patient and eye. Left column, before SDM; right column, after SDM. BA6: best logMAR visual acuity within 6° of fixation. GMA: global macular logMAR visual acuity. VA: visual area. Note improvements in all indices following panmacular SDM. From: *Luttrull JK, Samples JR, Kent D, Lum BJ: Panmacular subthreshold diode micropulse laser (SDM) as neuroprotective therapy in primary open-angle glaucoma. Glaucoma Research 2018-2020, pp. 281-294 Edited by: John R. Samples and Paul A. Knepper © 2018 Kugler Publications, Amsterdam, The Netherlands*

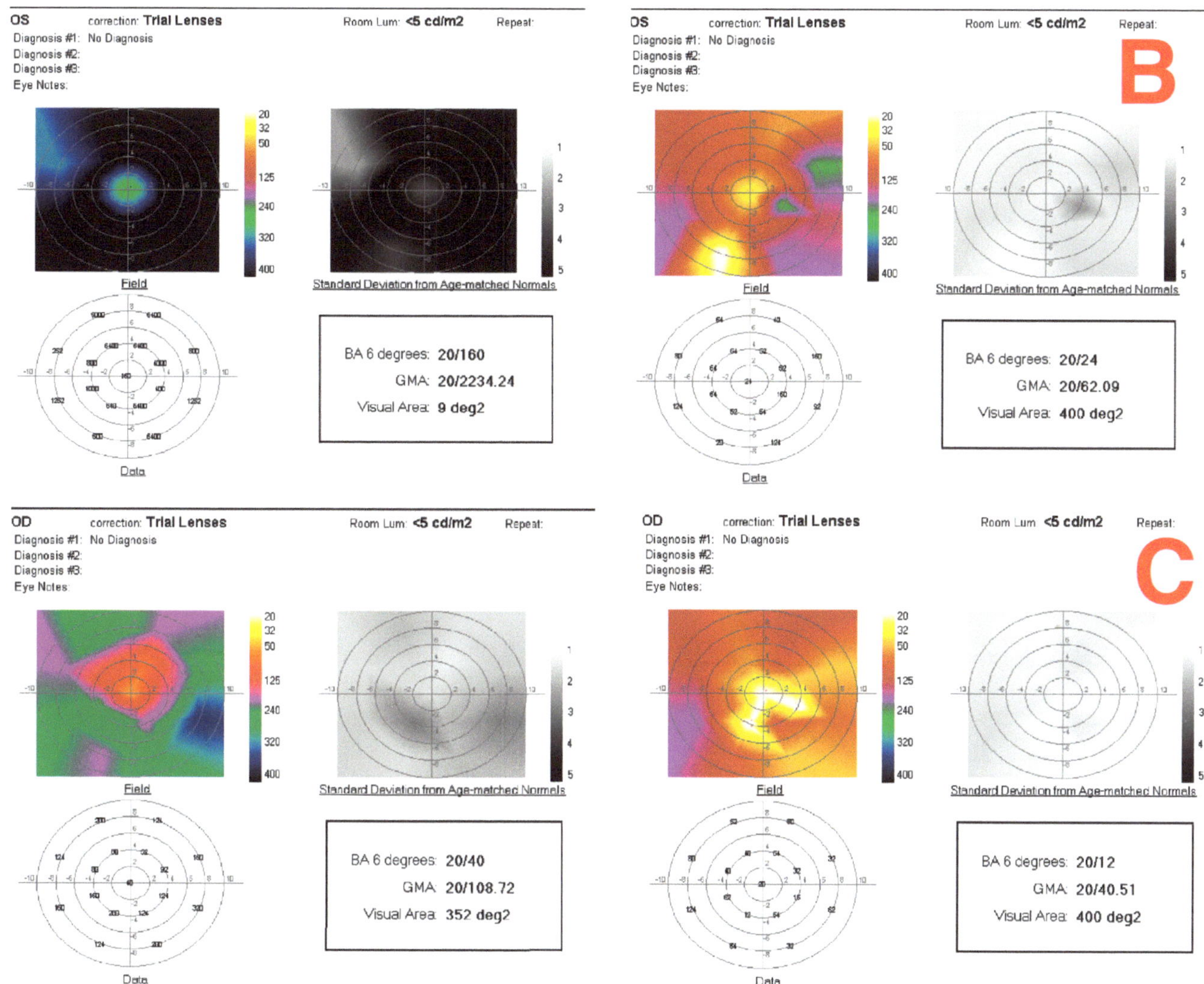

Fig. 69. (Continued)

Table 11. Demographics of propensity scored groups including dry AMD ICD-10 code matching.

AREDS Category	SCA Group	VPT Group
	230,854	660
Early	87,757 (38.0)	212 (32.1)
Intermediate	114,751 (49.7)	353 (53.5)
Non central GA	11,545 (5.0)	45 (6.8)
Central GA	16,801 (7.3)	50 (7.6)
Age (mean, SD)	76.36 (9.65)	76.67 (10.03)
AREDS use	90,038 (39.0)	312 (47.3)
Smoking	12,725 (5.5)	14 (2.1)
HTN	137,428 (59.5)	348 (52.7)
Encounters (mean, SD)	3.46 (4.53)	9.12 (8.33)
Conversions without encounter matching	305/6600 (4.62)	15/660 (2.27)
Conversions with encounter matching	959/6600 (14.53)	15/660 (2.27)

Table 12. VEP indices (in eyes before and after treatment with panmacular SDM MRT for open-angle glaucoma with glaucomatous optic neuropathy)

Variable	Mean (SD)	Median (IQR)	*p*-value
AMP, low contrast (N_{miss} = 7)	0.57 (4.15)	0.90 (−1.80, 2.60)	0.33
AMP, high contrast (N_{miss} = 6)	1.59 (4.59)	0.85 (−0.90, 3.00)	0.001
LAT, low contrast (N_{miss} = 7)	−2.27 (21.69)	−1.00 (−12.70, 6.80)	0.27
LAT, high contrast (N_{miss} = 5)	−0.78 (16.76)	−0.90 (−7.80, 5.90)	0.72

Summary of calculated difference (post- minus pre-SDM treatment). This table shows the mean and median differences for the covariates of interest. Each row shows the difference (post- minus pretreatment) in amplitude (AMP) or latency (LAT) at two contrast options. In order to test whether the mean difference is different from zero, a linear mixed models predicting the measure was performed, using an indicator for time as a covariate, also adjusting for left or right eye, and including a random patient intercept. The *p*-values are those associated with the time (pre- vs. posttreatment) regression coefficient. A significant *p*-value indicates that the mean difference is significantly different from zero. Only the high contrast amplitude (AMP, High Contrast) is significantly different pretreatment versus posttreatment. This method accounts for intereye correlation
SD = standard deviation. IQR = inter quartile range. N_{miss} = number of missing values. AMP = P1 wave amplitude in microvolts. From: Luttrull JK, Samples JR, Kent D, Lum BJ. Panmacular subthreshold diode micropulse laser (SDM) as neuroprotective therapy in primary open-angle glaucoma. In: Samples JR, Knepper PA, eds. *Glaucoma Research 2018-2020*. Kugler Publications; 2018:281-294.

not previously been observed, such that the occasional notations of trend improvement are sufficiently rare as to be considered statistical "noise" (Miki et al 2014, Mohammadzadeh et al 2022).

Thus, the author noted with some curiosity that NFL layer thicknesses and trends in many eyes managed by VPT (panmacular SDM MRT in a program of long-term periodic maintenance therapy for neuroprotection) appeared to improve. To investigate this observation, a retrospective study of three groups of eyes was undertaken. The first group were 70 eyes in a referring glaucoma practice managed conventionally with an emphasis on IOP control. The second group were 77 eyes with OAG from the referring glaucoma practice whose IOP was managed by the same glaucoma specialist, but who were referred for and managed with the addition of VPT for associated early to intermediate AMD. The third group were 69 eyes without OAG managed with VPT for early to intermediate AMD alone. Long-term trends in average retinal, NFL, and GCC thickness were recorded. In the VPT groups, this OCT data was restricted to the time period during which a Topcon Maestro 2 spectral-domain OCT machine (Topcon Inc, Freemont, CA) was available for recording. In the conventionally managed OAG group, longer term OCT data was available (Luttrull and Bhavan 2022).

The conventionally and VPT managed OAG groups were similar, except that the conventionally managed eyes were younger (avg 73 years) than the VPT OAG group (avg 80 years) reflecting AMD has the primary referring diagnosis in the VPT OAG group. The AMD alone group (no OAG) averaged 77 years of age. The differences in the annual rate and direction of the retinal layer thickness trends (positive = thickening / improvement, negative = thinning / worsening) is shown in Fig. 70. Note that improvements in NFL and GCC trends in the conventionally managed OAG eyes are rare, as expected. However, OAG and AMD eyes managed by VPT demonstrated high percentages of eyes with positive thickness trends (67% and 80%, respectively), indicating improved NFL and GCC layer thicknesses over time. While eyes with OAG and no VPT lost average GCC and NFL thickness and with time, OAG eyes managed with VPT lost minimal GCC and average NFL layer thicknesses actually increased. Such findings clearly exceed the definitions of neuroprotection and neuroenhancement, suggesting MRT-induced neuroregeneration (Johnson et al 2022). To our knowledge, this is the first observation of consistently progressive NFL or GCC layer improvement/thickening in any setting, either in normal aging, or disease, let alone in OAG (Celebi and Mirza 2013, Miki et al 2014, Mohammadzadeh et al 2022) (Table 13) (Fig. 70).

It is unclear what these increases in NFL and GCC thickness represent. It is known that axonal degeneration and death precede both GC death and visual field loss (Wei et al 2019). For this reason MRT-induced neuroregeneration appears to be one possible explanation for this observation. This is consistent with the improvements in MVFT and automated perimetry in eyes with both OAG

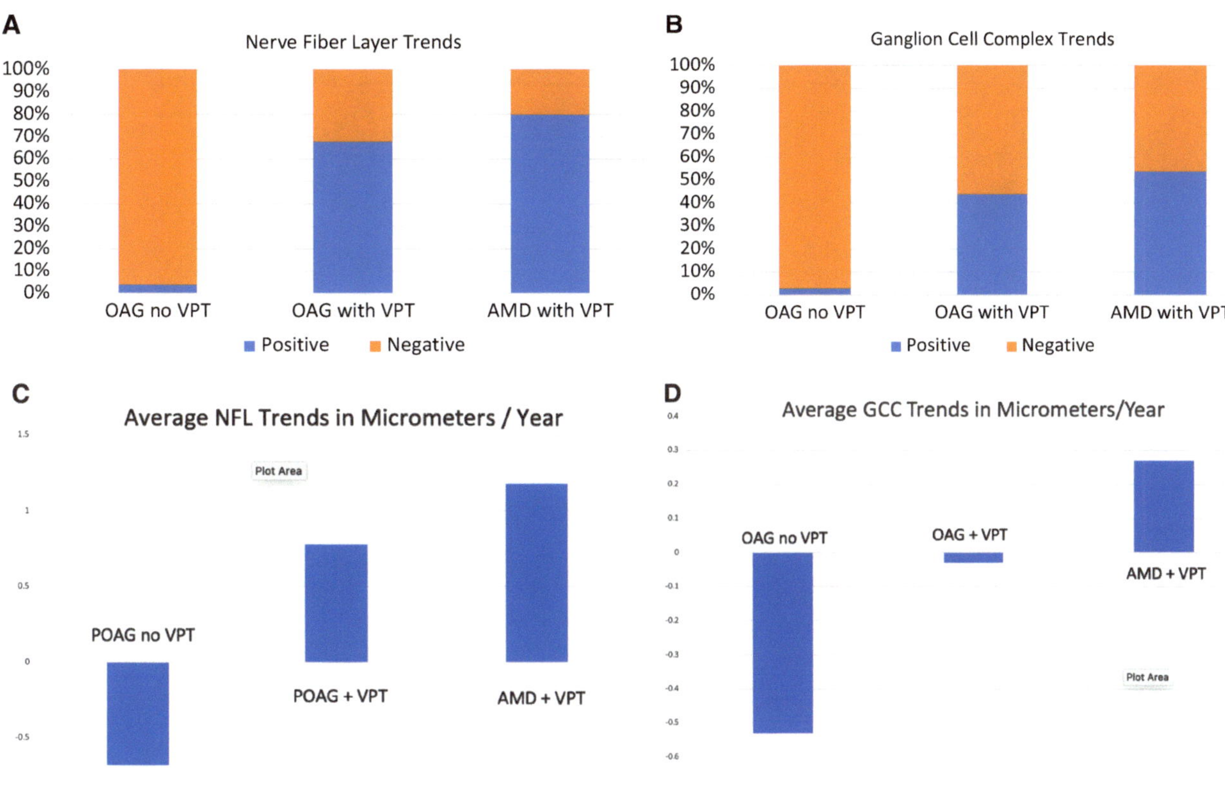

Fig. 70. Bar graphs showing the direction of retinal layer thickness trends (micrometers / year) over time. (A) Columns = per cent of eyes improved (progressively thickening layer with time) (blue) vs. per cent of eyes worsened (progressively thinning layer with time) (red). (A) Nerve fiber layer; (B) Ganglion cell complex layer. Note predominant thinning and worsening of both NFL and GCC in OAG managed conventionally without SDM MRT vision protection therapy (VPT). Note high percentage of eyes with improving and thickening layers in eyes with OAG, and eyes with AMD without OAG, managed with the addition of VPT. (C) Average nerve fiber layer thickness trends in um/year. (D) Average ganglion cell complex layer thickness trends in um/year

and AMD treated with VPT due to neuroenhancement (Figs. 19, 20, 22, 68, 69, 71, and 72). If so, humans and mice may share this facility, as Lu and associates have previously shown posttraumatic optic nerve regeneration mediated by activation of OSK genes (Oct4, Sox2 and Klf4 genes) in mouse retinal ganglion cells to restore youthful, presenile, DNA methylation patterns leading to axonal regrowth. Interestingly, this is thought to have occurred by an epigenetic "reprogramming" mechanism that is also a potential feature of the reset mechanism of MRT (Lu et al 2020, Luttrull and Bhavan 2022). Confirmed, the implications for the management of CPRs in general, OAG in particular, and neurodegenerative diseases across the board, would be significant.

Key point: MRT is the first and as yet only robustly neuroprotective treatment for OAG. MRT is the first and as yet only treatment to reverse OAG progression indicated by reversals in vision loss, visual field loss, and nerve fiber layer and ganglion cell complex loss independent of IOP.

Summary: The iconic models for MRT application

In DR, AMD and OAG we have iconic models of the major CPRs and MRT responses that then lend themselves to other different, but analogous, clinical settings and applications. Discussion of some of these applications follows.

Key point: As predicted by reset theory, MRT improves all major CPR neurodegenerations via neuroprotection to reverse progression and reduce risks of vision loss. These serve as iconic models for other treatment indications.

Table 13. Summary table: effect of VPT on OCT retinal layer thickness trends

Demographics	POAG, no VPT	POAG + VPT[a]	AMD, no POAG,+ VPT
Number of pts	37	45	37
Male	12	22	12
Female	25	23	29
No. eyes	70	77	69
Phakic	30	19	29
Pseudophakic	40	58	40
Age Avg, Med, SD	73, 73 (11)	80, 81 (8.8)	77, 78 (6.7)
Obs. interval (days) Avg, Med, SD	3330, 3463 (2027)	447, 480 (105)	516, 505 (56)
Days VPT Avg, Med, SD	NA	1217, 1036 (764)	1558, 1304 (850)
VA initial Avg, Med, SD	49, 30 (76)	34, 30 (15)	38, 30 (31)
VA final Avg, Med, SD	44, 25 (101)	44, 30 (41)	47, 30 (94)
IOP initial Avg, Med, SD	19, 19 (4.2)	16, 15 (4.4)	17, 15 (7)
IOP final Avg, Med, SD	14, 15 (3.7)	15, 14 (3.4)	15, 15 (2.7)
Topical meds per eye Avg, Med, SDM	1.6, 2 (0.6)	1.4, 1 (0.77)	NA
NFL trend (um/yr) Avg, Med, SD	−0.68, −0.60 (0.62)	+0.78, +0.75 (1.96)	+1.18, +0.83 (2.16)
NFL slope + No / %	3 (4%)	52 (68%)	55 (80%)
NFL slope −	67 (96%)	25 (32%)	14 (20%)
GCC trend (um/yr) Avg, Med, SD	−0.53, −0.43 (0.51)	−0.03, −0.12 (2.1)	+0.27, +0.08 (1.67)
GCC slope + No. / %	2 (3%)	34 (44%)	37 (54%)
GCC slope − No. / %	68 (97%)	43 (56%)	32 (46%)

Demographics of patients and trends of nerve fiber layer (NFL), ganglion cell complex layer (GCC), and retinal thickness changes over time
[a]36/45 (80%) patients with early to intermediate AMD in addition to POAG

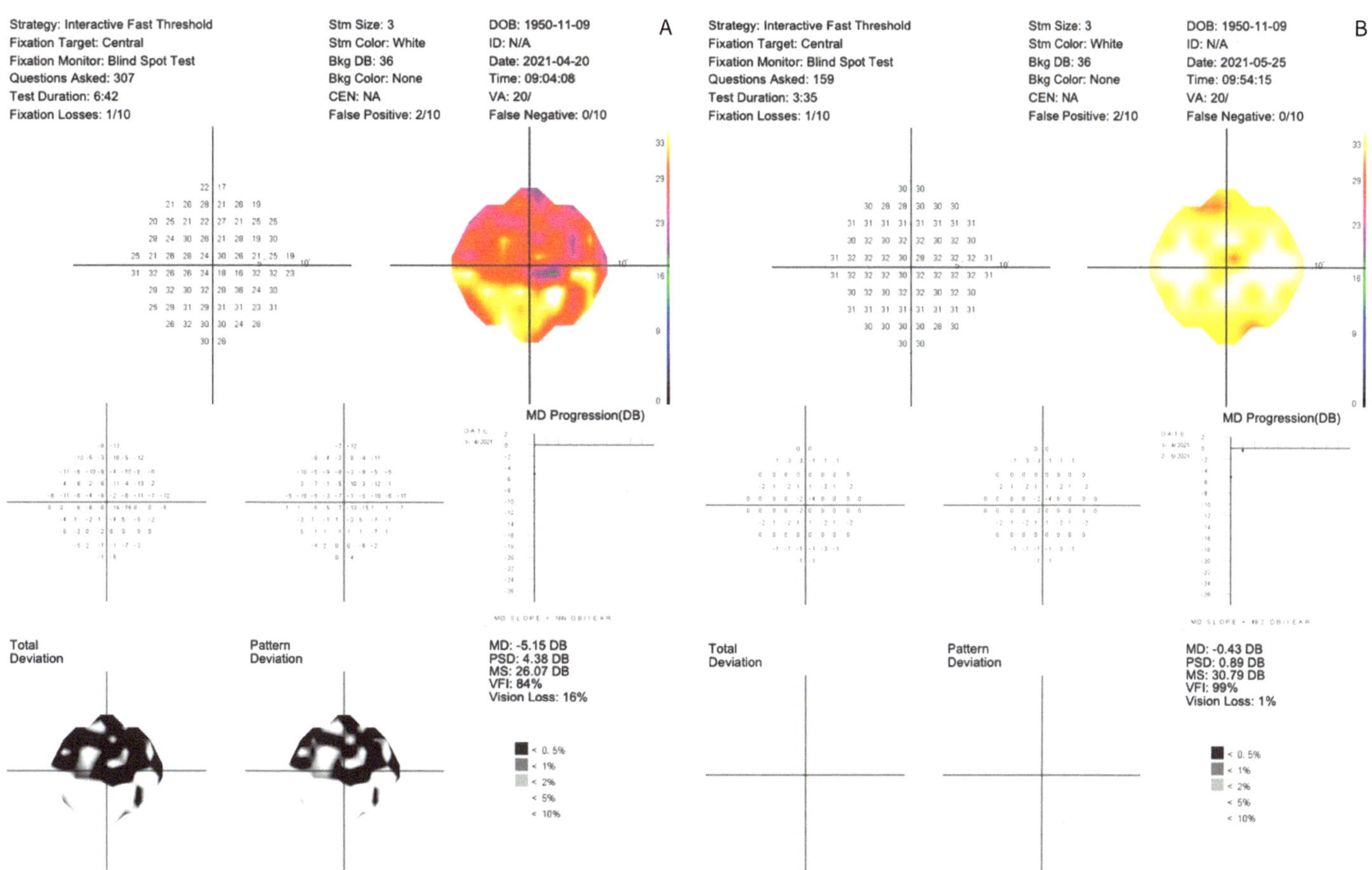

Fig. 71. 71 yo Hispanic woman with epiretinal membrane and history of OAG OU and central retinal vein occlusion OS with glaucomatous optic neuropathy and visual field loss OD. VA 20/25+ OU. 10-2 visual field (report modified to display a false-color map) of right eye before (A) and after one week after (B) SDM MRT. Note reduction in scotoma size due to recovery of visual and retinal / optic nerve function following MRT treatment.

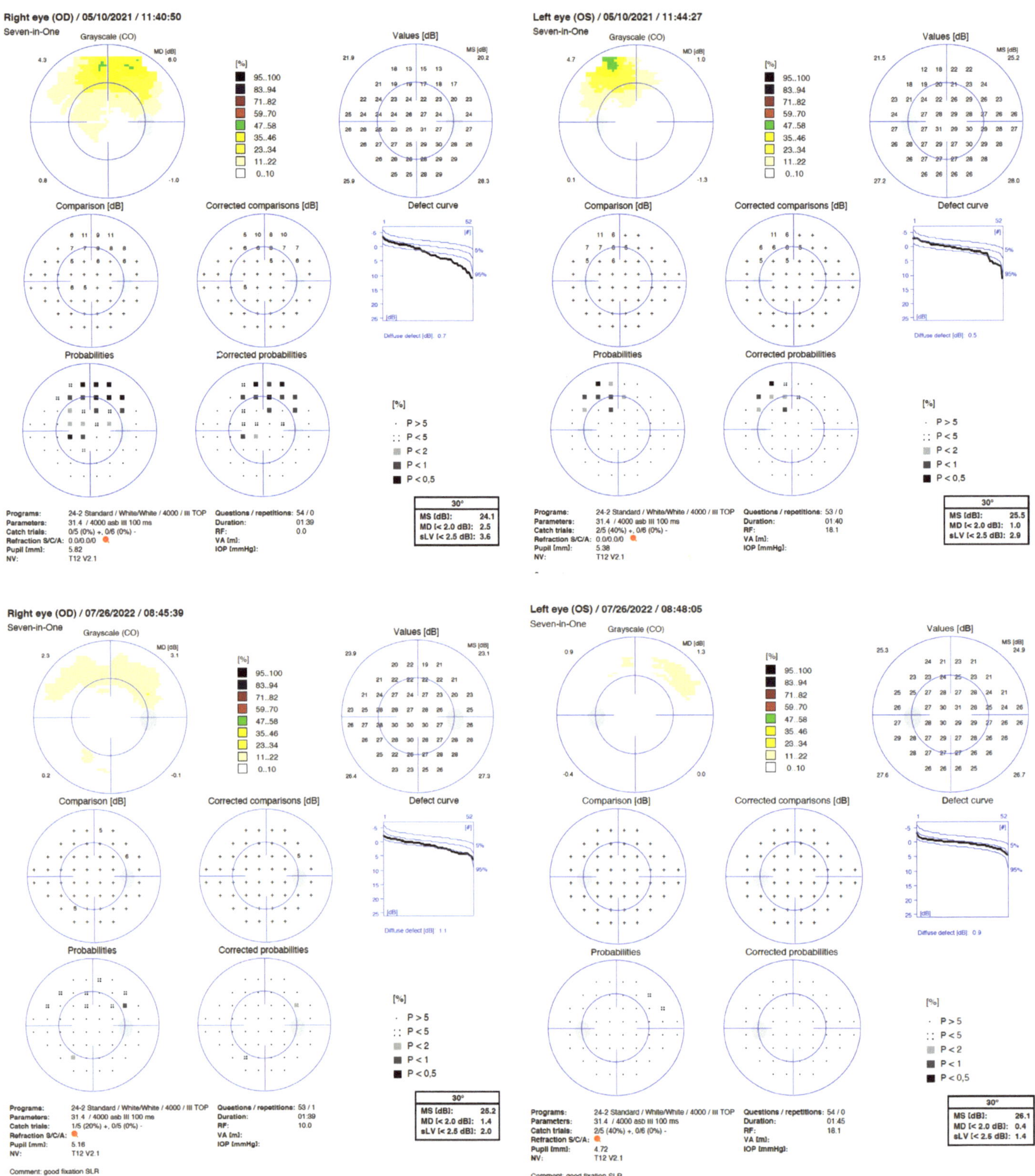

Fig. 72. Octopus (Haag-Streit, Mason, OH, USA) automated perimetry of the author, a 66 year old male with open angle glaucoma (top) May 2021 and (bottom) one day following his 20th session of panmacular SDM MRT as vision protection therapy in August 2022. Note improvement in arcuate visual field defects in both eyes indicating improved visual and retinal / optic nerve function with reversal of the disease process. VA 20/15 OU before and after SDM.

13. Analog Indications for Modern Retinal Laser Therapy: Extending the Treatment Concepts of the Iconic Chronic Progressive Retinopathies

You should take the approach that you're wrong. Your goal is to be less wrong.

—Elon Musk

Inherited retinal diseases (IRDs)

As with AMD, OAG, and DR, the goal of MRT in IRDs is to improve visual function and slow disease progression by improving retinal function and maintaining those improvements over time. IRDs vary widely in type and severity. Reset theory suggested that MRT should improve retinal and visual function in all IRDs, irrespective of cause. Subsequent retinal function testing by electrophysiology, and various types of visual function testing, has confirmed this to be the case (Luttrull and Margolis 2016, Luttrull 2018) (Figs. 16-23 and 73-81). Clinical experience finds that the half-life of MRT treatment effects is shorter in some IRDs than AMD and

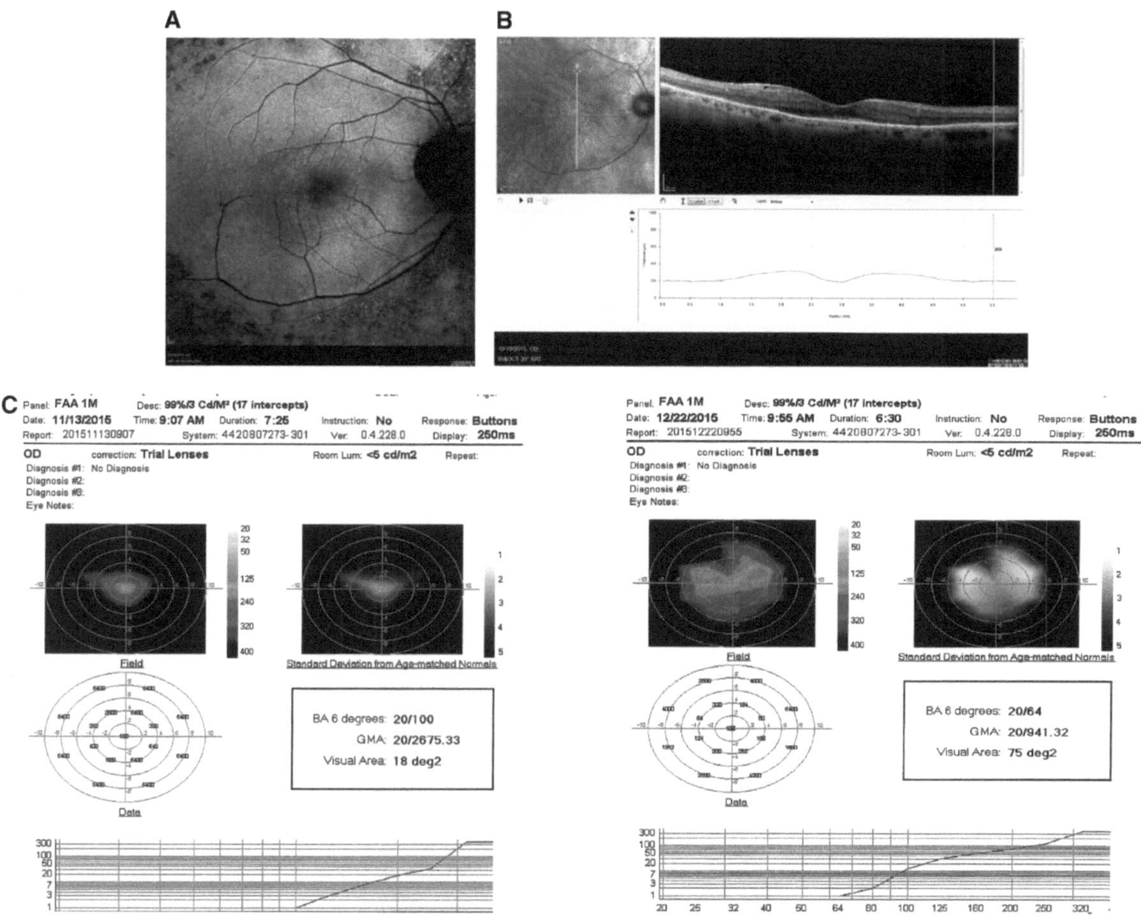

Fig. 73. (A) Fundus photograph of right eye 69-year-old man with retinitis pigmentosa on presentation, October 2015. (B) OCT at that time showing atrophy and loss of the RPE and photoreceptor layer outside the fovea. (C) ORP (Omnifield Resolution Perimetry) of the right eye on the same day before (left) and 1 month after (right) panmacular SDM. Note improvement in all indices with enlargement of the recordable visual area. SDM MRT as vision protection therapy Q6-8 weeks was begun. VA on presentation October 2015, 20/50 OD and 20/60 OS. VAs on most recent visit August 2022, 20/60 OD and 20/50 OS. BA6 = best logMAR visual acuity within 6° of fixation; GMA = global macular logMAR visual acuity. *From: Luttrull JK. Improved retinal and visual function following subthreshold diode micropulse laser (SDM) for retinitis pigmentosa. Eye (London) Feb 2018 PAP open access https://doi.org/10.1038/s41433-018-0017-3*

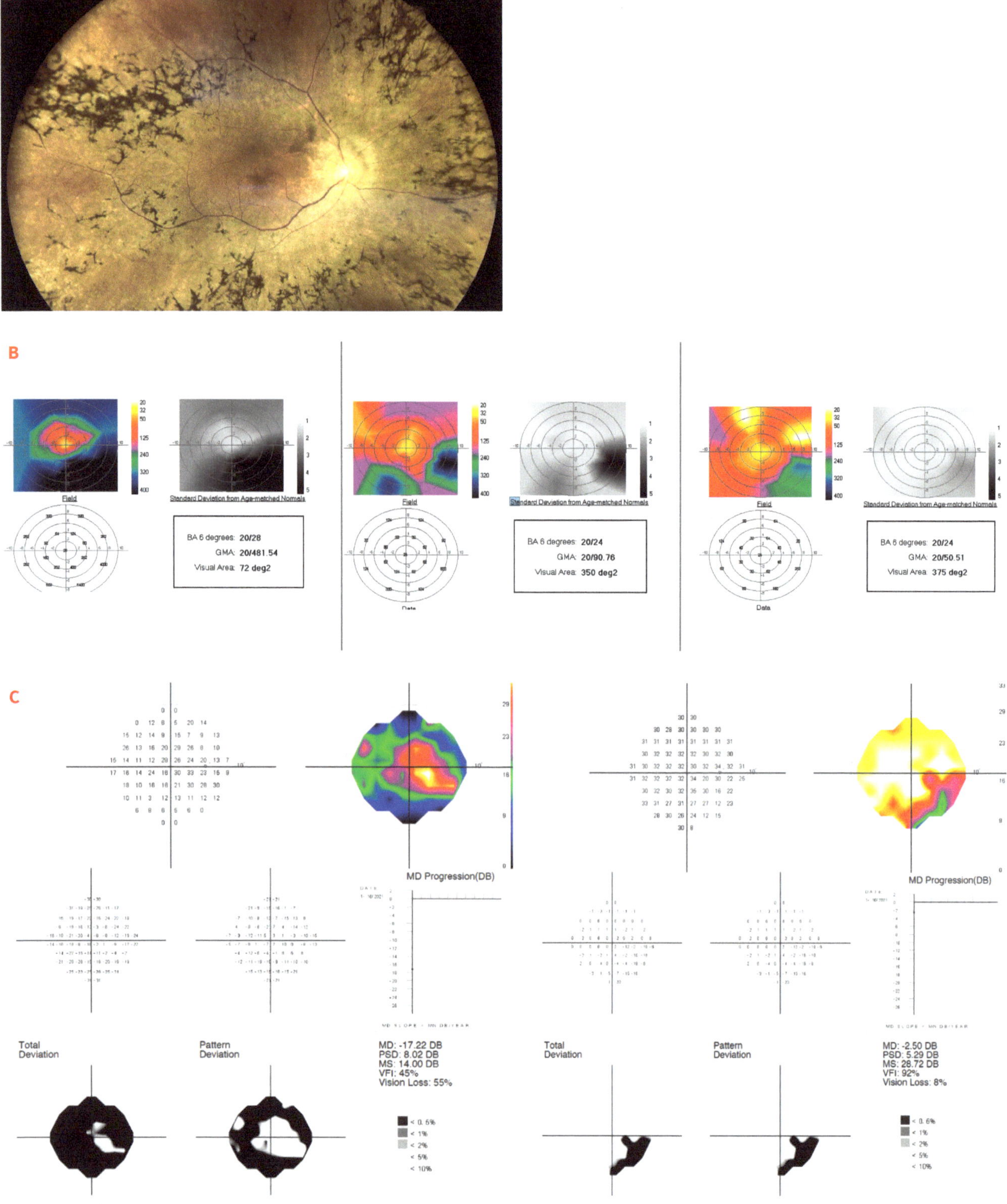

Fig. 74. (A) Fundus photo of the right eye of a 53 year old woman, carrier of X-linked retinitis pigmentosa, treated with vision protection therapy for 7 years in hopes of slowing disease progression. VA on presentation and at last visit both VA 20/30 OU. (B) Mesopic visual function on presentation (left), one month (middle) and two months after (right) first panmacular SDM treatment for visual protection in 2015. Note improved mesopic acuity and visual field post SDM treatment. (C) (Left) 10-2 automated perimetry of left eye in 2021 after no treatment for 4 months. (Right one) week after repeat panmacular SDM. Note function improved visual function after resumption of VPT.

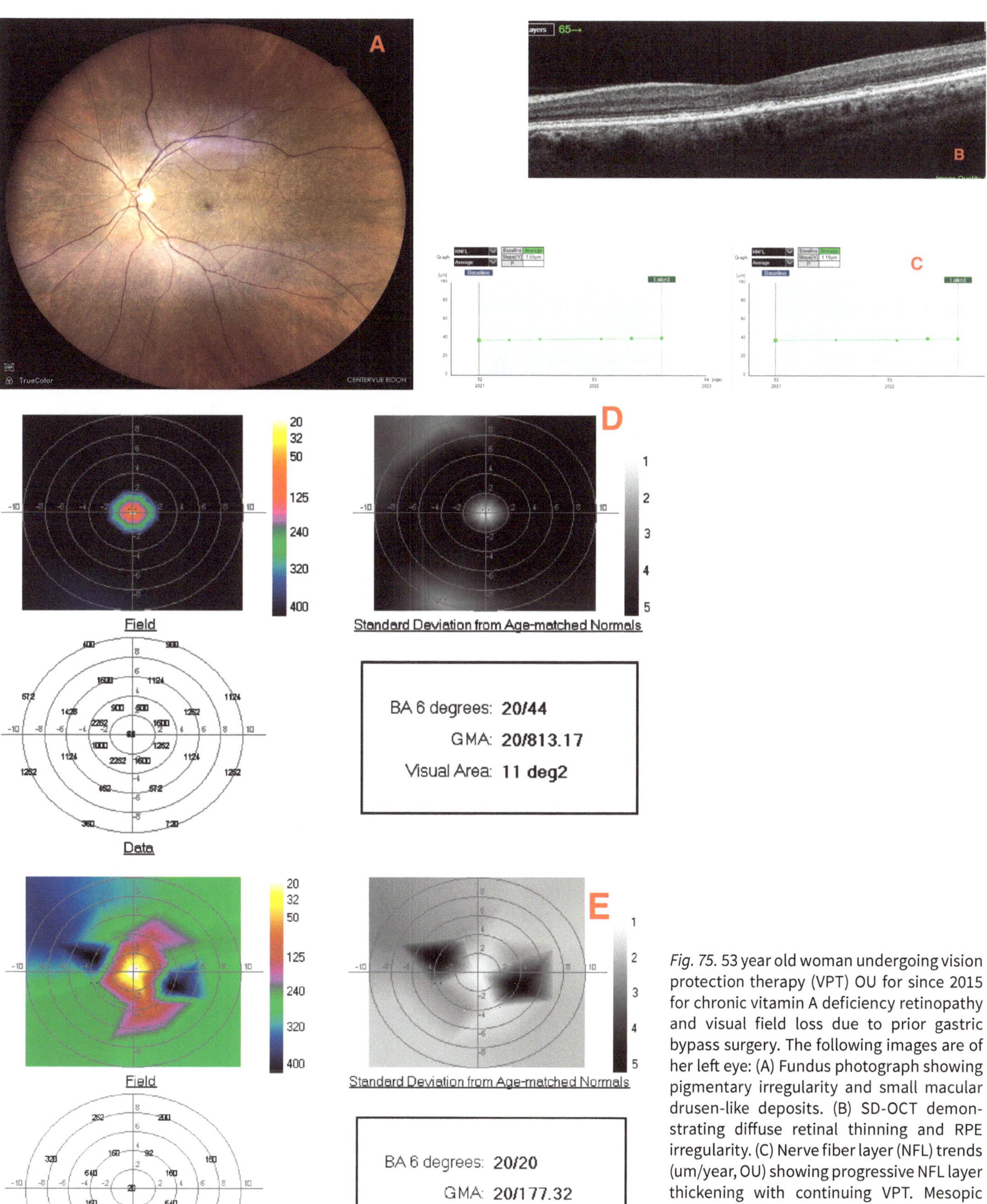

Fig. 75. 53 year old woman undergoing vision protection therapy (VPT) OU for since 2015 for chronic vitamin A deficiency retinopathy and visual field loss due to prior gastric bypass surgery. The following images are of her left eye: (A) Fundus photograph showing pigmentary irregularity and small macular drusen-like deposits. (B) SD-OCT demonstrating diffuse retinal thinning and RPE irregularity. (C) Nerve fiber layer (NFL) trends (um/year, OU) showing progressive NFL layer thickening with continuing VPT. Mesopic visual function (D) at presentation and (E) after first panmacular SDM MRT treatment. VA 20/20 OU at presentation in 2015, and on last visit August 2022.

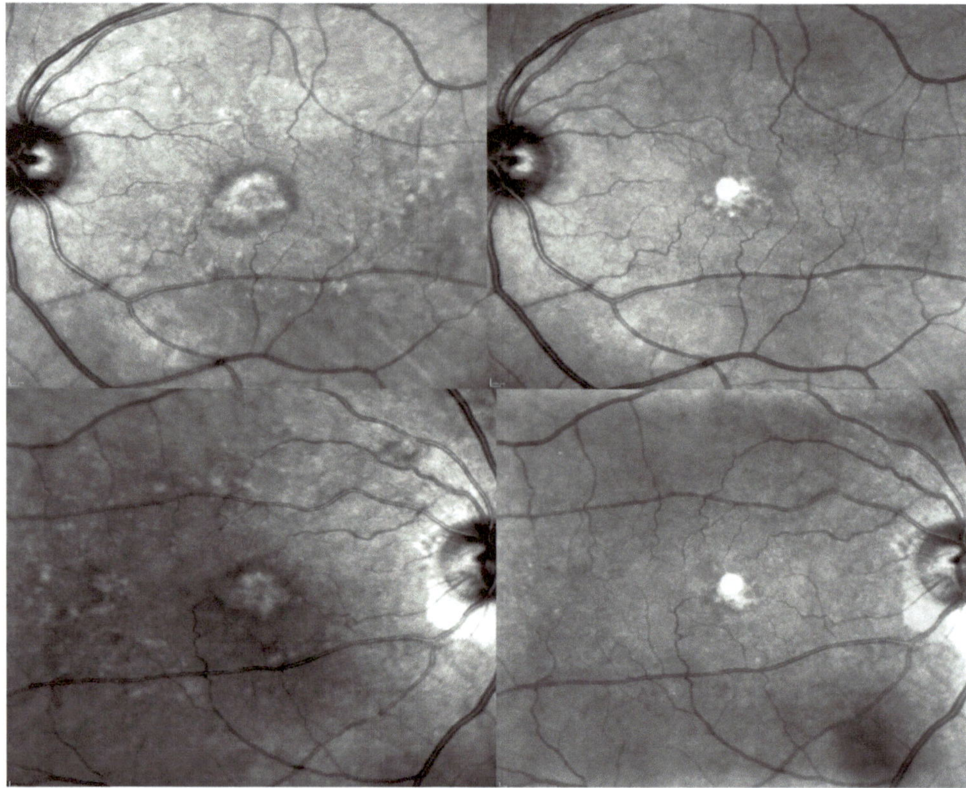

Fig. 76. 71 year old woman with pattern dystrophy of the retinal pigment epithelium and complaint of increasing difficulty in low light. Left, prior to panmacular SDM MRT. Right, 3 months after treatment. Note marked resolution of pigmentary abnormalities. VA 20/30 OD and 20/40 OS before and after treatment. Symptoms improved following treatment.

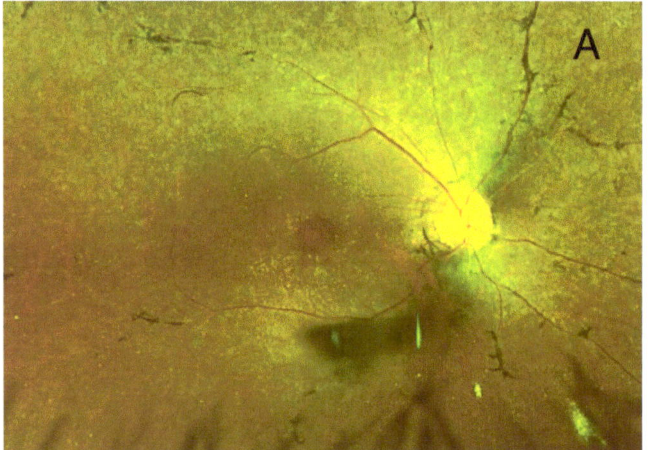

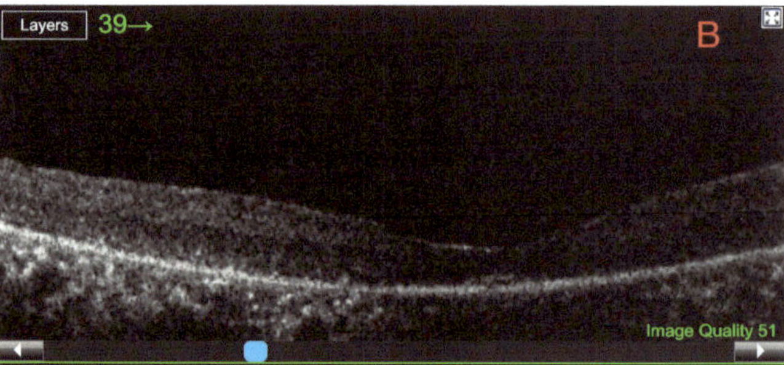

Fig. 77. 42 year old Hispanic woman presented with the complaint of progressive visual loss and disabling bright-light amaurosis and photophobia. VA 20/30 right eye and 20/200 left eye. There was no history of familial visual loss. (A) Fundus photograph of right eye showing appearance of retinitis pigmentosa. (B) SD-OCT of right eye showing retinal thinning and loss of RPE and PROS outside the fovea. Genetic testing revealed an OCA2 gene, associated with autosomal recessive oculocutaneous albinism. The patient elected to begin SDM MRT as vision protection therapy. After her first VPT treatment the patient reported resolution of bright-light amaurosis/photophobia and improved functional ability. VPT was continued.

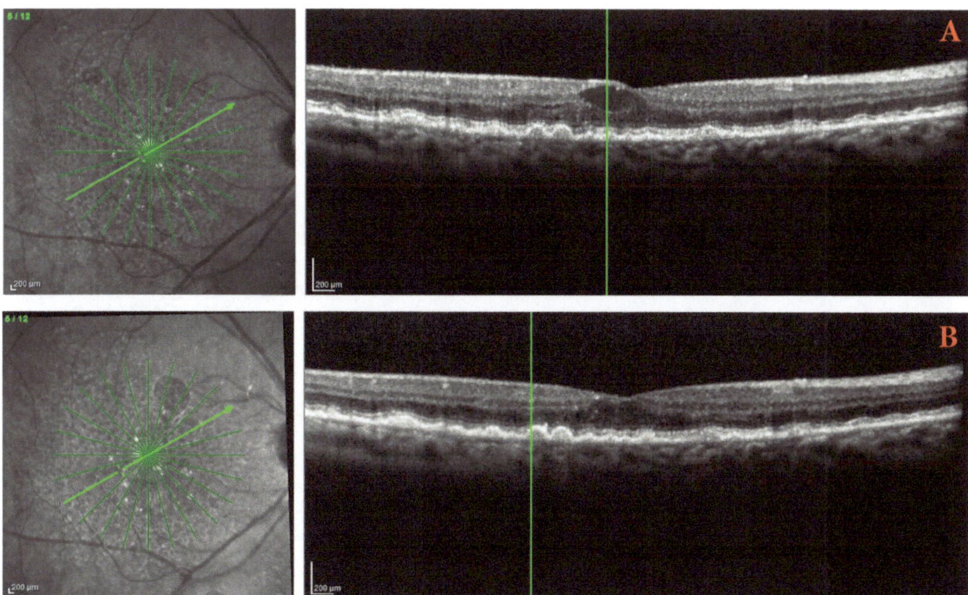

Fig. 78. 88 year old woman with intermediate AMD, reticular pseudodrusen, and type 2 idiopathic microvascular telangiectasis. (Top) OCT of right eye showing drusen, pseudodrusen, telangiectatic vessel and CME. VA 20/60. (Bottom) 6 months later, after two panmacular SDM sessions, CME has resolved. VA improved to 20/30.

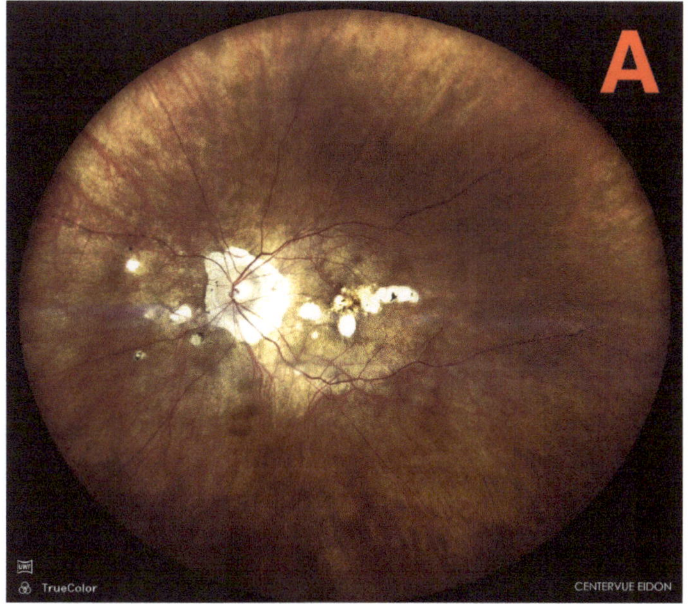
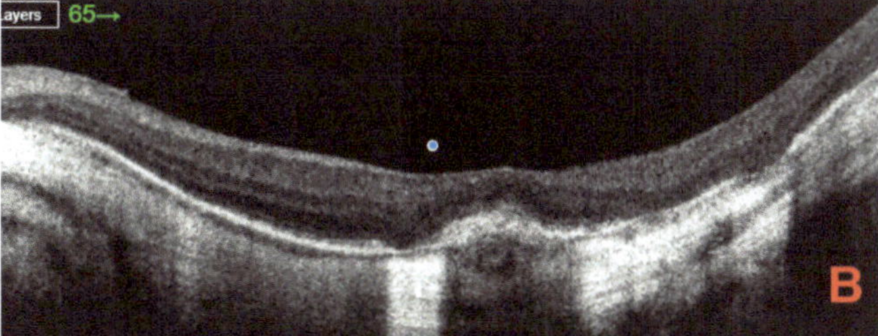

Fig. 79. Fundus photograph (A) of left eye August 2022 of a 53 year old woman with degenerative myopia and ocular histoplasmosis presenting in 2018 with visual loss and subfoveal choroidal neovascularization, VA 20/400. Anti-VEGF injections were begun along with SDM MRT as vision protection therapy to reduce the risk of recurrent exudation and attempt to slow progression of the geographic atrophy. After 3 injections, the last in August 2018, her VA was 20/400 and remained 20/400 until August 2019, when it began to gradually improve as VPT was continued. After 4 years of vision protection therapy her VA had improved to 20/30 OS. (B) SD-OCT of left eye at that time, August 2022, showing subfoveal fibrosis, myopic macular thinning, and parafoveal geographic atrophy.

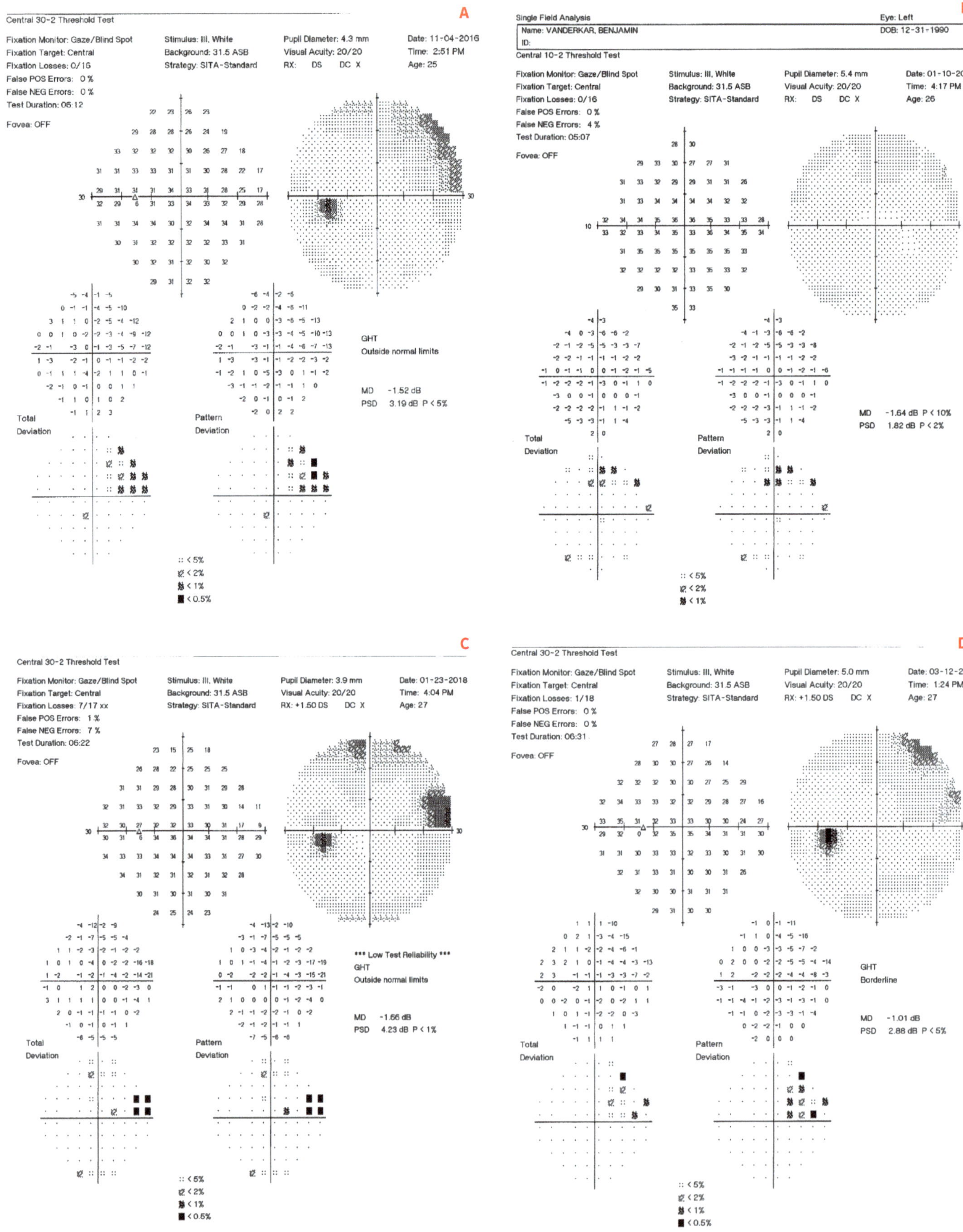

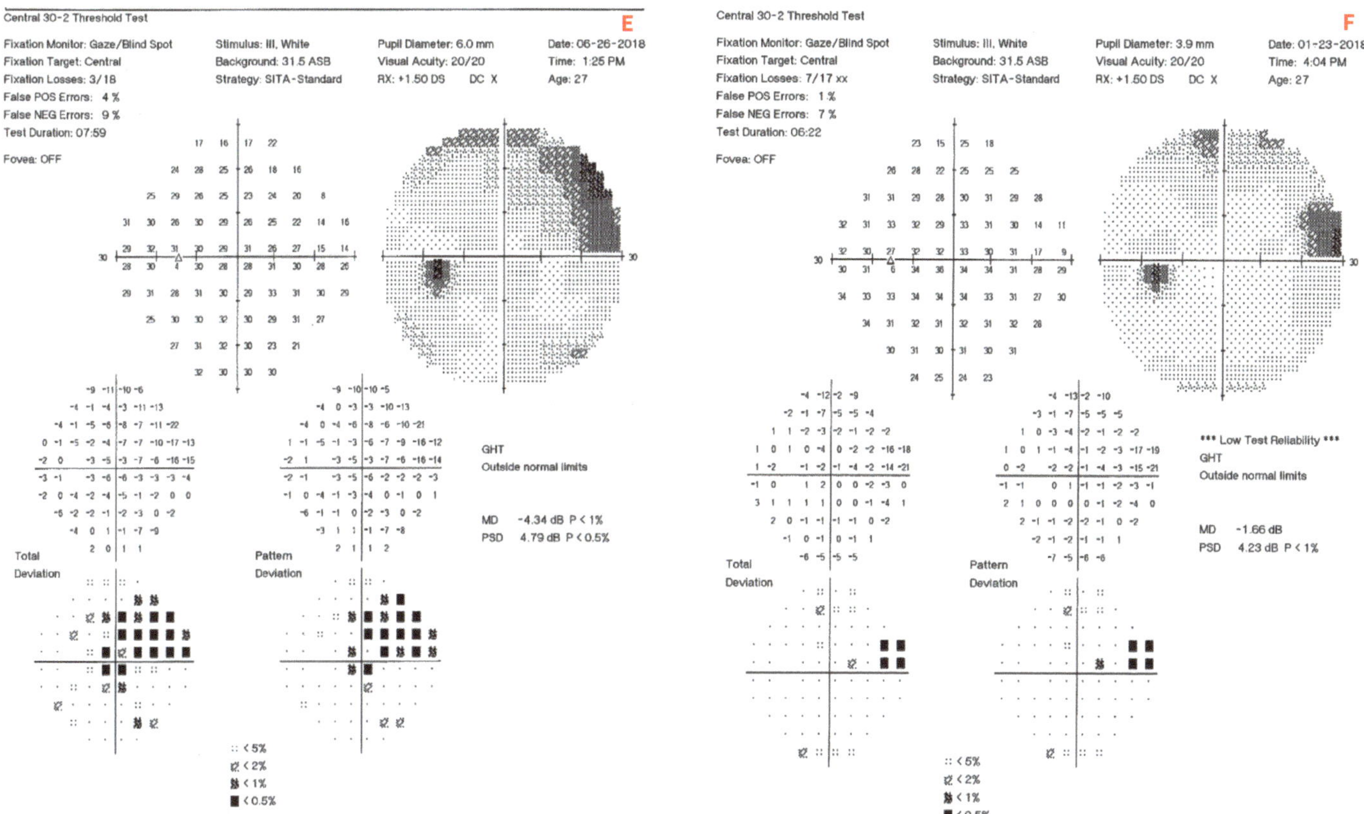

Fig. 80. SDM MRT used as provocative test: Because MRT has no effect on normal retina and normal retinal function, it can be used to detect retinal dysfunction. In this patient, SDM MRT was used for suspected Stargardt's disease in a 26 year old male with a family history of autosomal dominant Stargardt's disease. Asymptomatic with 20/15 VA uncorrected OU and a single small fleck-like lesion in the left eye. 10-2 automated perimetry (A) before and (B) one month after panmacular SDM MRT of the left eye. Note defects in left eye improved after MRT. (C) One year later 30-2 automated perimetry demonstrating recurrent defects in the left eye. (D) 6 weeks after repeat panmacular SDM MRT OS demonstrating improvement of the VF again in response to treatment. (E) Three months later, recurrent worsening of visual field. SDM MRT repeated. (F) Again, note recurrent VF improvement one month following retreatment with MRT.

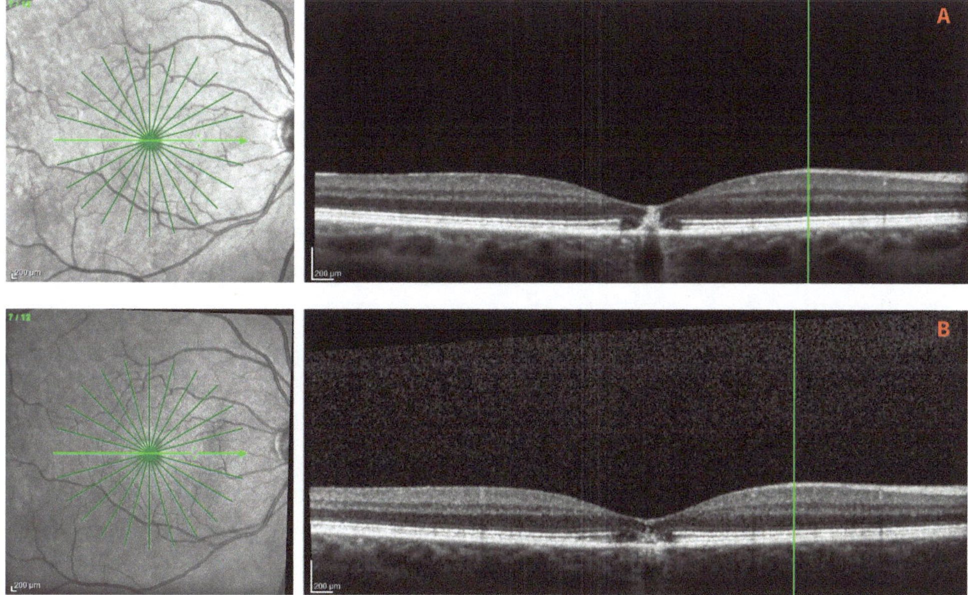

Fig. 81. 62 yo woman presenting with the complaint of blurred vision in her right eye due to adult pseudovitelliform foveal dystrophy. (Top) on presentation and (bottom) two years after starting SDM MRT VPT. VA had been diminished to 20/80 for two years. With VPT the VA gradually improved to 20/30 where it has remained with VPT for the past 5 years.

DR. This difference appears to simply reflect the greater disease severity and faster rates of progression, such as x-linked retinitis pigmentosa. Thus, MRT needs to be performed more frequently, as often as every 6 weeks, to maintain maximum treatment effects (Luttrull and Margolis 2016, Luttrull 2018, Luttrull and Kent 2019). At or about this time, patients often report waning of treatment-associated visual improvements and the perceived need for retreatment. By 3 to 4 months, retinal function testing will often return to the pretreatment baseline. Some have expressed concern about the possibility of retinal burns over pigment clumps and bone spicules common to RP (M. Marmor, personal communication 2016). This does not occur with SDM/MRT, which employs 810 nm. However, burns over pigment clumps may be a real concern with 577 nm and shorter wavelengths, even at a 5% DC, due to higher energies and higher pigment absorption (Chang and Luttrull 2020).

It is noteworthy that despite these MRT-elicited improvements in all disorders, including IRDs, MRT has no direct effect on the neurosensory retina or retinal photoreceptors, the primary disease locus in many IRDs, as longer wavelengths such as 810 nm have no uptake in the NSR. Instead, the improvements in retinal and visual function produced by MRT in all disorders, including primary photoreceptor disorders, indirectly in the NSR as the result of improved RPE function. In photoreceptor disorders, one factor contributing to RPE dysfunction may be due to the RPE being overtaxed by the increased demands of accelerated photoreceptor degeneration and death that may cause photoreceptor toiletry to decompensate and ultimately fail. Once the RPE ER UPR's ability to maintain proteostasis is sufficiently exhausted, apoptosis ensues. Survival and function of the NSR cannot survive failure and death of the underlying RPE. In this regard, the situation is not altogether different from other CPRs, where the stressors may instead be metabolic disease, or age. By improving RPE function with MRT, the ability of the RPE to continue to provide essential support to the neurosensory retina appears to improve, thus slow, and even temporarily reverse, disease progression measured by retinal and visual function testing. It is hoped that by maintaining these neuroprotective effects and neuroenhancement through regular periodic retreatment with MRT, visual loss may be avoided or significantly delayed

(Kolomyer and Zarbin 2014, Luttrull and Margolis 2016, Johnson et al 2022). Prospective study is necessary to confirm and further characterize long-term benefits of MRT in various IRDs. However, the robust results of SDM MRT in DR and AMD are encouraging in this regard. In the meantime, in the absence of adverse treatment effects or other effective therapies, it is difficult to argue against use of MRT to safely improve retinal and visual function in these relentlessly progressive and potentially blinding disorders in hopes of realizing long-term benefits.

Key point: MRT improves retinal and visual function in inherited retinopathies. The more severe, such as X-linked RP, the more frequently treatment is required to provide maximum treatment benefits if disease progression is to be slowed.

Central serous chorioretinopathy

Despite typically manifesting clinically as focal disease, CSR is a panchorioretinal disease that is typically bilateral and often associated with diffuse choroidal thickening ("pachychoroid") and diffuse RPE dysfunction (Spaide et al 2022). In this light, the approach to MRT treatment of CSR is the same as other CPRs, that of broad confluent geographic treatment, such as panmacular treatment, rather than focal or local treatment (Luttrull 2016) (Figs. 82-85). Review of the literature demonstrates the importance of applying MRT principles to the management of CSR, as the success of treatment of low-intensity laser treatment, sublethal to the RPE, parallels treatment area and density (Lanzetta et al 2008, Chen et al 2008, Roisman et al 2013, Malik et al 2015, Luttrull 2016, Gawęcki et al 2017, Battaglia-Parodi and Iacono 2018, Van Rijssen et al 2019, Luttrull AJO 2020). (See Chapter 5 "Treatment Density" for key discussion on the importance of treatment density and area for CSR treatment.) In acute, or "simple", CSR, MRT performed according to International Retinal Laser Society Guidelines typically results in complete resolution of subretinal fluid following MRT within 4 to 8 weeks (Luttrull 2016, Keunen et al 2020) (Fig. 83).

Subretinal fluid predominates in simple CSR and CME is rare, while "leaks" at the RPE are generally small and focal. While simple CSR is easily treated successfully, chronic, or "complex" CSR is generally more difficult. Chronic, or complex, CSR is usually characterized by minimal, poorly localized and ill-defined leakage. In complex CSR, CME predominates over subretinal fluid and is often seen alone, in the absence of subretinal fluid. RPE abnormalities in chronic/complex CSR are generally more widespread, indicating accumulated damage from chronic disease that is likely recurrent and often multifocal (Luttrull 2016, Spaide et al 2022). Whether the multifocality of complex chronic CSR is the result of multiple recurrences, or simply reflects more severe disease in general, is unclear. MRT in chronic complex CSR can also be highly effective. However, in contrast to simple CSR which generally resolves from a single treatment, treatment of complex CSR may need to be applied periodically as needed to suppress recurrent exudation (Luttrull 2016, 2020) (Figs. 82-85). Slowing of GA in AMD suggests that regular periodic treatment in complex CSR may also prevent or slow progression of secondary RPE damage often present in chronic CSR, and that may lead to irreversible visual loss from GA or CNV (Luttrull et al 2020). The safety of MRT makes it the logical first choice for treatment for either acute or chronic CSR, allowing complete treatment,

treatment of foveal leaks, prompt treatment, and safe retreatment for recurrences (Fig. 81). Because MRT is absent retinal damage, MRT is also effective and safe after failed photodynamic therapy or other prior treatments. With respect to the timing of MRT, while most cases of acute/simple CSR resolve spontaneously, several studies have shown that long-term visual and anatomical results are improved by prompt/early treatment to hasten resolution of SRF. It is important to remember that the traditional approach of deferred treatment of acute CSR was informed not only by the likelihood of eventual spontaneous resolution, but also the risks and adverse effects of RPC. The safety of MRT allows prompt treatment of CSR to hasten resolution, minimizing retinal damage and maximizing visual recovery and preservation without adverse effects (Luttrull 2016, Gawęcki et al CJM 2019 and BMC 2019).

Serous macular detachments associated with the dome-shaped macula that may occur in highly myopic eyes represent a subset of eyes with CSR-like disease that is especially resistant to any type of treatment. However, MPL has been reported to be effective in some of these eyes, often requiring multiple treatments over time. In light of the treatment safety of MRT and lack of

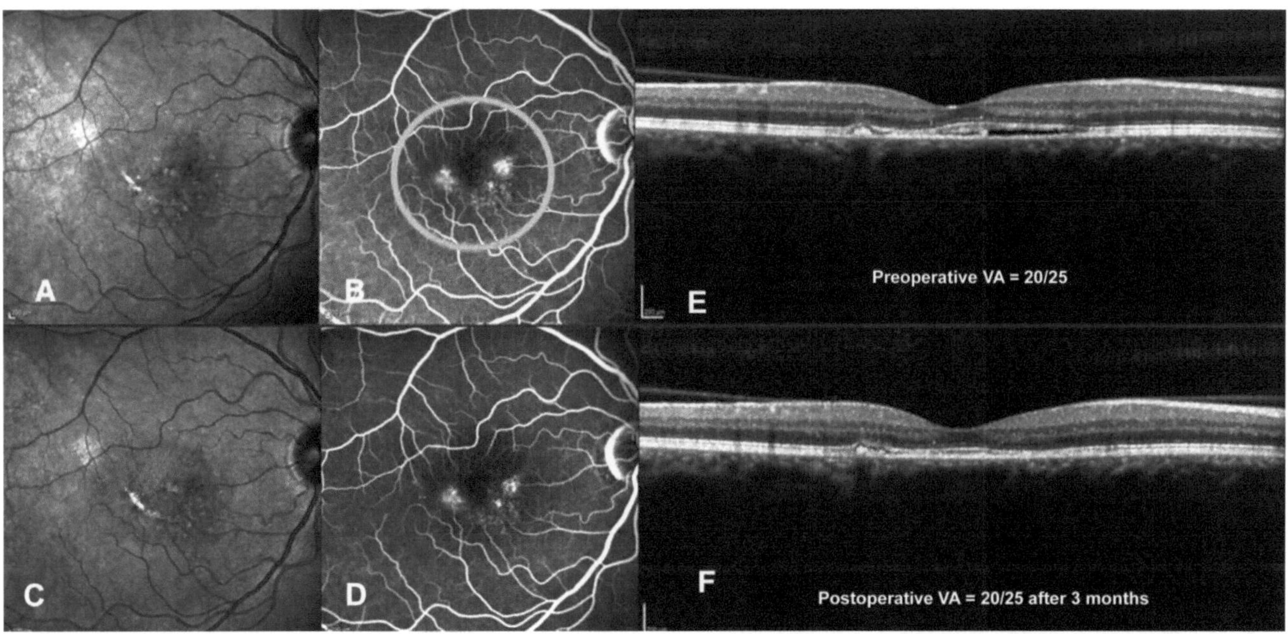

Fig. 82. Preoperative fundus photograph (A) and late-phase intravenous fundus fluorescein angiogram (B) of an eye with active CSR. The superimposed circle approximates the area of confluent SDM spot application at the time of treatment. (Panmacular treatment had not yet become the default for macular disease.) Postoperative fundus photograph (C) and late phase fundus fluorescein angiography (D). Note absence of leakage and absence of laser-induced retinal damage. Optical coherence tomograms of the same eye (E) before and (F) after SDM treatment. Note resolution of subretinal fluid and absence of laser-induced retinal damage. From: *Luttrull JK. Low-intensity / high-density subthreshold diode micropulse laser (SDM) for central serous chorioretinopathy. Retina. 2016 Sep; 36 (9):1658-63*

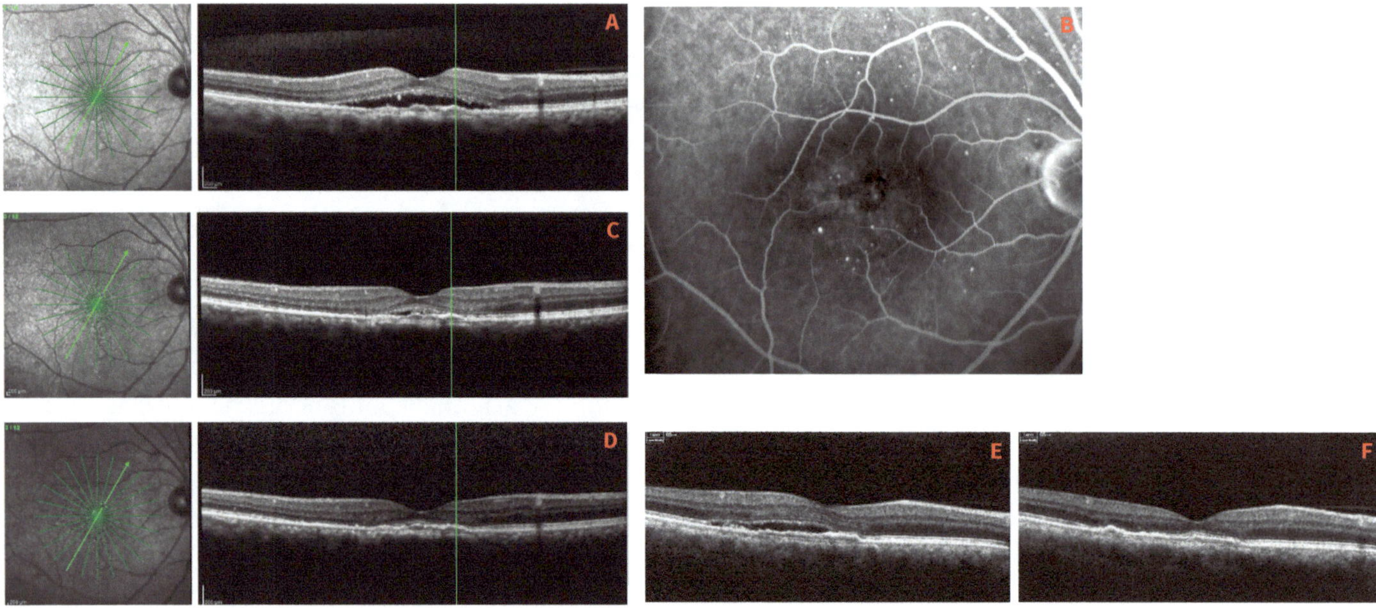

Fig. 83. 52 yo male with chronic central serous chorioretinopathy active and persistent in the right eye for 3 years without treatment. (A) OCT on presentation. (B) FFA on presentation showing absence of defined leakage. VA 20/50. Panmacular SDM MRT was performed. (C) One month after initial SDM. Note reduction in subretinal fluid. VA 20/30. (D) 5 months following initial treatment, including retreatment 3 months after initial treatment, showing further improvement. VA 20/30. (E) Two years following presentation with recurrent subretinal fluid. VA 20/40. (F) One month following retreatment with resolution of subretinal fluid. VA 20/30.

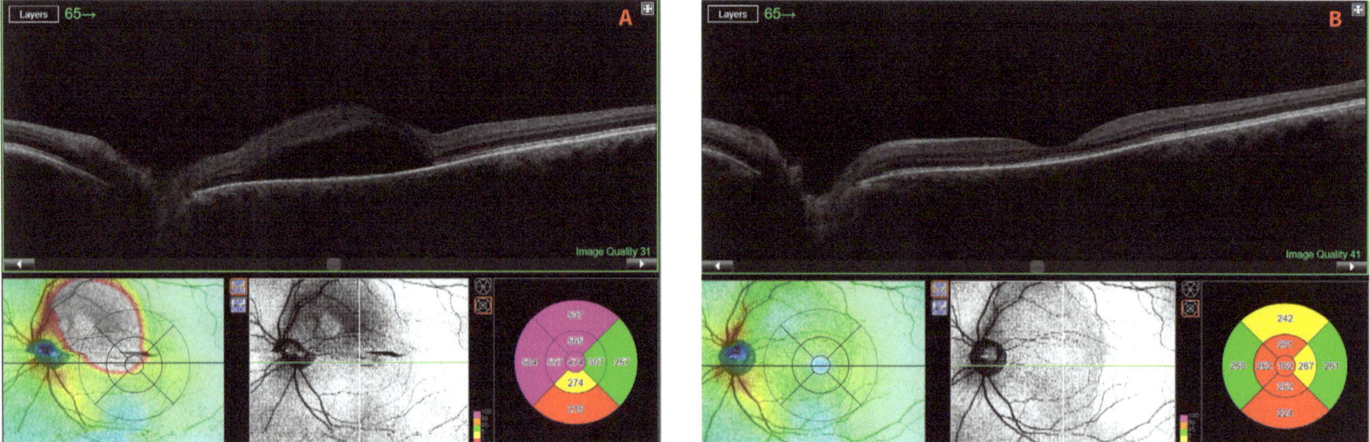

Fig. 84. SDM 38 year old male with a history of multiply recurrent central serous chorioretinopathy for 10 years in his right eye, treated with panmacular SDM for recurrences June and November 2018 with resolution of subretinal fluid on each episode. Top OCT shows another episode of recurrent exudation May 2022. VA 20/100. Bottom OCT shows complete resolution of subretinal fluid one month later. VA 20/30.

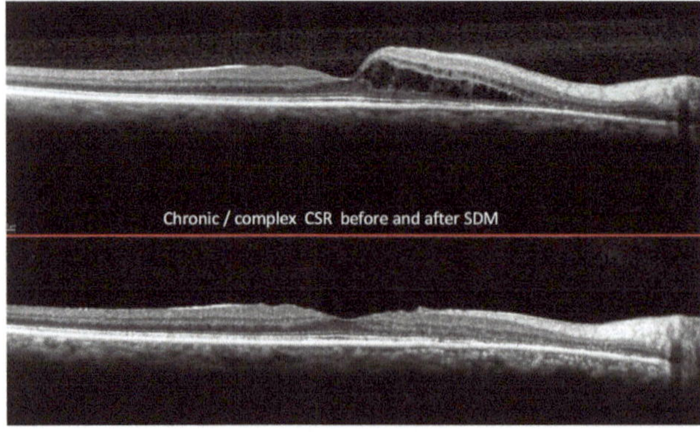

Fig. 85. 73 yo male with chronic / recurrent CSR OU characterized by chronic recurrent CME and secondary pigmentary disturbance over a 40 year period. OCT shows recurrent CME (top) resolved following panmacular SDM MRT (bottom). VA 20/30 before and after treatment.

other clearly effective treatments, MRT is a reasonable first-line approach in these eyes (Minowa 2021).

Treatment failure with MRT for CSR is sufficiently rare that it should alert one to the possibility of misdiagnosis, the most common being posterior polypoidal choroidopathy (PPCV) or primary or secondary CNV. If uncertain, anti-VEGF injection is a useful provocative test as CSR does not respond to VEGF inhibitors, while PPCV and CNV generally do.

Key point: MRT is highly effective for both acute (simple) and chronic (complex) CSR. Treatment failure is usually due to misdiagnosis or inadequate treatment due to insufficient treatment area and density.

Nondiabetic retinovascular disease

Retinal vein occlusion

Over 20 years of clinical experience have shown that retinal vein occlusions (RVO) represent the least gratifying of all conventional indications for MRT, as it had been for PC before it (Luttrull and Spink 1997, Parodi et al 2006, Eng and Leng 2020, Heyreh 2021). This appears attributable to the pathophysiology of disease, which, rather than like the chronic progressive retinopathies for which MRT is highly effective, is instead an acute and often catastrophic failure of inner retinal blood flow and oxygenation. In this setting, the generally poor response to laser treatment indicates that the target

RPE has a limited influence on the disease process. If the ischemic damage is sufficient, the retinal microvasculature may become irreversibly damaged with loss of retinal perfusion and retinal ischemia. In the absence of ischemia, varying degrees of microvascular incompetence often develop resulting in macular edema. If the swelling is sufficiently severe and chronic, microvascular damage may develop which is unresponsive to any intervention. In these cases, secondary pigmentary degeneration and atrophy may develop contributing to visual loss and further reducing the potential for recovery (Heyreh 2021). Optimal management of ME due to RVO currently requires early and continued long-term intravitreal drug therapy. This is not to say that there is no role for MRT in RVO, however. Several studies have shown that the combination of laser and drug therapy can reduce the number of intravitreal injections required, and this in itself is a benefit (Parodi et al 2008, Terashima et al 2019). In milder cases, MRT alone may be sufficient. Ischemic RVOs with retinal or disc neovascularization and vitreous hemorrhage can be managed effectively with MRT to the areas of ischemia, precluding the need for intravitreal injections or retinal ablation, analogously to PDR. MRT may also be of value to attempt to prevent or slow secondary pigment atrophy arising from chronic recurrent ME, analogous to the slowing of ARGA by MRT (Luttrull et al 2020). Perhaps the greatest value of MRT in RVO is to maintain and preserve maximal macular health and function despite the chronic / recurrent ME to improve the long-term visual prognosis (Figs. 86-88).

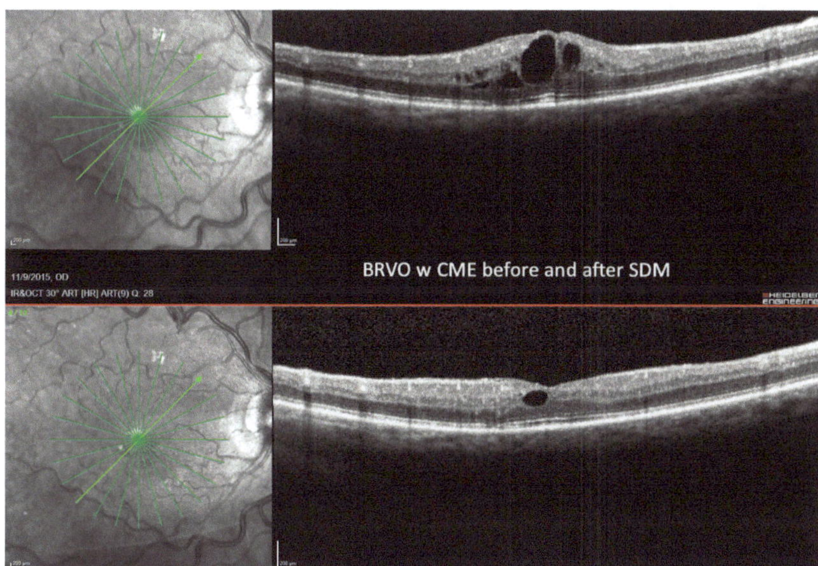

Fig. 86. Eye with macular edema due to BRVO (impending CRVO) before (top) and after (bottom) panmacular SDM MRT. Note substantial resolution of the macular edema after SDM.

SDM for Lucentis non-response

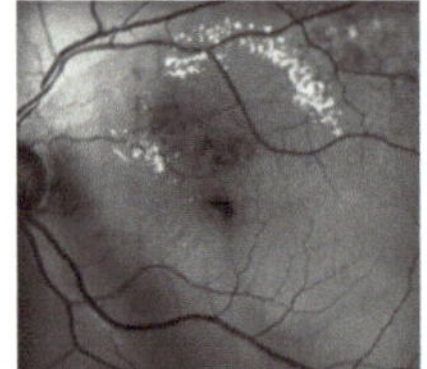

Red-free photo: BRVO
1 month post Lucentis

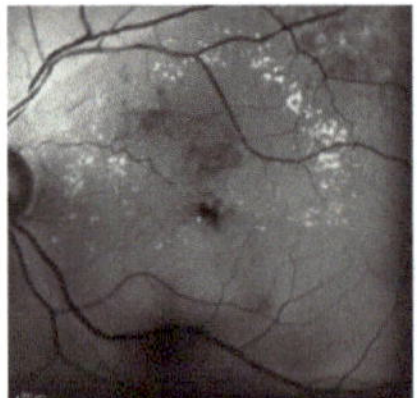

Red-free photo: BRVO
7 months post SDM

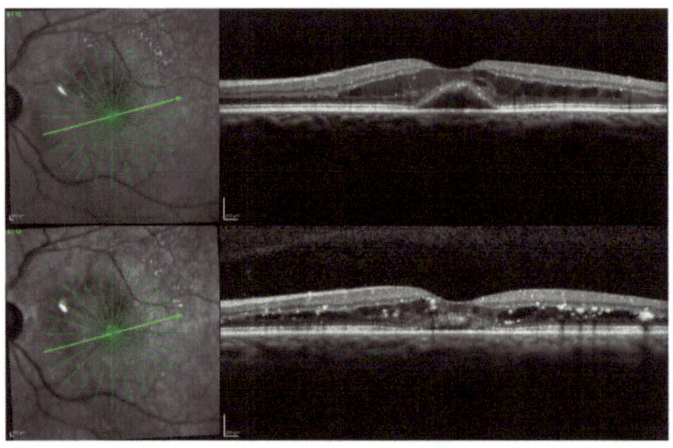

Top: SD-OCT 1 month post Lucentis. CFT 390 µm, VA 20/50-.
Unimproved. SDM performed.

Bottom: 7 months* post SDM. CFT 282 µm, VA 20/40+.
***Progressive improvement in ME from 6 weeks** post SDM by
SD-OCT.

Fig. 87. Eye with macular edema and serous macular detachment due to BRVO unresponsive to bevacizumab and ranibizumab injections, improved following panmacular SDM MRT. The presence of a serous macular detachment associated with macular edema is highly suggestive of a significant inflammatory component to the macular swelling. Often, such eyes do not respond well to anti-VEGF medications, but can respond well to MRT, which is anti-inflammatory.

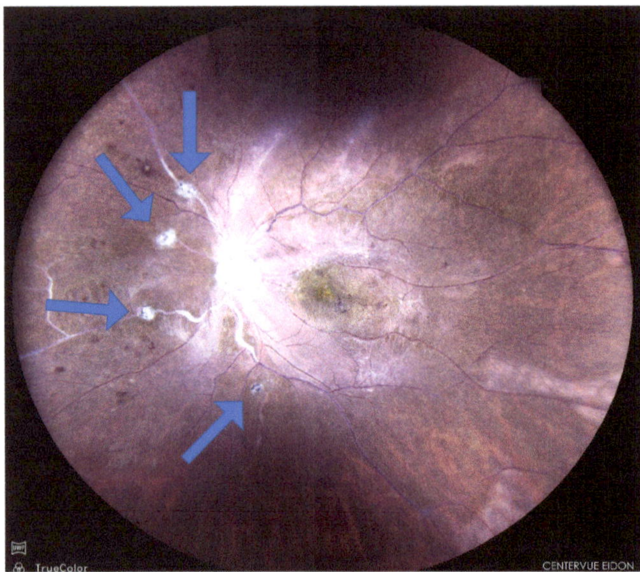

Fig. 88. Fundus photograph of left eye of 67 yo Asian male with a central retinal vein occlusion, macular edema, and epiretinal membrane. Treated with periodic panmacular SDM MRT, anti-VEGF and intravitreal dexamethasone implants since 2018 with VA 20/80. June 2020 the patient underwent pars plana vitrectomy with multiple transvenous chorioretinotomies (arrows) to create chorioretinal anastomoses for successful bypass of the CRVO, along with macular epiretinal membrane peeling. Postoperatively, periodic panmacular SDM was continued with decreased frequency of intravitreal dexamethasone injections and elimination of anti-VEGF injections. June 2022 VA 20/40. This case illustrates that continuing SDM MRT may help reduce the need for intravitreal injections, complement any other intervention including drugs and/or surgery, and help preserve macular and visual function in the face of chronic / recurrent disease such as fluctuating CME associated with an RVO.

Key point: MRT is generally ineffective as monotherapy for RVO except for NV, or mild cases of ME. However, along with drug therapy MRT can reduce the injection burden in eyes with ME and help maximize and preserve retinal and visual function

Retinal artery occlusion

The fundamentally neuroprotective nature of MRT suggests a possible role in limiting visual loss from retinal arterial occlusions (RAO) (Luttrull and Kent 2019). Logic would suggest that earlier treatment in the acute phase of the occlusion should be more effective than later treatment. In some cases, scotoma size and density can be reduced by MRT in branch retinal artery occlusion (BRAO) even long after the occlusion. Such improvements are generally short lived, weeks to months, but can be renewed by retreatment if the patient finds the improvements from treatment helpful and elects to continue treatment (Fig. 89).

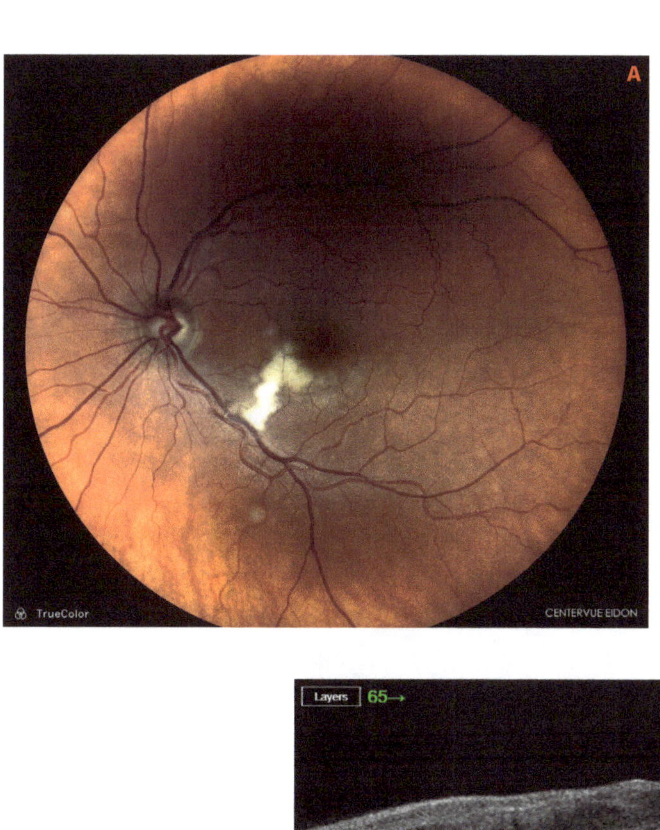

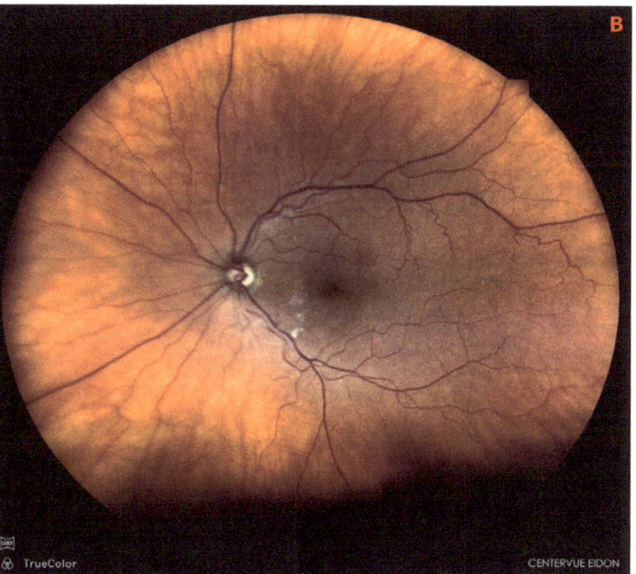

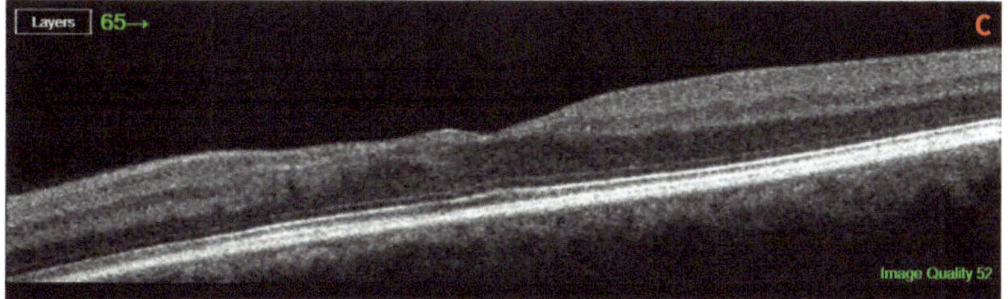

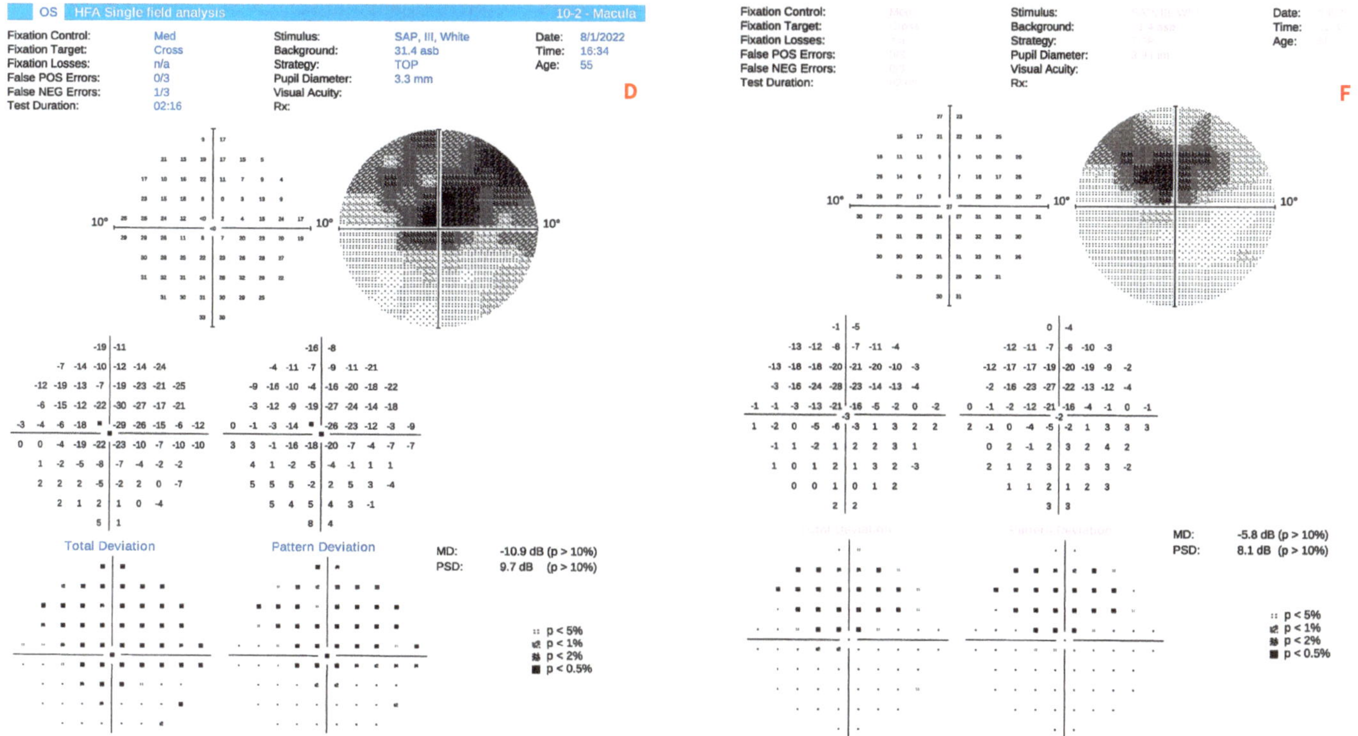

Fig. 89. (A) Fundus photograph of left eye of 54 year old male complaining of a central scotoma in his left eye 2 weeks following thoracic trauma. Note Purtcher's retinopathy. VA 20/70 (B) 8 weeks later, fundus photograph shows resolution of the retinal infarcts. (C) OCT reveals retinal atrophy in areas previously infarcted. VA 20/50-. (D) Octopus 10-2 automated perimetry showing scotoma associated with retinal infarcts on the same day as the upper right fundus photograph, after resolution of the acute retinal infarct. . Panmacular SDM MRT performed. (E) Octopus 10-2 one week following SDM MRT. Note reduced size and density of the scotoma.

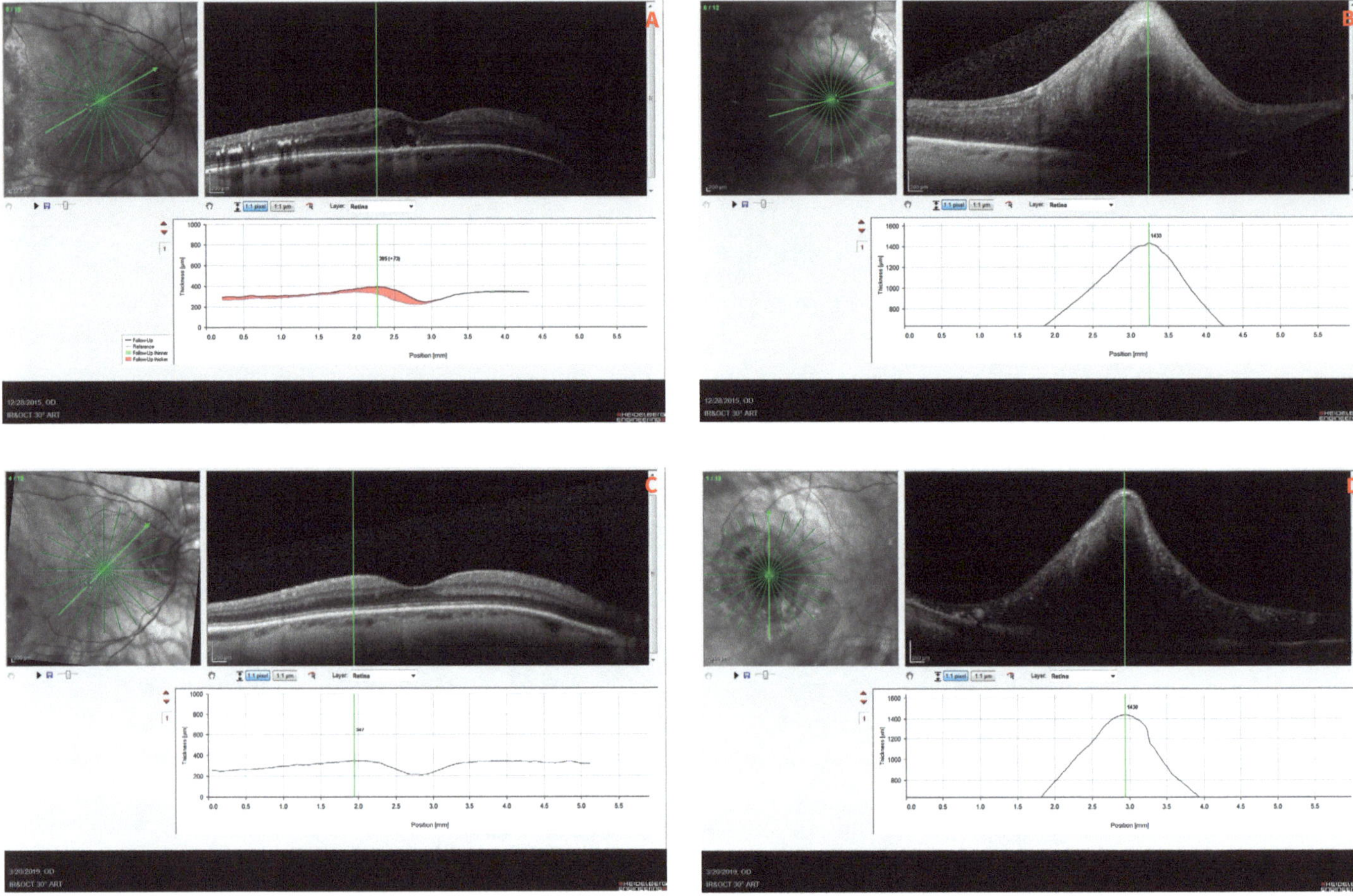

Fig. 90. OCTs of right eye of an 81 year old woman with macular edema due to an acquired retinal hemangioma before (A and B), and 4 months after a single treatment session of SDM MRT (C and D). Note resolution of CME and reduction in lesion height. VA improved from 20/30 to 20/25. Exudation from the lesion did not recur in 6 years of post-treatment observation.

The following case suggests MRT might be of benefit in rare cases of central retinal artery occlusion (CRAO) as well: An 85-year-old Caucasian male presented with a history of sudden visual loss 6 weeks previously in his left eye. The VA had not improved since onset. Examination found a VA in the left eye of finger-counting, and a CRAO with pale retina and a markedly delayed arterial perfusion by FFA. Panmacular SDM was performed for neuroprotection. One month later, the VA had improved to 20/200. SDM was repeated. One month later, the VA had improved to 20/30 and remained 20/30 until last seen 3 months later, 5 months after initial SDM treatment. While clearly anecdotal, the time course and unusually good outcome of this case suggests neuroprotection elicited by MRT may have played a role in this patient's remarkable visual recovery. Thus, in the absence of other effective therapies and in light of the devastating visual loss that often results from CRAO, MRT for neuroprotection in the acute phases of the occlusion may be worth considering.

Acquired retinal vascular lesions

Lesions such as capillary hemangiomas and smaller areas of Coat's disease, may be responsive to MRT, suggesting MRT as a reasonable first-line retina-sparing approach to treatment. As with every MRT indication, the lack of treatment associated tissue damage and inflammation may reduce adverse treatment effects and visual loss that can result from acutely increased exudation, fibrosis, tissue contraction, and bleeding that may occur from such lesions after conventional RPC. The effects of MRT in these settings are often long-lasting, avoiding or minimizing the treatment burden often imposed by intravitreal drug therapy (Fig. 90).

Macular scarring

Post-photocoagulation (PC) / post-inflammatory macular scarring and non-age-related geographic atrophy
Macular damage from macular PC leads to eventual visual loss in as many as 60% of eyes treated for DME

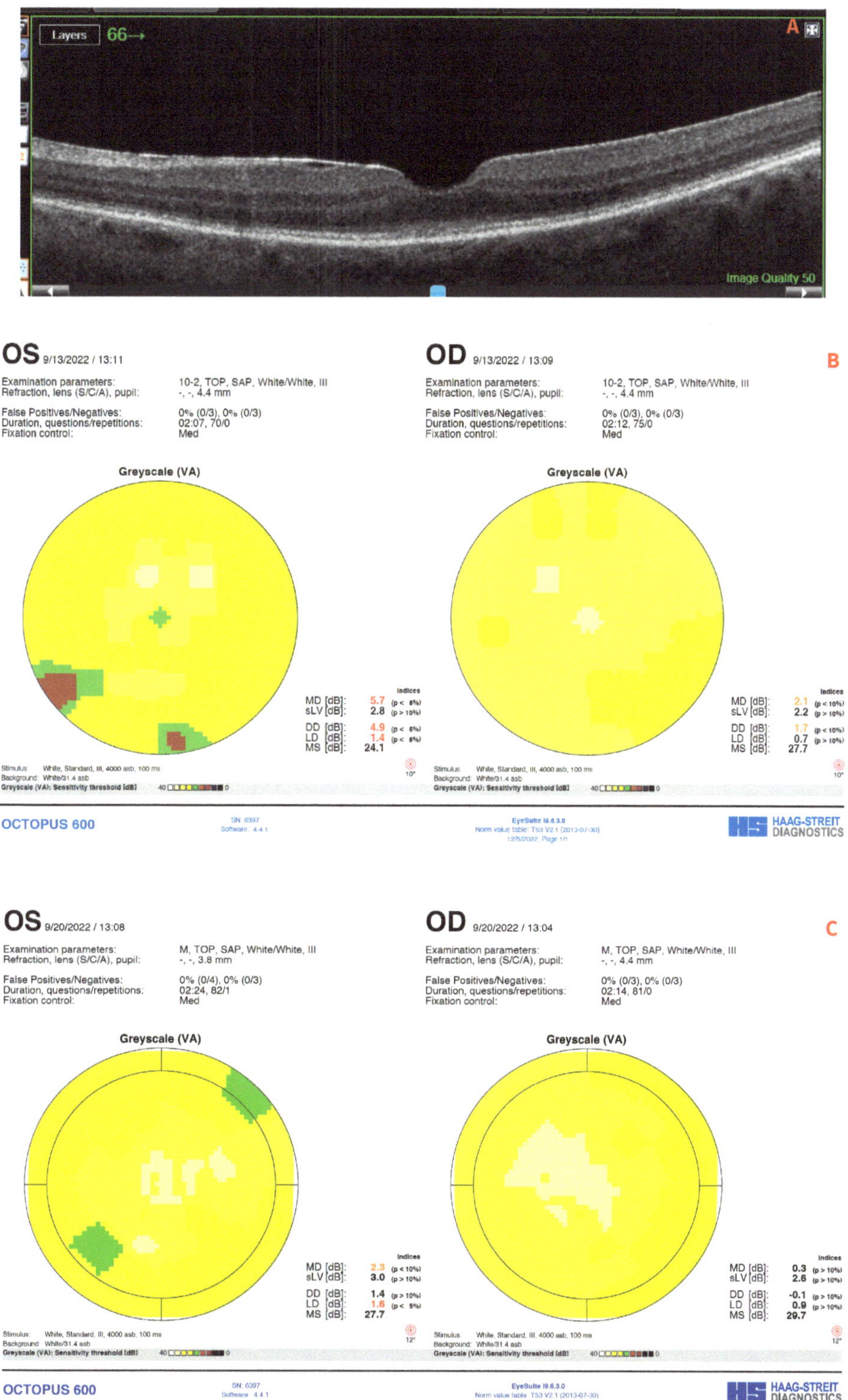

Fig. 91. Fundus photographs, OCTs, and automated perimetry of 61 year-old diagnostic radiologist with a history multiple evanescent white-dot syndrome (MEWDS) in OS>OD in 2019. He presented January 2021 with the complaint of poor night vision and a central scotoma in his left eye since MEWDS . VA 20/20 OD and 20/30 OS. Clinical exam showed a minimal pigment disturbance in fovea and mild epiretinal membrane. OCT showed disruption of the outer retinal layers and RPE beneath the fovea. SDM MRT was performed after which he reported improved night vision and diminution of central scotoma OS. He elected to continue regular periodic SDM MRT Q 4 months as VPT. During VPT he noted continued symptomatic improvement, with occasional recurrence of symptoms a few months after treatment, improvable by retreatment. (A) Fundus photograph and (B) OCT 18 months later, unchanged from presentation. (C) 10-2 automated perimetry before and (D) 1 week after most recent VPT treatment September 2022 showing reversal of recurrent scotoma OS following treatment. VA unchanged at 20/20 OD and 20/30 OS.

(ETDRS 1985, Morgan and Schatz 1989, Mainster 1999, Blumenkranz 2014, Jampol 2014) (Figs. 2-4, and 11). Most commonly this is due to gradual enlargement of these atrophic laser lesions into the fovea; and less often due to the development of secondary choroidal neovascularization (CNV) arising via laser damage to the Bruch's membrane/RPE barrier. The robust results of MRT for AMD suggest that MRT may be useful in reducing the risks of late visual loss in eyes with photocoagulation scars, from both scar progression and the risk of CNV (Luttrull, Sinclair et al 2018, 2020, Luttrull CO 2020, Luttrull and Gray 2022). In the same way, focal retinal scarring, progressive pigment atrophy, and/or secondary CNV in the macula associated with high or degenerative myopia, ocular histoplasmosis, retinal inflammation or infections, or other chorioretinopathies may also potentially benefit from regular periodic MRT as VPT in an attempt to limit progression of pigment atrophy, reduce the risk of secondary CNV, reduce the injection burden if already neovascular, improve VA, reduce associated scotomata or visual field loss, and improve mesopic and/or scotopic visual function (Figs. 79 and 91) (Ohno-Matsui et al 2018).

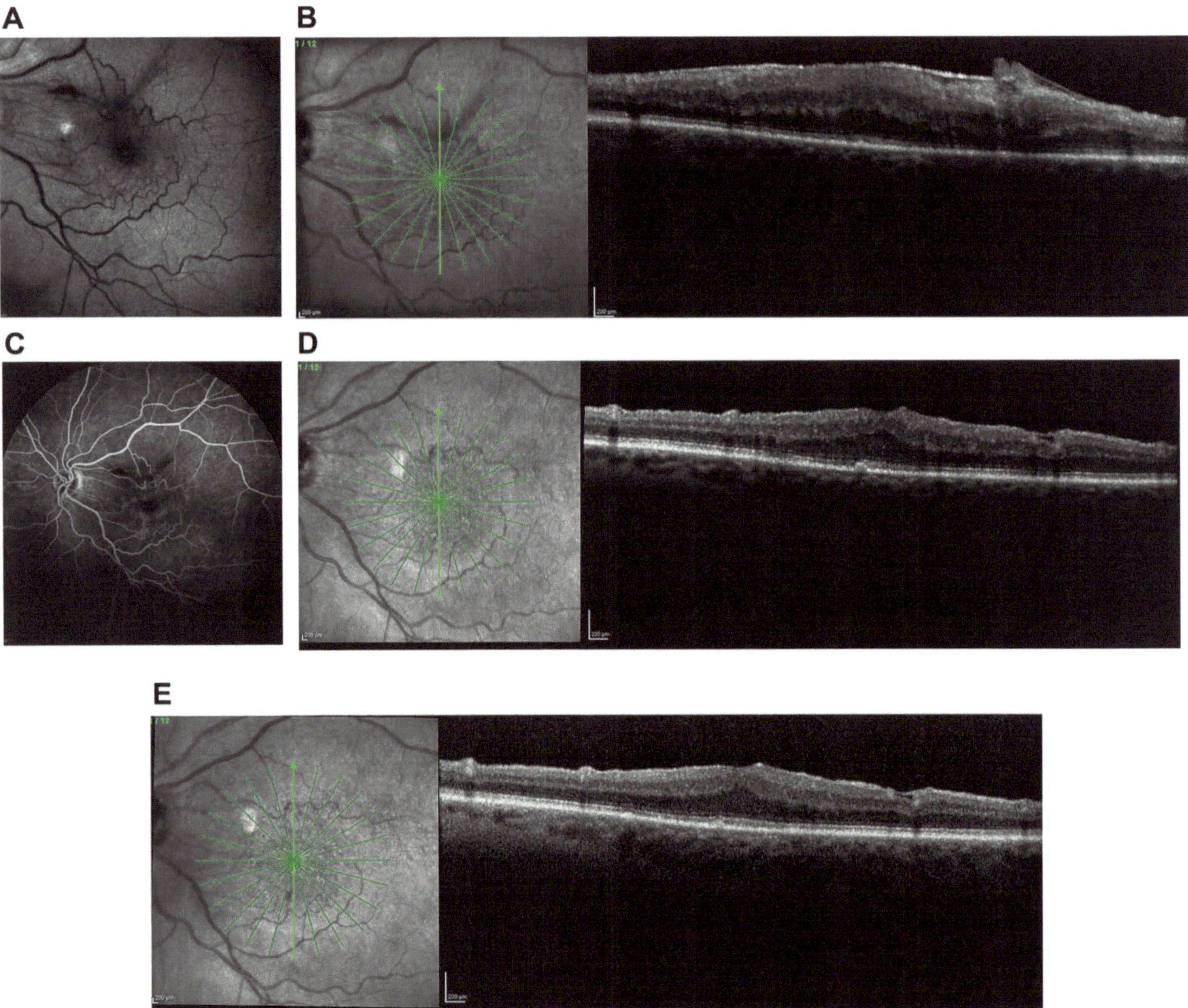

Fig. 92. F(A) Fundus photograph of a left eye with epiretinal membrane. Visual acuity = 20/400. (B) OCT of the same eye on the same date. Note marked macular thickening. (C) Late-phase intravenous fundus fluorescein angiogram of the same date. Note the paucity of angiographic leakage in the macula. (D) OCT of the same eye 13 months after membrane peeling. Note persistent macular thickening. Visual acuity = 20/200. SDM performed. (E) OCT 11 months after SDM. Note the reduction in macular thickening. Visual acuity improved to 20/30. From: *Luttrull JK. Subthreshold diode micropulse laser (SDM) for persistent macular thickening and limited visual acuity after epiretinal membrane peeling. Clin Ophthalmol, April 2020: 14; 1177-1188*

By repeatedly eliciting improvements in retinal and visual function in eyes with macular damage from various causes it is hoped and expected that progression of the macular damage, generally featuring RPE atrophy that tends to worsen with time, can be slowed or stopped and visual function maintained or improved.

Key point: If it looks like AMD, it may benefit from MRT in the same ways AMD does

Tractional maculopathies

Tractional disorders of the macula, such as vitreomacular traction, epiretinal membranes (ERM) and macular holes (MH) can be thought of as forms of macular injury leading to chronic macular dysfunction. Thus, these conditions may be amenable to MRT (Luttrull CO 2020). Typically, ERMs disturb macular function by exerting tangential, and less often anteroposterior, retinal traction. Often, this leads to macular thickening which is typically solid rather than cystic. Leakage on FFA may be absent, likely accounting for the fact that this type of tractional macular thickening is usually unresponsive to medicine. This thickening and dysfunction may persist after membrane peeling and limit VA improvement. If sufficiently chronic, secondary RPE damage may develop which can cause further progressive visual loss. MRT can improve both VA, further reduce macular thickening, and inhibit RPE atrophy in such eyes.

ERMs with significant visual loss are generally addressed by membrane peeling. However, in many eyes, visual function may be symptomatically affected despite retention of relatively good VA. Some patients with significant visual loss from ERM may not be good candidates for surgery for various reasons. In such eyes, even modest VA improvements achievable by MRT may be helpful and improve symptoms. Because of the ability of MRT to improve vision in the absence of morphologic change (MRT will not cause resolution of ERMs), a trial of panmacular SDM MRT may be reasonable in many eyes with ERM to try to improve visual acuity enough to avoid surgery. If MRT is ineffective or insufficient, membrane peeling can still be performed without any diminished expectation of success. MRT may also improve visual function and VA after anatomic repair of chronic macular holes (Figs. 92-95).

MRT may also improve visual acuity after macular surgery in cases of persistent visual loss and/or macular

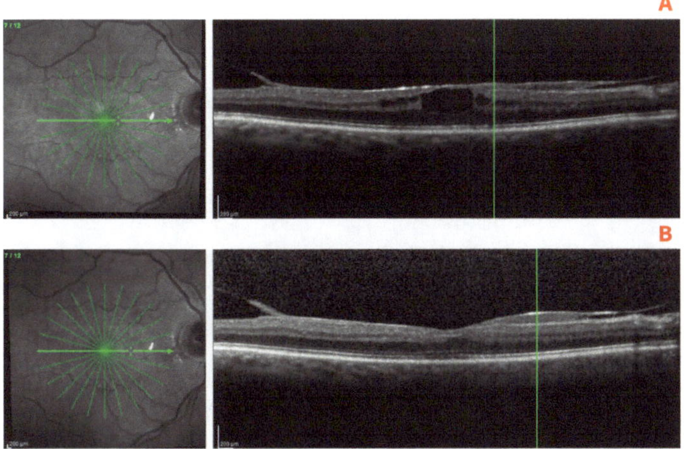

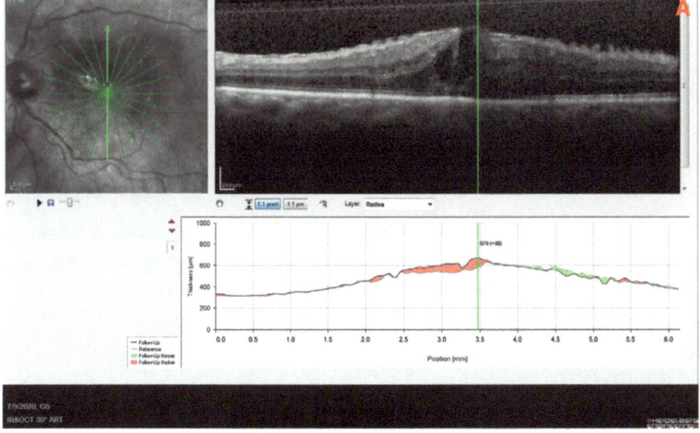

Fig. 93. 85 year old male with epiretinal membrane and vitreomacular traction with CME. (A) before SDM MRT. VA 20/60. (B) 14 months and 3 sessions of panmacular SDM later. Note resolution of CME. VA 20/50.

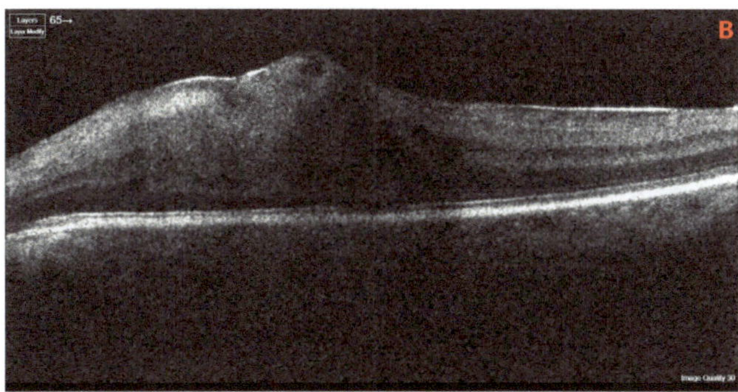

Fig. 94. OCT of 58 year old Hispanic woman with epiretinal membrane and macular edema following scleral buckling for a macula-on retinal detachment, before (left) and 6 months after (right) 2 sessions of SDM MRT. Visual acuity improved from 20/80 to 20/30 and maintained at 20/30 for 2 years until her most recent examination with continue MRT as vision protection therapy.

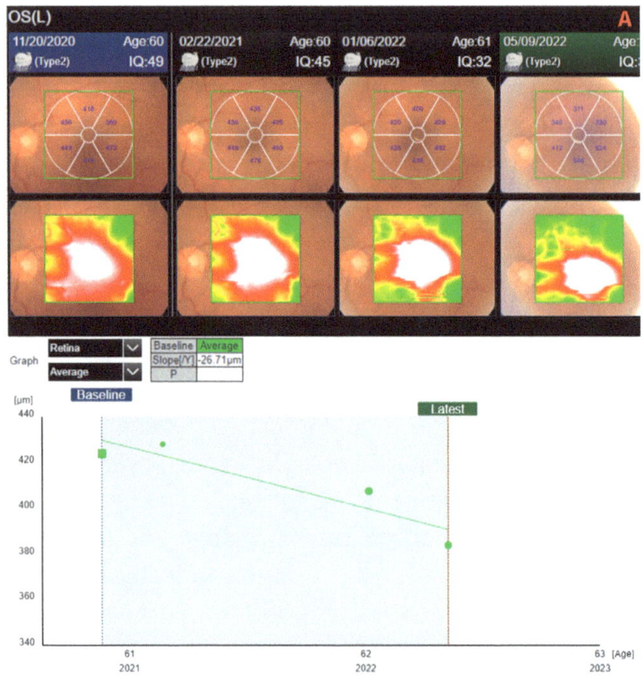
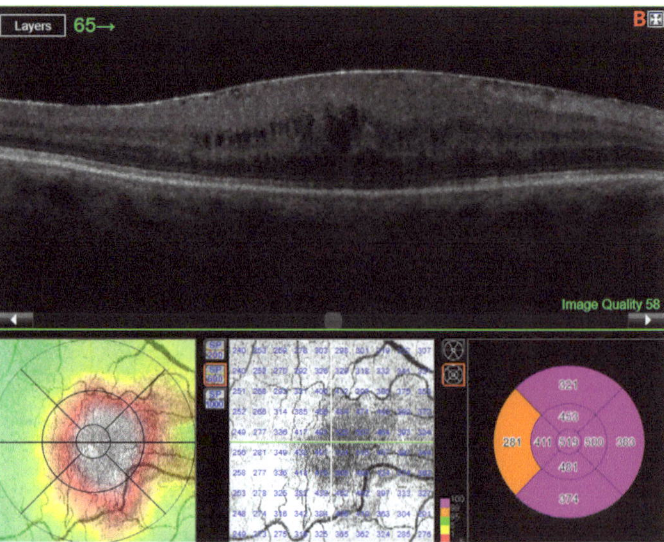
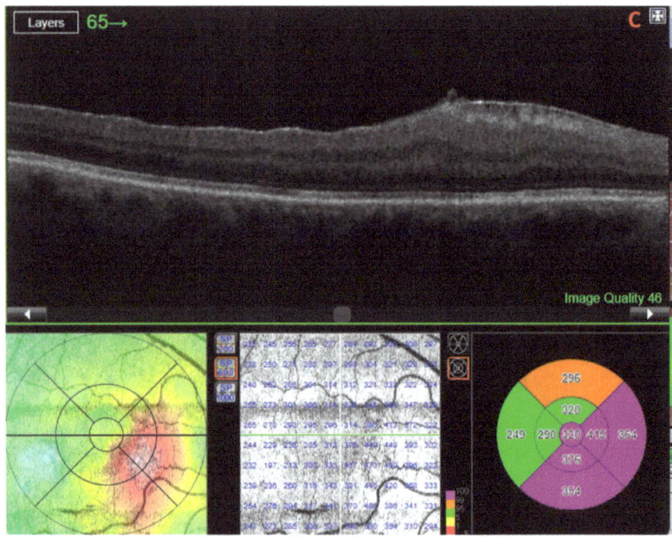
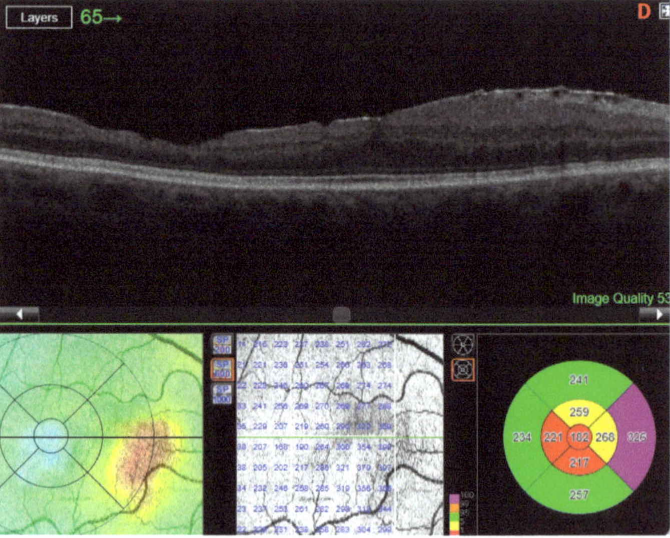
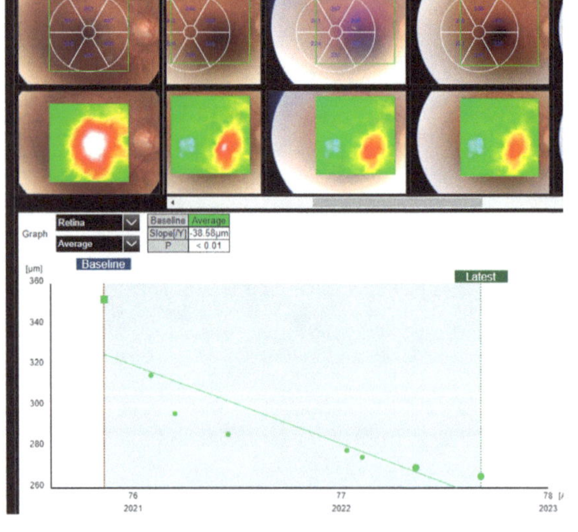

Fig. 95. (A) Longitudinal topographical OCT report of a left eye in 62 year old female with a new epiretinal membrane and macular edema first noted Nov. 2020. Patient declined membrane peeling. SDM MRT begun as VPT. Note progressive reduction in macular edema over time through May 2022 with VPT. VA stable at 20/60. (B) OCT of right eye of a different patient, a 75 year old male, showing an epiretinal membrane and macular edema 6 months following repair of a macula-on retinal detachment. VA 20/200. (C) OCT 4 months following membrane peeling, VA 20/100-2. Note resolution of CME. Panmacular SDM VPT begun. (D) OCT one year later, after 4 SDM treatments. Note further reduction in non-cystoid "solid" macular thickening. VA improved to 20/20. (E) Topographic macular thickening trends showing progressive decrease in macular thickening.

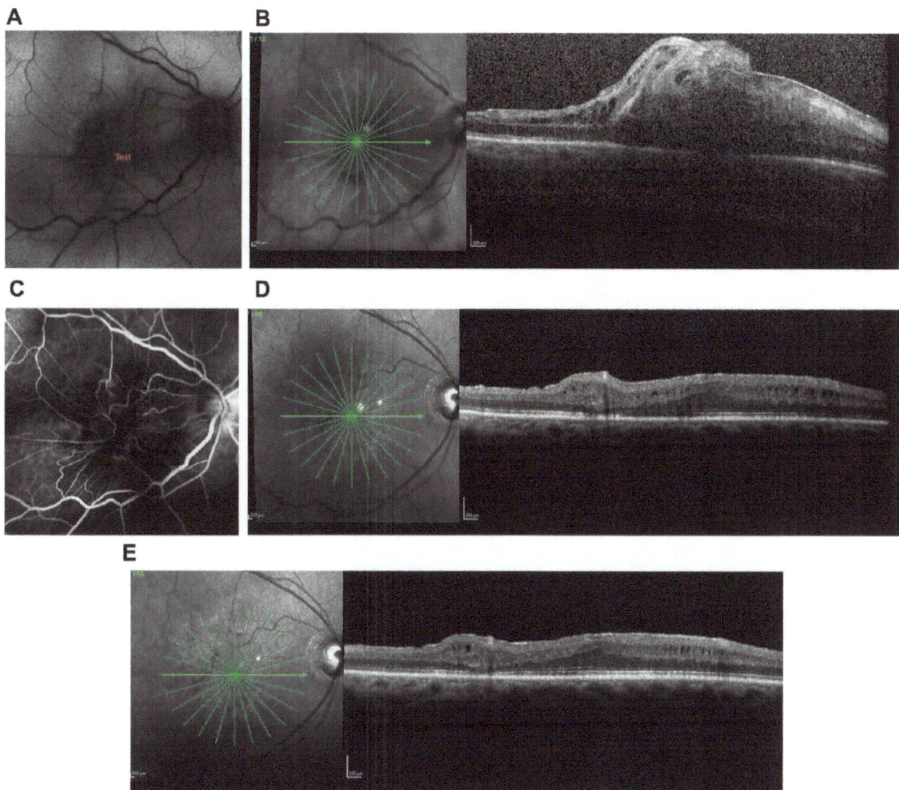

Fig. 96. (A) Fundus photograph of a right eye with epiretinal membrane prior to membrane peeling. Visual acuity = 20/400. (B) OCT of the same right eye with epiretinal membrane and marked macular thickening prior to membrane peeling. (C) Late-phase intravenous fundus fluorescein angiogram of the same eye prior to membrane peeling. Note the paucity of angiographic leakage within the macula. (D) OCT of the same eye 18 months following membrane peeling, at the time of SDM treatment. Visual acuity =20/80. (E) OCT of the same eye 6 months after SDM. Visual acuity = 20/30. From: *Luttrull JK. Subthreshold diode micropulse laser (SDM) for persistent macular thickening and limited visual acuity after epiretinal membrane peeling. Clin Ophthalmol, April 2020: 14; 1177-1188*

thickening (Luttrull CO 2020). A retrospective study identified 19 eyes of 18 consecutive patients treated with panmacular SDM MRT for persistent or recurrent visual loss following membrane peeling. After membrane peeling, VA improved from a mean Snellen acuity of 20/240 [logMAR 1.08] to 20/72 [0.56] (p = 0.0004). In the presence of persistent post membrane peeling macular thickening, visual acuities then gradually declined again to a mean of 20/91 [logMAR 0.66] by 4—109 months (avg. 41) post vitrectomy. At that point panmacular SDM was begun. At a mean 15 months post SDM, both visual acuities (to mean 20/68 [logMAR 0.53]) and maximum macular thicknesses were improved (p = 0.007 and p = 0.008, respectively) (Luttrull CO 2020) (Figs. 96-98).

Myopic foveal schisis may or may not be associated with traction. Although treatment is rarely indicated, when severe, the most common treatment is vitrectomy, the results of which are mixed. However, MRT of myopic foveal schisis may be also considered. Foveal schisis is often superimposed over pigmentary atrophy which is generally progressive and may also benefit from MRT to try slow progression of the pigmentary atrophy, as in AMD. In one such case, marked diffuse posterior myopic retinoschisis resolved completely following three sessions of SDM MRT, each three months apart (Fig. 99). Few cases of spontaneous resolution of nontractional myopic foveal schisis have been reported (Lai et al 2016).

Key point: MRT can improve eyes with ERMs, eyes following membrane peeling, and eyes with tractional macular edema and/or schisis with visual loss to avoid surgery, or to complement and improve the results of surgery

Post retinal reattachment

As noted at the outset, because MRT does not damage the retina it is not suitable for laser retinopexy to treat retinal breaks. However, following retinal detachment repair, VA may be limited by prior macular detachment, ERM, or limited by retained loculated subretinal fluid.

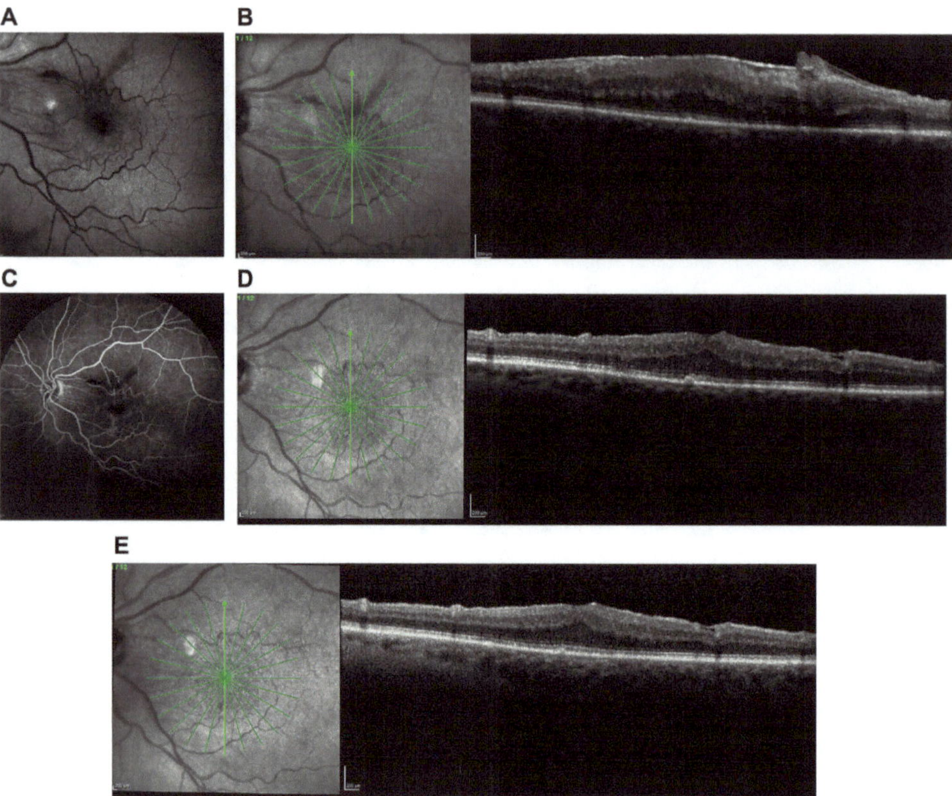

Fig. 97. (A) Fundus photograph of the left eye with epiretinal membrane. Visual acuity = 20/400. (B) OCT of the same eye on the same date. Note marked macular thickening. (C) Late-phase intravenous fundus fluorescein angiogram of the same date. Note the paucity of angiographic leakage in the macula. (D) OCT of the same eye 13 months after membrane peeling. Note persistent macular thickening. Visual acuity = 20/200. SDM performed. (E) OCT 11 months after SDM. Note the reduction in macular thickening. Visual acuity = 20/30. From: *Luttrull JK. Subthreshold diode micropulse laser (SDM) for persistent macular thickening and limited visual acuity after epiretinal membrane peeling. Clin Ophthalmol, April 2020: 14; 1177-1188*

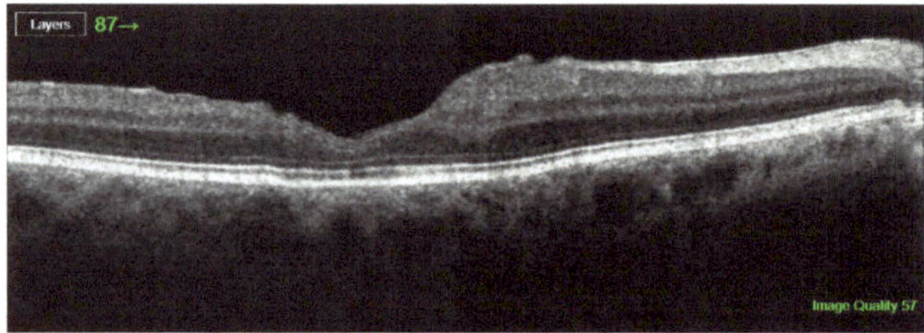

Fig. 98. 74 yo woman presenting with epiretinal membrane and BCVA of 4/400, right eye August 2018. Pars plana vitrectomy with membrane peeling was performed. January 2019 VA OD remained 5/200. SDM MRT vision protection therapy (VPT) begun. On return April 2019 VA was improved to 20/100+. In February 2020 VA OD had improved to 20/30, at which it was maintained through May 2022 (last visit). OCT shows right macula in May 2022, VA 20/30.

In such cases, by improving macular function, MRT may help to speed and improve visual recovery, including encouraging resorption of loculated submacular fluid (Landa 2018) (Figs. 100 and 101).

MRT for inflammatory retinal disease

Anti-inflammatory effects of MRT
As previously noted, infrared lasers, such as the 810 nm used in SDM MRT, reduce chronic inflammation, and are used for this purpose in other fields of medicine (Avci et al 2013, Berman and Nichols 2019). This may be another factor, in addition to safety, to recommend near infrared 810 nm over visible wavelengths for MRT. HSP activation is also anti-inflammatory (Kregel 2002, Caballero et al 2017, Midena et al 2019, De Cillà et al 2019, Midena et al 2019, Frizziero, Calciati, Torresin et al 2021). PC, while activating HSPs at spot margins, is net pro-inflammatory due to tissue destruction. This is easily demonstrated by increased local angiograph-

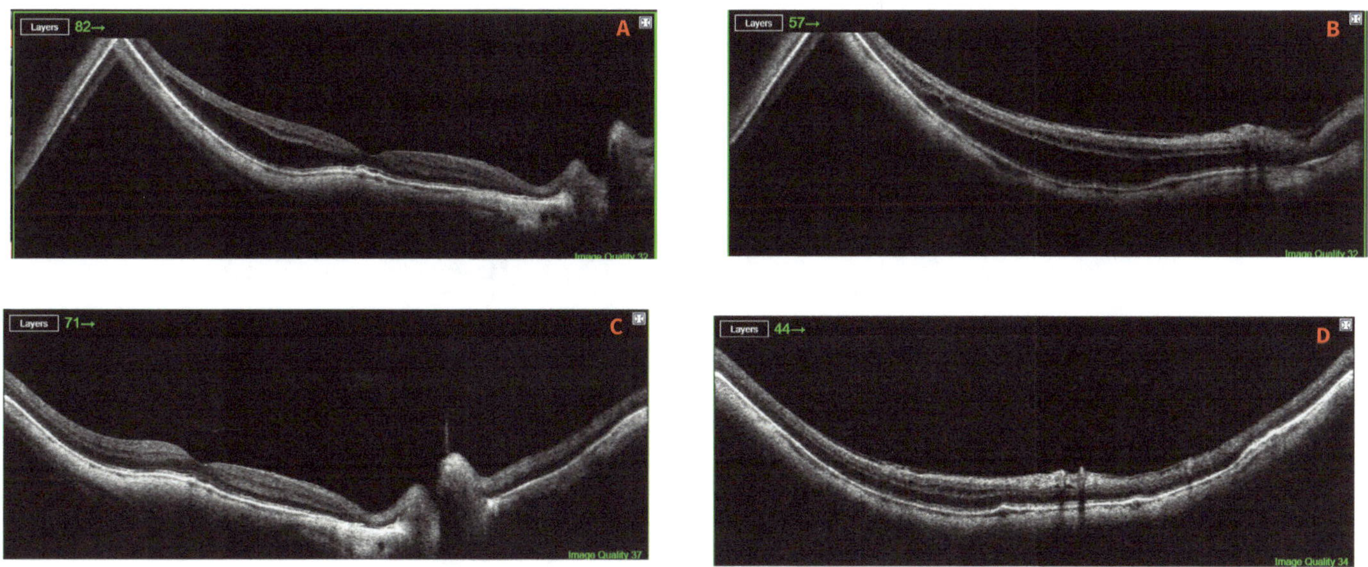

Fig. 99. OCTs of right eye 67 year old woman with unilateral high myopia before and after panmacular SDM MRT Q4 months x 3. Before SDM (Top row) note myopic macular schisis extending to the center of the fovea with and associated epiretinal membrane. After SDM (bottom row) note complete resolution of macular schisis. The epiretinal membrane remains. VA before and after treatment 20/40.

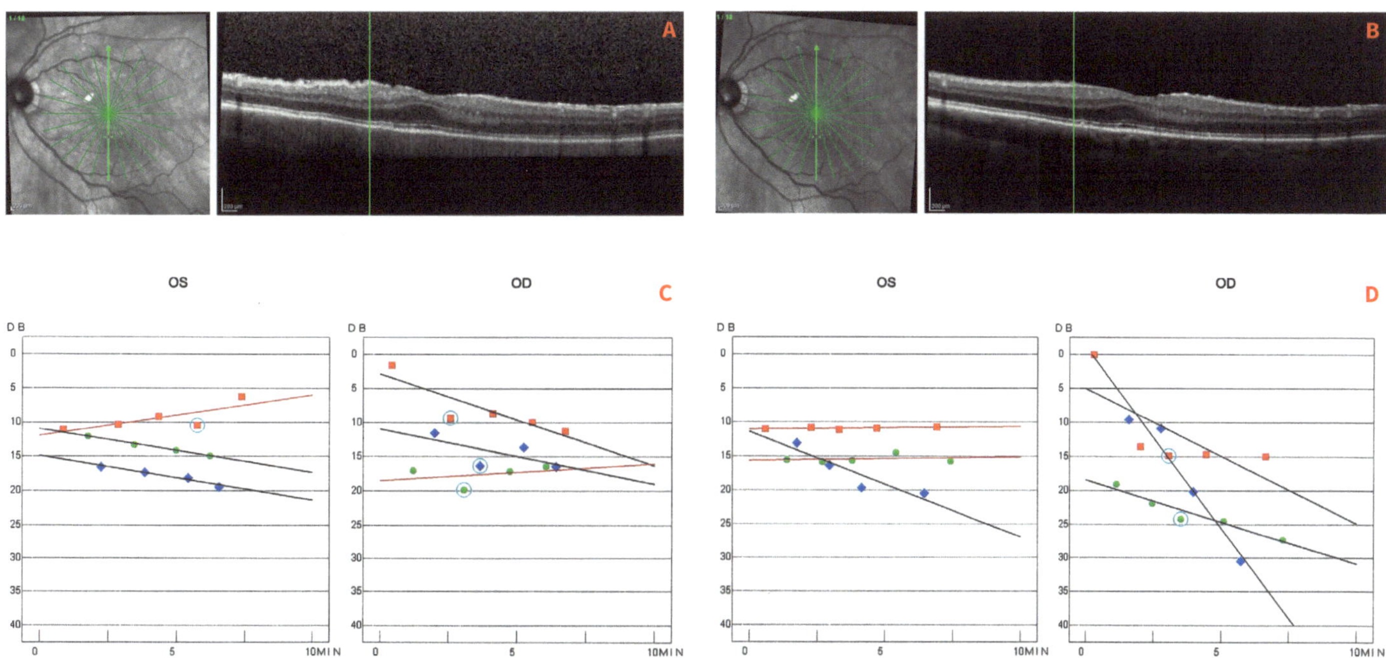

Fig. 100. 73 yo male 1 year post repair of macula-off retinal detachment in left eye with VA 20/50 and complaint of "dark" vision. (A) OCT before and (B) one month after panmacular SDM in the left eye only demonstrating slight reduction in thickness (C) Dark adaptometry (DA) before and (D) one month after SDM. Note improvement of DA in both eyes (increased slopes, particularly for blue response from parafoveal rods). Visual acuity improved to 20/25. Symptoms improved.

ic leakage early after PC for any indication (Luttrull and Dorin 2012, Chhablani et al 2018). Anti-VEGF medications can reduce microvascular leakage resulting from inflammation but are not otherwise anti-inflammatory. Steroids are anti-inflammatory, but not particularly anti-angiogenic and have significant use limitations such as for glaucoma and cataract. Only MRT is both anti-angiogenic and anti-inflammatory (Clark 1996, Luttrull and Kent 2019 and 2020). Thus, MRT can be helpful in the treatment of inflamma-

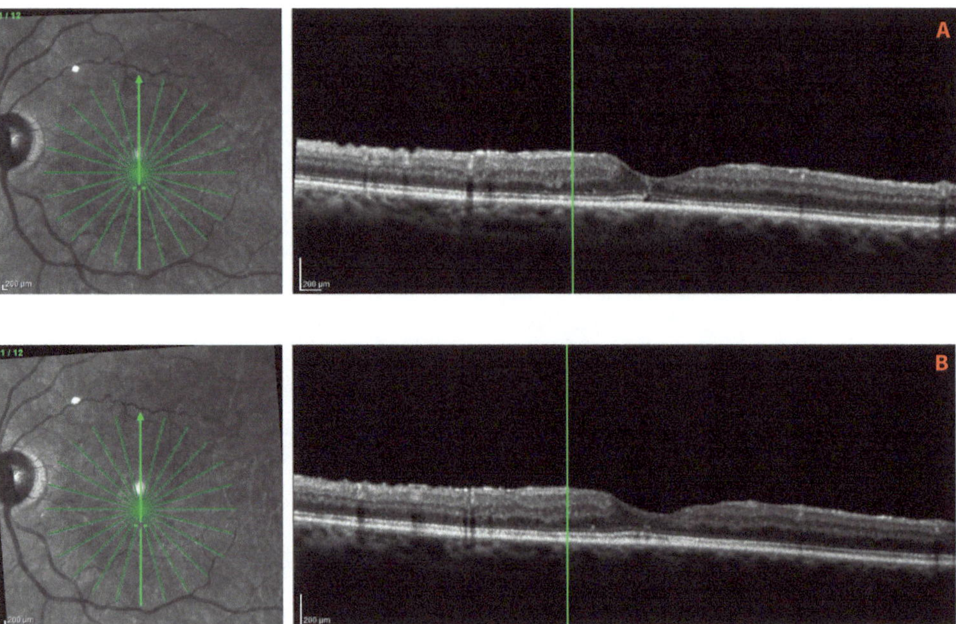

Fig. 101. Left eye of 70 year old male with type 2 diabetes s/p repair of macula-off retinal detachment two years prior; and repair of subsequent full thickness macular hole one year prior, to depicted OCT (top). VA unimproved at 20/200 since retinal detachment repair and macular hole closure. Panmacular SDM VPT begun Q 3-4 months with VA improved to 20/50 at six months, and 20/30 at one year, following initiation of SDM. Note absence of notable change in OCT (bottom) despite visual improvement.

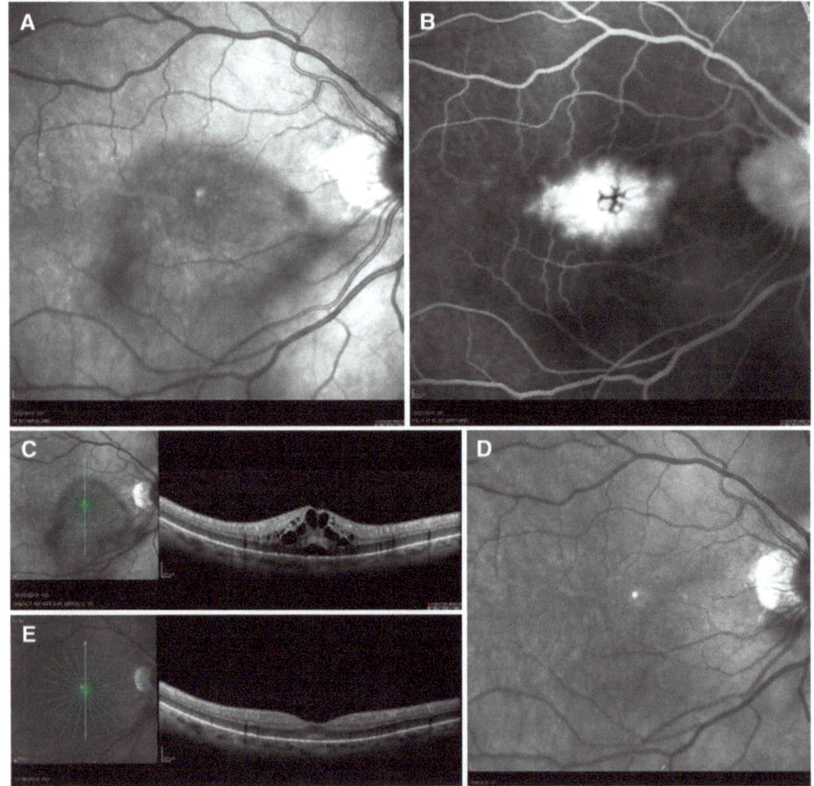

Fig. 102. Pseudophakic cystoid macular edema (CME) unresponsive to combination of topical steroid and nonsteroidal anti-inflammatory drops for 1 year. VA 20/200. Drops discontinued and panmacular SDM performed. (A) Infrared (IR), (B) late phase FFA and (C) Spectral-domain optical coherence tomography (OCT) prior to treatment with severe CME. (D) IR and (E) OCT 1 month following panmacular SDM. CME resolved. VA improved to 20/30. From: *Luttrull JK, Kent D. Laser therapy to prevent choroidal neovascularization. Choroidal Neovascularization. Chhablanni J, Ed. Springer Verlag. July 2020. DOI: 10.1007/978-981-15-2213-0_30*

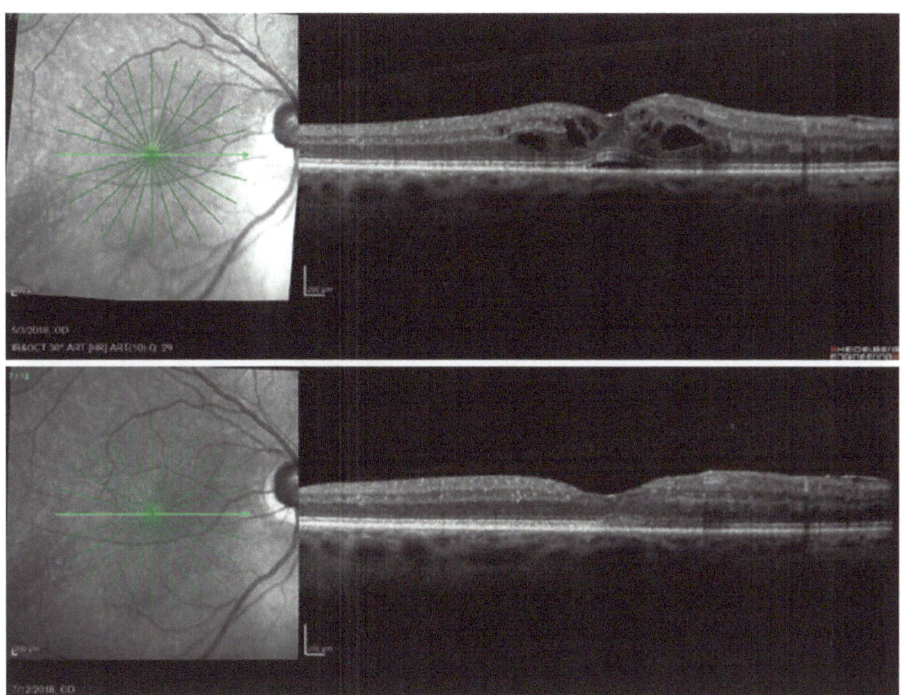

Fig. 103. Sarcoid uveitis with cystoid macular edema in the right eye. History of severe steroid response in the fellow eye. The CME OD was unresponsive to bevacizumab. Other VEGF inhibitors were refused by his medical insurance. Top: Prior to panmacular SDM treatment VA 20/30. Bottom, 1 month following panmacular SDM. VA 20/25. Note resolution of CME following SDM MRT. From: *Luttrull JK, Kent D. Laser therapy to prevent choroidal neovascularization. Choroidal Neovascularization. Chhablanni J, Ed. Springer Verlag. July 2020. DOI: 10.1007/978-981-15-2213-0_30*

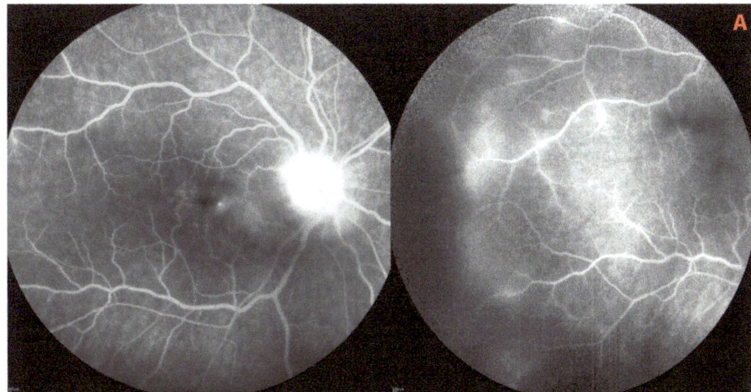

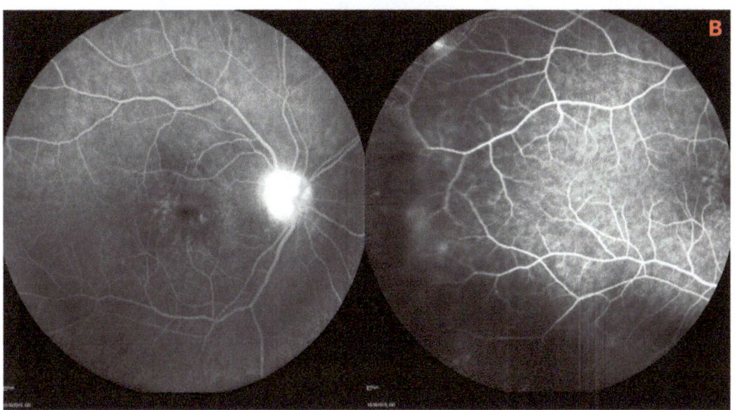

Fig. 104. Eye with idiopathic retinal vasculitis, vitriitis, and optic neuritis in patient with history of severe steroid respondent glaucoma. Total retinal SDM MRT (TRT) was performed as anti-inflammatory therapy. (Top) FFA before treatment. (Bottom) FFA 1 week following total retinal SDM laser. No topical, local or systemic medical treatment given. Note the decrease in inflammatory dye leakage from retinal vessels and optic nerve. VA prior to treatment 20/70; one week later, 20/50. From: *Luttrull JK, Kent D. Laser therapy to prevent choroidal neovascularization. Choroidal Neovascularization. Chhablanni J, Ed. Springer Verlag. July 2020. DOI: 10.1007/978-981-15-2213-0_30*

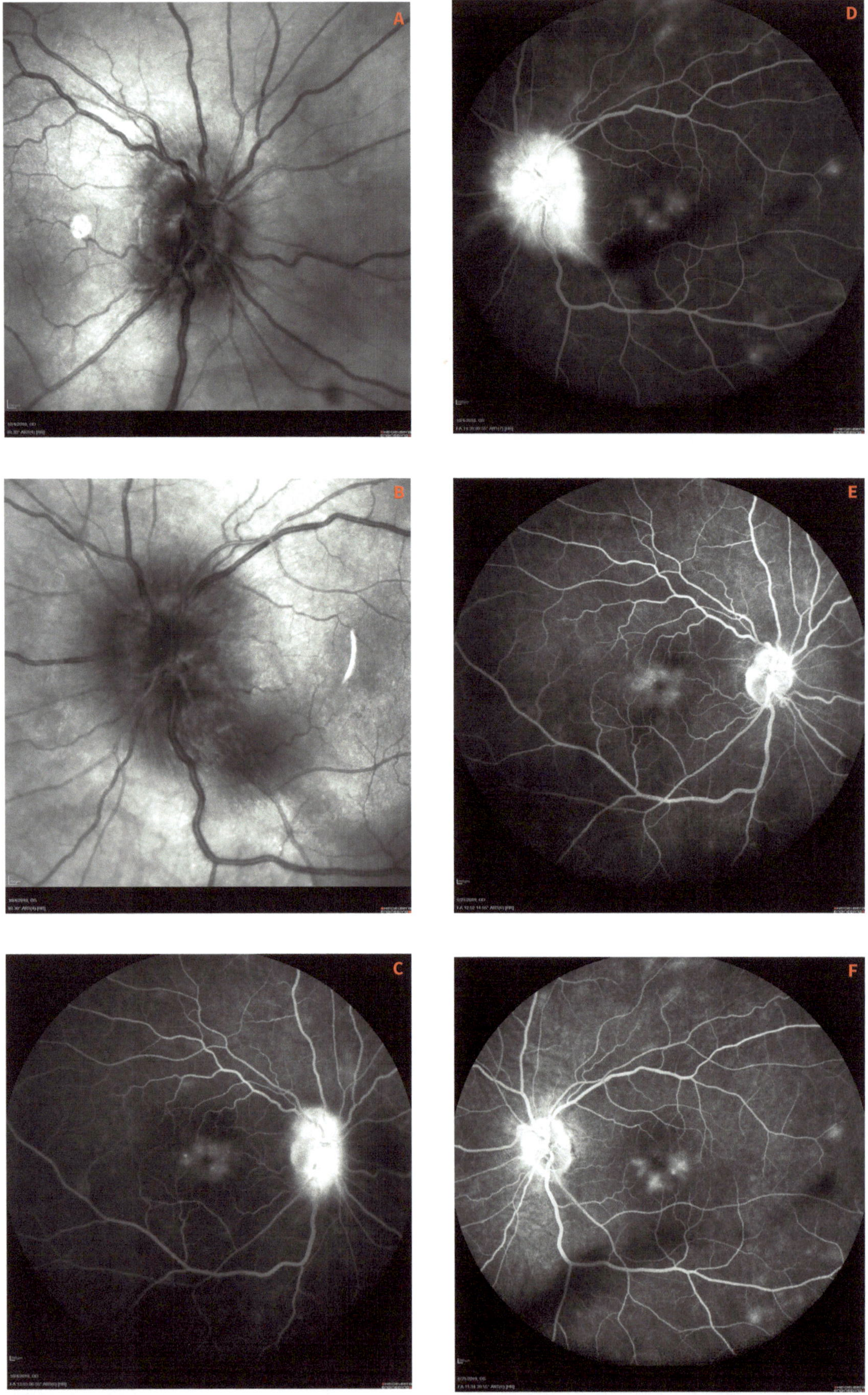

Fig. 105. 67 yo woman with type 2 diabetes mellitus with severe non proliferative diabetic retinopathy and acute adult diabetic papillopathy OU. Fundus photographs (A and B) showing optic nerve edema and FFA (C and D) leakage from optic nerve OU. VA 20/25 OD and 20/30 OS. Total retinal SDM MRT performed. FFA (E and F) 2 months later demonstrating resolution of optic nerve swelling. VA 20/30 OU.

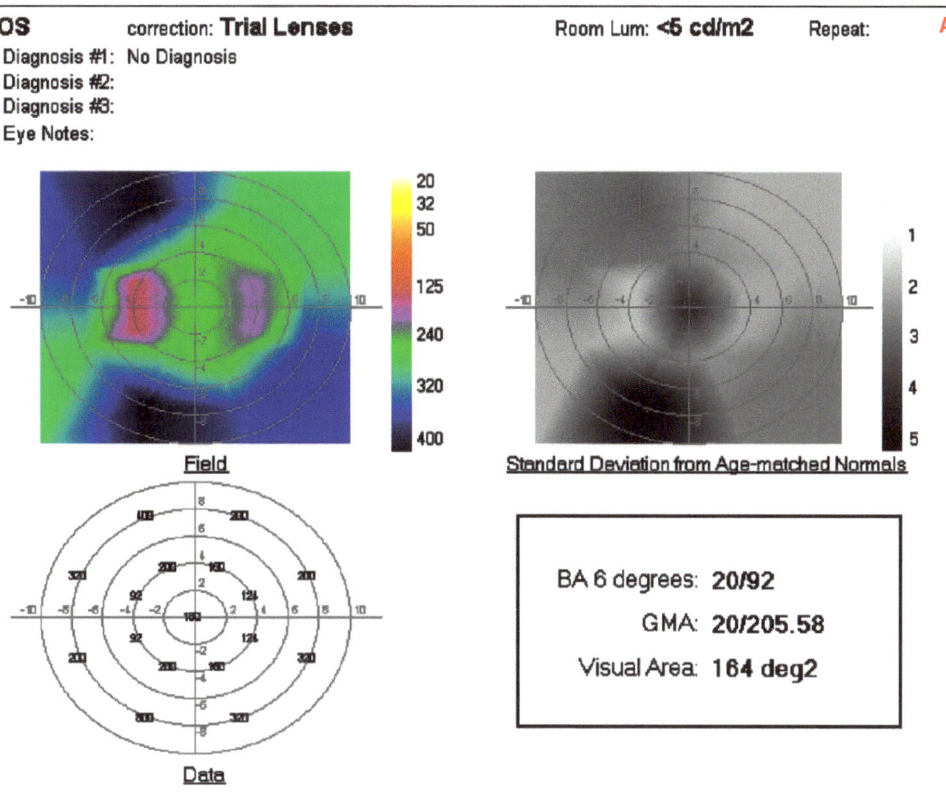

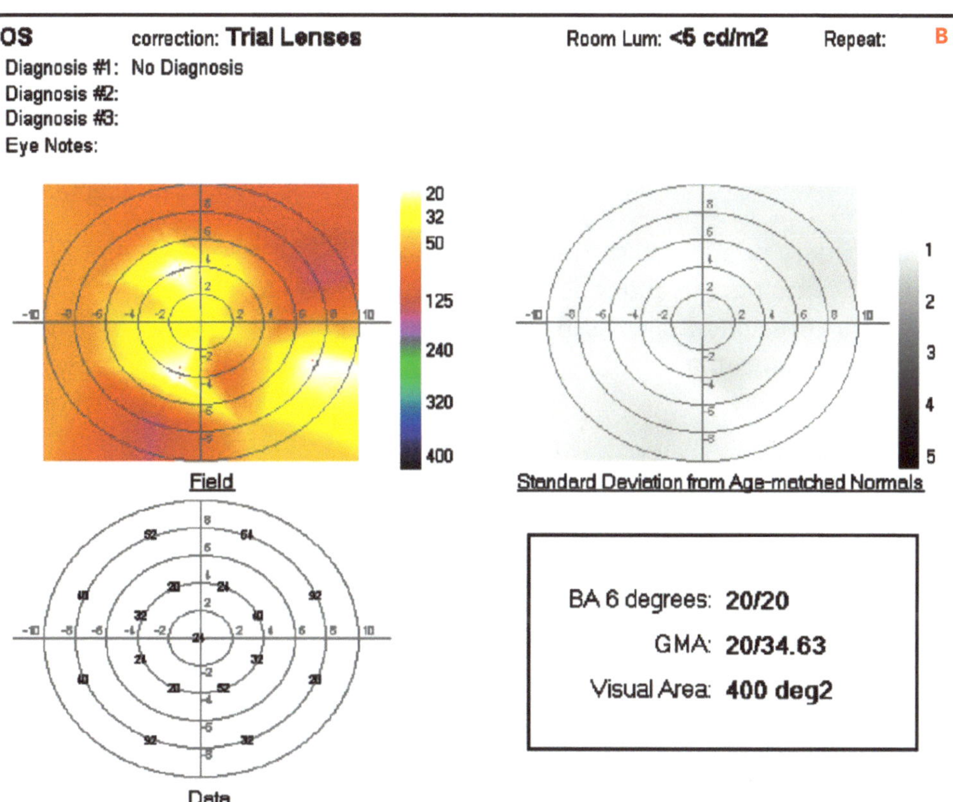

Fig. 106. (A) Omnifield mesopic visual field of left eye of 71 year old man 6 weeks post acute non-arteritic anterior ischemic optic neuropathy, presenting with complaint of a paracentral scotoma. Note inferior nasal paracentral scotoma. VA 20/20. One month after panmacular SDM MRT, patient reported resolution of scotoma OS, which was confirmed by repeat Omnifield MVT (B). Two months later (3 months following treatment) the scotoma recurred.

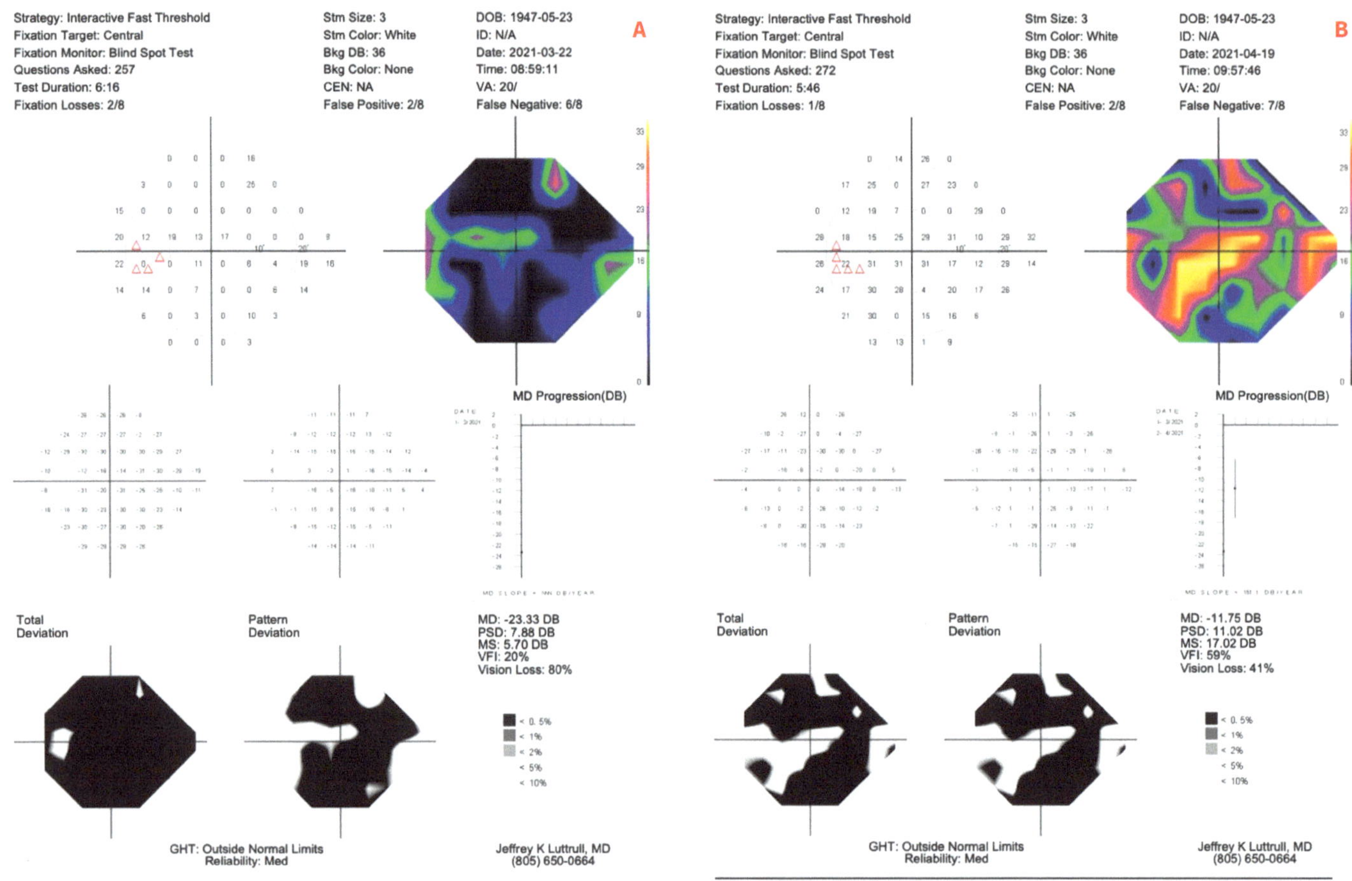

Fig. 107. 74 year old man with history of vision loss OU for 8 years due to non-arteritic anterior ischemic optic neuropathy. VA hand motions OD; 20/70 OS. (A) 10-2 automated perimetry OS on presentation. Panmacular SDM MRT performed. (B) Repeat 10-2 one month later. Note improved visual function. VA 20/60. SDM continued Q 3 months as vision protection, with improvement in visual acuity to 20/30 at 14 months post presentation with average nerve fiber layer thickness improvement, increased by 9.65um/year over period of VPT. The patient was then able to pass the vision requirement for a California driver's license.

tory retinal disease, as primary or adjunctive therapy, or in cases where other treatments are either absent, carry significant risks, or are precluded, such as in eyes prone to steroid-respondent glaucoma.

Cystoid macular edema

A common clinical example is inflammatory cystoid macular edema. This includes pseudophakic, uveitic, and diabetic macular edema, especially if associated with serous macular detachment (Figs. 30, 35, 102, and 103) (Midena et al 2019, Frizziero, Calciati, Midena et al 2021, Verdina et al 2021). Because anti-VEGF medication is not anti-inflammatory, it is often ineffective in this setting (Figs. 30, 33, and 35). Clinical experience shows that SDM (810 nm) MRT monotherapy is usually effective in these settings, avoiding the risks, adverse effects, and treatment burden of local, topical, and intravitreal medications.

Retinal vasculitis

The ability of MRT to reduce peripheral retinal micro- and macrovascular inflammation is well illustrated by FFA in DR, in which chronic neuroinflammation is a prominent component to the disease (Khetarpal et al 2017, Luttrull and Sinclair 2014, Luttrull and Kent 2019, Sinclair and Schwartz 2019, Pillar et al 2020) (Figs. 14, 26, and 51-55). Thus, MRT may aid management of generalized retinal vasculitis, especially in cases where the cause of the inflammation is unknown, precluding targeted therapy (Fig. 104). As retinal inflammatory disorders are often chronic and/ or relapsing, the absence of adverse treatment effects, long-lasting effects of MRT, and ability to retreat as often as necessary are aids to clinical management.

Key point: The anti-inflammatory effects of MRT are therapeutic for CPRs and this facility can be exploited for

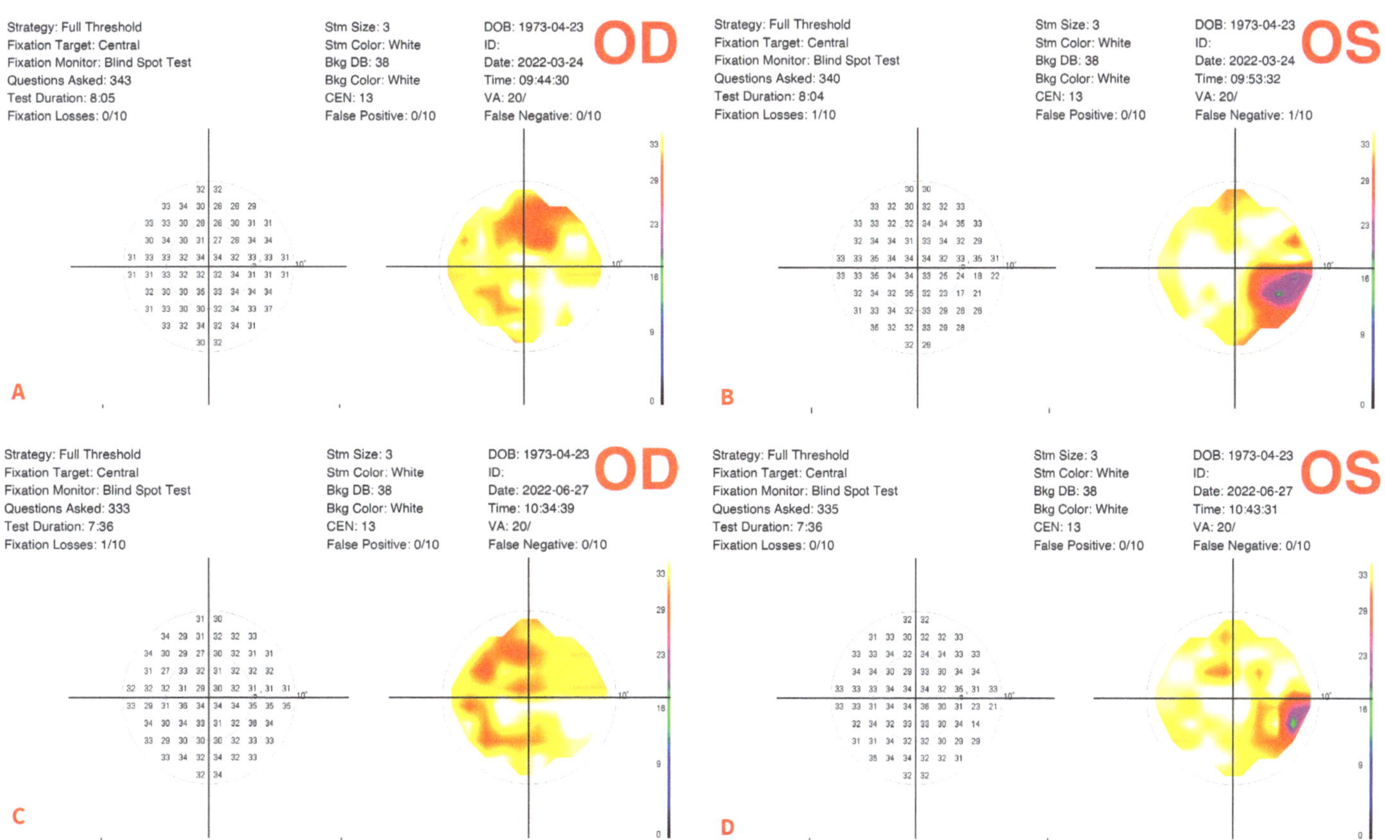

Fig. 108. 10-2 automated perimetry of 49 year old woman with optic nerve drusen. Top row, at presentation. Panmacular SDM MRT performed for neuroprotection. Bottom row, 3 months following treatment. Note improvement in both eyes following SDM MRT.

treatment of primary inflammatory retinal conditions as well

Nonglaucomatous optic nerve diseases

MRT for glaucomatous optic neuropathy has been discussed earlier. Following the same conceptual lines, the neuroprotective effects of MRT can be demonstrated in treatment of other optic nerve disorders as well (Figs. 105-108). Restoration of visual function to areas of the retina previously demonstrating no function, such as scotomata documented by visual field testing, is a common observation following MRT (Luttrull, Samples et al 2019). Such restoration has been observed in eyes with optic atrophy due to nonarteritic anterior ischemic optic neuropathy and multiple sclerosis and in eyes with optic nerve drusen (Figs. 103-106). This is yet another demonstration of the ability of MRT to restore function to previously non- or highly dysfunctional, preapoptotic cells, thus, at least temporarily reversing the disease process (Iwami et al 2014, Luttrull and Margolis 2016, Caballero et al 2017, DeCilla 2019, Luttrull and Kent 2019, Luttrull, Samples et al 2019, Frizziero, Calciati, Midena et al 2021).

Key point: MRT is neuroprotective for disorders of the optic nerve beyond glaucoma

14. Perspectives and Predictions for Modern Retinal Laser Therapy

MRT is elegant

Simplicity is the keynote of all true elegance.

—Coco Chanel

In MRT and the reset theory of retinal laser action, we have a nontargeted but disease-specific treatment that is agnostic to the primary cause of disease, pathoselective, functionally normalizing, restorative and therapeutically immunoactivating, that is predictable, highly effective, safe, and renewable, and able to reverse disease progression for all major causes of irreversible visual loss, and other commonly encountered macular disorders, besides. No currently known treatment modality has the potential to achieve what has already been demonstrated with MRT. The robust nature of the results, for wet AMD prevention to name just one, are such that prospect of a safer and more effective therapy appearing on the horizon is essentially nil. MRT is thus destined to become the most important clinical intervention to treat and prevent irreversible visual loss. This permitted by the unparalleled safety of MRT, which allows application in any clinical setting where treatment might be of benefit; and for the most effective treatment of all—prevention. MRT treatment effects are long lasting compared to drugs. MRT can minimize the drug burden and preclude the need for drugs altogether, especially if implemented early as the first-choice intervention to prevent disease progression and visual loss (Luttrull et al 2005, 2008, Luttrull and Sinclair 2014, Luttrull 2018, Luttrull, Sinclair et al 2018, 2020, Luttrull and Gray 2022). Finally, MRT can be repeated *pro re nata ad infinitum* to preserve and maintain treatment effects to optimize clinical outcomes, without loss of effectiveness. Acting physiologically, all known MRT effects are therapeutic. None are adverse. MRT is not limited by tolerance phenomena or other adverse effects that typically compromise drug and biologic therapies. MRT is simple, quick and painless, minimizing patient resistance to treatment and enhancing compliance. Automation will soon eliminate the final risk associated with treatment: physician error.

Preventive thinking

The ability to intervene as early as desired, conferred by treatment safety, is one of the most compelling and important attributes of MRT. Regarding retinal disorders, prevention has historically taken the form mainly of advice rather than active intervention. For doctors customarily thinking in terms of therapy, the issues and expectations of active preventive treatment can be disconcerting. First, unlike therapy, following ideal preventive treatment nothing changes. The earlier preventive treatment is performed, the more the preserved state will approximate normality. The more effective preventive treatment is, the less likely anything will change, and more likely normality will persist. This can lead to disappointment to all concerned, suspecting that treatment was either unnecessary, or did not do anything. Patients (and doctors) need to be counseled that lack of change is a good thing and is, in fact, the goal of treatment. It does not mean the treatment is ineffective. It means the opposite. It is important to remember that the "P" in CPR is progressive and the "D" in AMD is degeneration. The normal course of all the principal indications for MRT is worsening over time. Thus, to *not* worsen is to actually improve compared to the usual course of events. Second, how does one know that this particular patient with early, currently low-risk disease, will actually benefit from preventive treatment to reduce the risk of a possible future adverse event? The answer is that one cannot know. The earlier preventive treatment is instituted, the greater the number of patients who will be treated who may have done just fine without it. But which ones? Functional testing and provocative treatment is one way to rationally aid prediction. But the fact that preventive treatment necessarily includes many "unnecessarily" treated patients emphasizes the importance of preventive treatment being safe, quick, simple, noninvasive, convenient, durable, and patient-friendly as well as effective. And cost effective as well. Finally, in another challenge to instant gratification, preventing vision loss in some distant future lacks the emotional curb appeal of restoring sight with effective therapy, like fixing a retinal detachment or doing a vitrectomy for a vitreous hemorrhage. The result, however, is the same, if not better, because excellent vision is more easily preserved than restored.

MRT challenges

Published . . . to take part in a severe contest between intelligence, which presses forward, and an unworthy, timid, ignorance obstructing our progress.
—The Economist Magazine

A tree falls in the forest

With the introduction of anti-VEGF drug therapy, attention shifted quickly and heavily away from laser. Major studies continued to employ conventional PC to compare with drug therapy, long after LIRD was known to be an SAE. Because of the inherent adverse effects and poor visual results associated with PC, retinal laser treatment became largely relegated to rescue therapy (Chen et al 2018, Jorge et al 2018, Glassman, Wells et al 2020). Reflecting this shift in attention was the virtual disappearance of laser studies from the podium at major retinal meetings and from major journals. Similarly for institutional funding of laser studies. Since introduction of the first intravitreal anti-VEGF agents, well over 95% of all major retinal meeting podium presentations have concerned drug therapy, and far fewer than 1% concerned retinal laser treatment. In one period of over 5 years, over 95% of all podium presentations focused on one drug made by one company (AAO.org, ASRS.org, Lundh et al 2017). The pharmaceutical industry has used its unmatched resources to create an information vacuum in which no other sound but theirs is heard. The phenomenon of "regulatory capture" is well known. The current situation in ophthalmology—if not medicine in general—might thus be well-described as "professional capture" (Lundh et al 2017). Remarkably, despite this monomania retinal laser treatment has remained an essential treatment modality, with "subthreshold" and quasi-MRT approaches largely replacing RPC in clinical practice. At the same time, tremendous progress was being made elucidating the mechanisms of retinal laser action and the reset phenomenon, identifying, and demonstrating new treatment applications, and developing the concepts and techniques of MRT. Few are heard.

The prospect of domination of the nation's scholars by Federal employment, project allocation, and the power of money is ever present and is gravely to be regarded.
—Dwight D Eisenhower, 1955

Impediments to MRT adoption

In addition to the laser-like focus of attention on drug therapy, are three additional issues limiting wider use of retinal laser treatment in general, and adoption of MRT, in particular. First, because the response to MRT is physiologic, it takes time to manifest and may frustrate or worry those accustomed to the instant but short-lived gratifications of drug therapy. This requires experience to overcome. Second, is confusion over best practices—laser modalities, settings, and treatment techniques. Like any other surgery or procedure, each has a profound influence on treatment expectations, applications, and outcomes. There are better and worse ways to do anything (Battaglia Parodi and Iacono 2019, Keunen et al 2020, Luttrull AJO 2020, Van Rijssen et al 2020). But the variability of treatment approaches to "subthreshold" retinal laser leaves most in confusion about what to do, and how best to do it. This is clearly illustrated by the plethora of parameters and approaches reported in various studies. However, an answer is on its way.

The principles of MRT allow, for the first time, retinal laser treatment to become uniform and standardized to guarantee both safety and maximum efficacy. This was not a possibility with RPC, which was inherently dangerous, or any of the subsequent treatment approaches built on the concepts of RPC, such as short-pulse CW and nanosecond lasers. The variability of MPL approaches for "subthreshold" treatment has been likewise largely the result of thinking predicated on application of RPC principles to MPL (van Rijssen et al 2019). Because of the ability of MRT to provide uniform, standardized safe and effective treatment, the ultimate solution to eliminate nonuniformity and suboptimal treatment approaches is automation. MRT is ideally suited to automation. Automated delivery of MRT in a uniform fashion in all eyes of all patients without the possibility of surgeon error will be the next sea-change in the progress of retinal laser treatment to allow it to reach its full potential. In fact, the potential of MRT will not be realized absent this type of automation. The good news is that it is coming.

When the first microsecond pulsed lasers (MPL) were introduced clinically at the turn of the century, they were used according to RPC treatment concepts and techniques. Results were poor. Like golfers who blame the club, most novice users concluded it was the microsecond pulse mode, rather than its application, that was at fault. Many, now in senior positions of influence and authority, persist in this belief. One, the senior editor of a major American ophthalmology journal, explained his refusal to send a paper on MPL for peer review by stating simply: "Everyone knows it doesn't work." (Email communication to the author, 2017) This vignette illustrates what has been the most significant impediment to progress with retinal laser treatment: people not science (Bacon 1902, Rosenfeld and Feuer 2019). Planck, speaking as a realist rather than idealist concluded, as have many studies since, that scientific progress depends less on discovery than it does on the simple mortality of the *ancien regime* (Hull et al 1989).

Regardless, there has been considerable progress in the general understanding of retinal laser treatment since the days of RPC and introduction of MPL. In that time, two fundamental concepts of MRT have become broadly accepted. These include recognition that LIRD is nontherapeutic and thus to be avoided (a sea change from the RPC era); and the importance of avoiding microsecond pulse duty cycles above 5% in the macula to minimize the risk of retinal damage (Luttrull, Sramek et al 2012, Luttrull and Margolis 2016, Chang and Luttrull 2020, Keunen et al 2020). However, many still cling to the last vestiges of the RPC era. These include use of visible laser wavelengths and titration. These too will eventually be abandoned with more data and experience (Chhablani et al 2022). Third is the paucity of high-quality data and, in particular, large well-done RCTs. Those RCTs of microsecond pulse laser that have been done have generally been small and/or done using a variety of nonuniform treatment protocols generally uninformed by the current understanding of retinal laser biophysics, the mechanism of action, and current (MRT) treatment guidelines designed to optimize safety and effective-

ness (Chen et al 2018, Keunen et al 2020, Verdina et al 2021). As a testament to the reset mechanism of retinal laser action, despite the variability in techniques and laser parameters, the results of such studies have been remarkably consistent and positive (Lavinsky et al 2011, Chen et al 2018, Jorge et al 2018, Frizziero, Calciati, Torresin, et al. 2021). A principal problem is that RCTs are expensive. As previously noted, virtually all RCTs in medicine are sponsored and paid for by industry, mostly pharmaceutical companies. At the time of this writing, there are 43 RCTs for AMD and retinal vascular disease listed at http://clinicaltrials.gov/. Forty-one (possibly 42—it is unclear) of the 43 of these are industry-sponsored (95+%) (Schott et al 2010). Compared to the resources of the pharmaceutical industry, retinal laser companies are small, generally poorly capitalized, and unable to fund RCTs even if they wanted to (Lundh et al 2017).

Evidence for MRT
The forest versus the trees

In the absence of large RCTs, what is the evidence to support MRT? One may reasonably argue that the evidence for MRT consists of nothing but a cacophony of small studies of varying degrees of quality, applying nonuniform treatment approaches, dominated by a small group of investigators, producing little high-quality information. To paraphrase Barth, "anecdote writ large" (Barth 1919). However, if one steps back to see a larger picture, the view one gets is different. As the preceding discussion and illustrations describe, MRT robustly improves retinal and visual function virtually wherever and whenever applied. It is safe and renewable. It has no adverse effects. Many of the supportive studies are small, and few are RCTs. However, taken together the evidence is clear and highly consistent. Where long-term evidence exists, it demonstrates robust long-term benefits from MRT absent adverse effects. Working physiologically and homeotropically, the neuroprotective and neuroenhancing effects of MRT cut across a wide spectrum of disparate diseases united by the fundamental property of RPE dysfunction induced by disease-specific stressors, leading to a specific menu of intracellular protein misfolding and the inevitable consequences, reversible by MRT. There is no evidence to the contrary.

The power of prediction

Following on the elegance of the MRT mode of action is the ability of the reset theory—which is the direct product of SDM MRT—to both explain the effects of any type of retinal laser treatment in any clinical setting (RPC, subthreshold, short-pulse CW, nanosecond, MRT), and to accurately predict new, novel applications for MRT. Indeed, the ability to both explain and predict are essential attributes of any useful theory. It was the inability to explain that was the failure of the various theories for the mechanism of action retinal laser assuming the prerequisite of LIRD (Fazlollah 1961, Mainster 1999). As noted earlier, the reset theory predicts MRT should be effective for a wide variety of retinal disorders that would seem to have little in common, other than their shared status as neurodegenerations (Luttrull and Dorin 2012, Luttrull et al 2015, Luttrull and Margolis 2016). Many reset theory predictions had no precedent in prior retinal laser use; whilst others—like reversal of anti-VEGF drug tolerance in wet AMD—had no precedent in medicine (Luttrull et al 2015, Luttrull and Margolis 2016, Luttrull 2018, Luttrull, Samples et al 2018). Without exception, predictions arising directly and only from reset theory have been confirmed. Further, the treatment responses in these novel applications predicted by reset theory have not been marginal; instead, they have been robust and highly significant across the board.

From chaos, order

Reflecting on the above, to the extent that the many various treatment protocols of the various studies of "subthreshold" retinal laser treatment reflect current International Retinal Laser Society Guidelines for MRT, we see a clear pattern: Low-intensity treatment is safest, and high-density treatment is most effective (Luttrull et al 2005 and 2007, Lavinsky et al 2011, Luttrull, Sramek et al 2012, Keunen et al 2020, Luttrull AJO 2020, Frizziero, Calciati, Torresin, et al. 2021). Despite current nonuniformity, studies that incorporate both to precepts of MRT the greatest degree report the best clinical and visual results. There are no exceptions and to this rule (Chen et al 2018, Verdina et al 2021). Many more studies are needed as there is much yet to be learned. This further study is clearly justified by what is already known. Automation, by standardizing, optimizing, and making treatment uniform in all respects will improve the value of such future studies.

The future and MRT

Nuclear-powered vacuum cleaners will probably be a reality in 10 years.
　　　—Alex Lewyt, president of vacuum cleaner company Lewyt Corp., in the *New York Times* in 1955.

There are more things in heaven and earth, Horatio, than are dreamnt of in your philosophy.
　　　　　　　　　　—Shakespeare, *Hamlet*

Homeotrophic hormetic medicine

MRT and reset theory represent the foundation of a new area of medicine that employs highly controlled tissue-sparing activation of the immune system initiated by thermal HSP activation to treat and prevent disease. This can be described as pulsed electromagnetic hormesis (PEH). While thermal HSP activation has been exploited medically to enhance wound healing and reduce inflammation, particularly in dermatology and cosmetic surgery, SDM MRT is the first clinical intervention to engage these processes to treat and prevent disease. Reset theory predicts that the effects of such HSP activation should be both therapeutic and preventative in virtually any tissue for virtually any disorder, but of most benefit to those that are chronic and progressive. Reset theory further predicts that the reset effect can be produced by any form of electromagnetic radiation and applying the PEH method appropriate for the target tissue, such as laser for skin and the hematologic system, ultrasound for solid soft tissues, and radiofrequency for the brain and bone marrow. Reset-triggering PEH, by reversing aging and the drivers of chronic disease generically, holds tremendous promise for stopping or slowing many of the most common currently pharmacologically and biologically untreatable diseases, including Alzheimer's disease, idiopathic pulmonary fibrosis, and many, many others.

Prevention of acquired myopia

Particularly intriguing is the use of MRT to prevent acquired myopia. Because progressive acquired myopia is mediated by chemical factors almost certainly arising from and modulated by the RPE, this dysfunctional, abnormal adaptation to near work should be amenable to reset correction. To this end, PC for retinopathy of prematurity (ROP) has been found to inhibit myopia development (Al-Ghamdi et al 2004). While there is retinal destruction from PC in ROP, there is also HSP activation. Thus, it is possible, if not likely, that normalizing retinal function with MRT to correct the myopic stimulus, and maintaining this normalization, may be able to minimize if not prevent acquired myopia in children, provided treatment is started early and continued (Al-Ghamdi et al 2004, Feigl et al 2011, Luttrull et al 2015, Luttrull and Margolis 2016, Karouta et al 2021).

Prevention and treatment of ocular senescence

The future always arrives as low-quality data. Such is the case for MRT prevention of ocular senescence. An interesting and not infrequent report from patients treated with MRT as vision protection therapy is that, typically after a year or two of treatment, they are no longer reliant on spectacles for near, or distance vision. Reset theory suggests a way to understand how this might happen. First, MRT normalizes retinal function regardless of the cause. While aging is not properly a disease, there is clearly much progressive dysfunction involved. Normal age-related deterioration in macular function is well-known and this is reversible by MRT (Feigl et al 2011, Luttrull and Bhavan 2023, Nape et al 2022). Second, the RPE-derived chemical mediators of both the dysfunction and MRT treatment response circulate throughout the eye, detectable in both the vitreous and aqueous fluids (Midena et al 2019). Because RPE-derived cytokines are potent mediators of ocular function, it is not unreasonable to expect that normalization of senescent dysfunction could lead to reversal of senescent changes, such as loss of visual sensitivity and even presbyopia. Might cataract be delayed as well? Doubtful, but it will be interesting to find out.

New treatment platforms

All current retinal laser treatment platforms were designed to perform high-risk and inherently destructive treatments, such as PC. As the goal of MRT is to avoid the things current lasers are designed to do, current laser platforms are ill-suited to MRT. The low-intensity/high-density treatment paradigm of MRT is also perfectly suited to automation. As noted above, the first retinal treatment system designed expressly to perform MRT is expected in 2024. The ability to perform optimized MRT quickly, easily, safely, and effectively in a uniform fashion without the potential for surgeon error promises to fundamentally alter use of retinal laser treatment going forward in ways that are difficult to overestimate.

Diagnostic testing and treatment thresholds

The coming transformation of treatment for the CPRs has a number of interesting ramifications. One is the role of diagnostic testing. One of the main indications for diagnostic testing is not simply to determine the disease, but to determine if it is in a particular state that justifies the risks of any treatment that might be available. The ability to treat in complete safety, eliminating even the risk of surgeon error, and to treat very quickly, comfortably, and with great ease will make earlier treatment both more desirable for physicians, and more acceptable to patients. Thus, the most common diagnostic tests in the future may be simply questions, such as, "Do you have diabetes?" "Are you over 35 years old?" "Does your child spend too much time on his phone and not enough time outdoors?" The answer of "Yes" to any one of these questions, and others like them, would then be followed by "Please look straight ahead and try not to blink for just a moment. There. Done." A treatment will have been determined to be indicated and then performed just as quickly. By shifting heavily toward effective preventive treatments, the need for and thus the role of diagnostic testing will considerably diminish, as well as the role of expensive, intensive, and invasive treatments of all kinds. Preventive treatment for the CPRs (let us add childhood myopia and aging to the mix as well) will transition from the fraught gravitas of dealing with a precarious and serious medical condition with potentially painful and frightful treatments and grave outcomes, to simple hygiene; something one does on a regular basis to keep things working well and to prevent problems, like a periodic tooth cleaning with the hygienist—but far quicker and more comfortable.

MRT as disruptor

If you have read this far, congratulations. If you started with the Preface and enjoyed a good, derisive laugh, my hope is that my assertion of the importance of MRT no longer seems so absurd.

The effect of the discovery of electricity, and the way its use has come to govern every part of our lives, is profound in the extreme. Compared to a world without electricity (reflect for a moment on the impact of the last brief power outage) its presence in our lives can only be described as disruptive. Thus, while disruption may occur in an instant—Eureka! — at times the full impact of that epiphany may take fruition slowly. Some time has passed since Franklin flew his kite in a storm, to the electrified world it introduced. In its infancy, innovation is never popular. This is because innovation is, by definition, an existential threat to established interests. Resistance is the rule. In ophthalmology, one need only reflect on the histories of iconic innovations like intraocular lenses, phacoemulsification, refractive surgery, and macular hole surgery to see the typical evolution from dismissal, to ridicule, to warm loving embrace (Hull et al 1989, Christiansen 1997, Pandey et al 2004). Expect the same for MRT.

Acknowledgments

The author thanks Nicholas Boucher of Vestrum Health, Inc, for providing data, data mining, filtering and propensity scoring for the real-world data studies; and Gerry Gray, PhD, of Regulatory Pathways, Inc, for the statistical analysis and methods for the real-world data studies on neovascular AMD conversion.

References

Age-Related Eye Disease Study Research Group. A randomized, placebo-controlled, clinical trial of high-dose supplementation with vitamins C and E, beta carotene, and zinc for age-related macular degeneration and vision loss: AREDS report no. 8 [published correction appears in *Arch Ophthalmol.* 2008 Sep;126(9):1251]. *Arch Ophthalmol.* 2001;119(10):1417-1436. doi:10.1001/archopht.119.10.1417

Akduman L, Olk RJ. Subthreshold (invisible) modified grid diode laser photocoagulation in diffuse diabetic macular edema (DDME). *Ophthalmic Surg Lasers.* 1999;30(9):706-714. doi:10.3928/1542-8877-19991101-04.

Akerfelt M, Morimoto RI, Sistonen L. Heat shock factors: integrators of cell stress, development and lifespan. *Nat Rev Mol Cell Biol.* 2010;11(8):545-555.

Al-Barki A, Al-Hijji L, High R, et al. Comparison of short-pulse subthreshold (532 nm) and infrared micropulse (810 nm) macular laser for diabetic macular edema. *Sci Rep.* 2021;11(1):14. doi:10.1038/s41598-020-79699-9.

Al-Ghamdi A, Albiani DA, Hodge WG, Clarke WN. Myopia and astigmatism in retinopathy of prematurity after treatment with cryotherapy or laser photocoagulation. *Can J Ophthalmol.* 2004;39(5):521-525. doi:10.1016/s0008-4182(04)80142-x.

Almanza A, Carlesso A, Chintha C, et al. Endoplasmic reticulum stress signalling – from basic mechanisms to clinical applications. *FEBS J.* 2019;286(2):241-278. doi:10.1111/febs.14608.

Ambati J, Atkinson JP, Gelfand BD. Immunology of age-related macular degeneration. *Nat Rev Immunol.* 2013;13(6):438-451.

American Association of Ophthalmology. Preferred Practice Patterns; 2021. https://www.aao.org/education/summary-benchmark-detail/summary-benchmarks-full-set-2020

American National Standards Institute. *American National Standard for the Safe use of Lasers, ANSI Z136.1-2000.* American National Standards Institute; 2000.

American Society of Retina Specialists. Preferences and Trends Survey; 2021.

Amoaku WM, Ghanchi F, Bailey C, et al. Diabetic retinopathy and diabetic macular oedema pathways and management: UK Consensus Working Group. *Eye (Lond).* 2020;34(suppl 1):1-51. doi:10.1038/s41433-020-0961-6.

Anglemyer A, Horvath HT, Bero L. Healthcare outcomes assessed with observational study designs compared with those assessed in randomized trials. *Cochrane Database Syst Rev.* 2014;2014(4):MR000034. doi:10.1002/14651858.MR000034.pub2.

Arden GB, Vaegan, Hogg CR. Clinical and experimental evidence that the pattern electroretinogram (PERG) is generated in more proximal retinal layers than the focal electroretinogram (FERG). *Ann N Y Acad Sci.* 1982;388:580-607. doi:10.1111/j.1749-6632.1982.tb50818.x.

Asea A, Kraeft SK, Kurt-Jones EA, Stevenson MA, Chen LB, Finberg RW, et al. HSP70 stimulates cytokine production through a CD14-dependant pathway, demonstrating its dual role as a chaperone and cytokine. *Nat Med.* 2000;6(4):435-442.

Austin PC, Stuart EA. Moving towards best practice when using inverse probability of treatment weighting (IPTW) using the propensity score to estimate causal treatment effects in observational studies. *Stat Med.* 2015;34(28):3661-3679. doi:10.1002/sim.6607

Avci P, Gupta A, Sadasivam M, et al. Low-level laser (light) therapy (LLLT) in skin: stimulating, healing, restoring. *Semin Cutan Med Surg.* 2013;32:41-52.

Bacon F. *Novum Organnum.* Devey J, ed. P. F. Collier & Sons; 1902.

Baker A. "Simplicity". *Stanford Encyclopedia of Philosophy.* California: Stanford University; 2010 (2004). ISSN 1095-5054.

Baldwin RL. Energetics of protein folding. *J Mol Biol.* 2007; 371:283-301. doi:10.1016/j.jmb.2007.05.078.

Banach M, Konieczny L, Roterman I. Secondary and supersecondary structure of proteins in light of the structure of hydrophobic cores. *Methods Mol Biol.* 2019;1958:347-378. doi:10.1007/978-1-4939-9161-7_19.

Bandello F, Brancato R, Menchini U, et al. Light panretinal photocoagulation (LPRP) versus classic panretinal photocoagulation (CPRP) in proliferative diabetic retinopathy. *Semin Ophthalmol.* 2001;16(1):12-18. doi:10.1076/soph.16.1.12.4223

Bandello F, Brancato R, Trabucchi G, Lattanzio R, Malegori A. Diode vs argon green laser panretinal photocoagulation in proliferative diabetic retinopathy: a prospective study in 44 eyes with long follow-up time. *Graefes Arch Clin Exp Ophthalmol.* 1993;231(9):491-494. doi:10.1007/BF00921112.

Banitt MR, Ventura LM, Feuer WJ, et al. Progressive loss of retinal ganglion cell function precedes structural loss by several years in glaucoma suspects. *Invest Ophthalmol Vis Sci.* 2013;54(3):2346-2352. doi:10.1167/iovs.12-11026.

Barnes J, ed. Aristotle, Physics. Translated in *The Complete Works of Aristotle*, Volume 1. The Revised Oxford Translation. Princeton University Press; 2014.

Barth K. *The Epistle to the Romans (Der Römerbrief. Zweite Fassung, 1922).* Hoskyns EC, trans. Oxford University Press; 1933, 1968.

Battaglia PM, Iacono P. Re: van Dijk et al.: Half-dose photodynamic therapy versus high-density subthreshold micropulse laser treatment in patients with chronic central serous chorioretinopathy: the PLACE trial (Ophthalmology. 2018;125:1547-1555). *Ophthalmology.* 2019;126(4):e29-e30. doi:10.1016/j.ophtha.2018.11.004.

Beckham JT. *The Role of Heat Shock Protein 70 in Laser Irradiation and Thermal Preconditioning*. PhD dissertation. Vanderbilt University Press; 2008.

Berbudi A, Rahmadika N, Tjahjadi AI, Ruslami R. Type 2 diabetes and its impact on the immune system. *Curr Diabetes Rev*. 2020;16(5):442-449. doi:10.2174/1573399815666191024085838.

Berman MH, Nichols TW. Treatment of neurodegeneration: integrating photobiomodulation and neurofeedback in Alzheimer's dementia and Parkinson's: a review. *Photobiomodul Photomed Laser Surg*. 2019;37(10):623-634. doi:10.1089/photob.2019.4685.

Blau HM, Daley GQ. Stem cells in the treatment of disease *N Engl J Med*. 2019;380:1748-1760. doi:10.1056/NEJMra1716145.

Bloom, A. The Closing of the American Mind: How Higher Education Has Failed Democracy and Impoverished the Souls of Today's Students. New York: Simon & Schuster; 1987. ISBN 978-0-671-47990-9.

Blumenkranz MS. The evolution of laser therapy in ophthalmology: a perspective on photons, patients, physicians and physics: the LXX Edward Jackson Memorial Lecture. *Am J Ophthalmol*. 2014;158(1):1-25. doi:10.1016/j.ajo.2014.03.013.

Bosco A, Crish SD, Steele MR, et al. Early reduction of microglia activation by irradiation in a model of chronic glaucoma. *PLoS One*. 2012;7(8):e43602. doi:10.1371/journal.pone.0043602.

Boswell J. *The Life of Samuel Johnson*. Hibbert C, ed. Penguin Classics; 1986.

Bourne RR, Stevens GA, White RA, et al; Vision Loss Expert Group. Causes of vision loss worldwide, 1990-2010: a systematic analysis. *Lancet Glob Health*. 2013;1:339-349. doi:10.1016/S2214-109X(13)70113-X.

Brader HS, Young LH. Subthreshold diode micropulse laser: a review. *Semin Ophthalmol*. 2016;31(1-2):30-39. doi:10.3109/08820538.2015.1114837.

Brain P. *Galen on Bloodletting: A Study of the Origins, Development, and Validity of His Opinions, with a Translation of the Three Works*. Cambridge University Press; 1986:1.

Brandvold KR, Morimoto RI. The chemical biology of molecular chaperones--implications for modulation of proteostasis. *J Mol Biol*. 2015;427(18):2931-2947. doi:10.1016/j.jmb.2015.05.010.

Bressler NM, Beck RW, Ferris FL 3rd. Panretinal photocoagulation for proliferative diabetic retinopathy. *N Engl J Med*. 2011;365(16):1520-1526. doi:10.1056/NEJMct0908432

Bressler SB, Ayala AR, Bressler NM, et al; for the Diabetic Retinopathy Clinical Research Network. Persistent macular thickening after ranibizumab treatment for diabetic macular edema with vision impairment. *JAMA Ophthalmol*. 2016;134(3):278-285. doi:10.1001/jamaophthalmol.2015.5346.

Brooks F. Marci Tullii Ciceronis; De Natura Deorum. Methuen & Company; 1896.

Brown DM, Nguyen QD, Marcus DM, et al; RIDE and RISE Research Group. Long-term outcomes of ranibizumab therapy for diabetic macular edema: the 36-month results from two phase III trials: RISE and RIDE. *Ophthalmology*. 2013;120(10):2013-2022. doi:10.1016/j.ophtha.2013.02.034.

Burton DGA, Faragher RGA. Obesity and type-2 diabetes as inducers of premature cellular senescence and ageing. *Biogerontology*. 2018;19(6):447-459. doi:10.1007/s10522-018-9763-7.

Caballero S, Kent DL, Sengupta N, et al. Bone marrow-derived cell recruitment to the neurosensory retina and retinal pigment epithelial cell layer following subthreshold retinal phototherapy. *Invest Ophthalmol Vis Sci*. 2017;58(12):5164-5176. doi:10.1167/iovs.16-20736.

Caesar CJ. *The Gallic War* 7.78.3.1. Digital version in the Packard Humanities Institute Latin Texts online: O. Seel (ed.), C. Iuli Caesaris commentarii rerum gestarum, Bibliotheca scriptorum Graecorum et Romanorum Teubneriana, Lipsiae; 1961.

Cao Y, Langer R. A review of Judah Folkman's remarkable achievements in biomedicine. *Proc Natl Acad Sci U S A*. 2008;105(36):1320-13205. doi:10.1073/pnas.0806582105.

Casson RJ, Raymond G, Newland HS, Gilhotra JS, Gray TL. Pilot randomized trial of a nanopulse retinal laser versus conventional photocoagulation for the treatment of diabetic macular oedema. *Clin Exp Ophthalmol*. 2012;40(6):604-610. doi:10.1111/j.1442-9071.2012.02756.x

Celebi AR, Mirza GE. Age-related change in retinal nerve fiber layer thickness measured with spectral domain optical coherence tomography. *Invest Ophthalmol Vis Sci*. 2013;54(13):8095-8103. doi:10.1167/iovs.13-12634.

Celkova L, Doyle SL, Campbell M. NLRP3 Inflammasome and Pathobiology in AMD. *J Clin Med*. 2015;4(1):172-192.

Chalmin F, Ladoire S, Mignot G, Vincent J, Bruchard M, Remy-Martin JP, et al. Membrane-associated Hsp72 from tumor-derived exosomes mediates STAT3-dependent immunosuppressive function of mouse and human myeloid-derived suppressor cells. *J Clin Invest*. 2010;120(2):457-471.

Chang DB, Luttrull JK. Comparison of subthreshold 577nm and 810nm micropulse laser effects on heat-shock protein activation kinetics: implications for treatment efficacy and safety. *Transl Vis Sci Tecnol*. 2020;9(5):23. doi:10.1167/tvst.9.5.23.

Charette SJ, Lavoie JN, Lambert H, Landry J. Inhibition of Daxx-mediated apoptosis by heat shock protein 27. *Mol Cell Biol*. 2000;20(20):7602-7612.

Chen G, Tzekov R, Li W, Jiang F, Mao S, Tong Y. Subthreshold micropulse diode laser versus conventional laser photocoagulation for diabetic macular edema: a meta-analysis of randomized controlled clinical trials. *Retina*. 2016;36(11):2059-2065. doi:10.1097/IAE.0000000000001053.

Chen SN, Hwang JF, Tseng LF, Lin CJ. Subthreshold diode micropulse photocoagulation for the treatment of chronic central serous chorioretinopathy with juxtafoveal leakage. *Ophthalmology*. 2008;115:2229-2234.

Chhablani J, Ong J, Rajendran A, et al. Subthreshold laser guidelines for retinal diseases. Eye. 2022;36(12):2234-2235. doi:10.1038/s41433-022-02136-w.

Chhablani J, Roh YJ, Jobling AI, et al. Restorative retinal laser therapy: present state and future directions. *Surv Ophthalmol*. 2018;63(3):307-328. doi:10.1016/j.survophthal.2017.09.008.

Chiang JF, Sun MH, Chen KJ, et al. Association with obstructive sleep apnea and diabetic macular edema in patients with type 2 diabetes. *Am J Ophthalmol*. 2021;226:217-225. doi:10.1016/j.ajo.2021.01.022.

Chidlow G, Shibeeb O, Plunkett M, Casson RJ, Wood JP. Glial cell and inflammatory responses to retinal laser treatment: comparison of a conventional photocoagulator and a novel, 3-nanosecond pulse laser. *Invest Ophthalmol Vis Sci*. 2013;54(3):2319-2332. Published 2013 Mar 28. doi:10.1167/iovs.12-11204

Christiansen C. *The Innovator's Dilemma*. 1st ed. Harvard Business Review Press; 1997.

Cicinelli MV, Cavalleri M, Querques L, Rabiolo A, Bandello F, Querques G. Early response to ranibizumab predictive of functional outcome after dexamethasone for unresponsive diabetic macular edema. *Br J Ophthalmol*. 2017;101(12):1689-1693. doi:10.1136/bjophthalmol-2017-310242.

Cimberle M. ASRS' ASRS' Global Trends survey shows growing homogeneity of retina treatment, part 1. *Ocul Surg News*, Feb 25, 2021

Citirik M. The impact of central foveal thickness on the efficacy of subthreshold micropulse yellow laser photocoagulation in diabetic macular edema. *Lasers Med Sci*. 2019;34(5):907-912. doi:10.1007/s10103-018-2672-9

Ciulla TA, Huang F, Westby K, Williams DF, Zaveri S, Patel SC. Real-world outcomes of anti-vascular endothelial growth factor therapy in neovascular age-related macular degeneration in the United States. *Ophthalmol Retina*. 2018;2:645-653. doi:10.1016/j.oret.2018.01.006.

Ciulla TA, Hussain RM, Pollack JS, Williams DF. Visual acuity outcomes and anti-vascular endothelial growth factor therapy intensity in neovascular age-related macular degeneration patients. A real-world analysis of 49, 485 eyes. *Ophthalmol Retina*. 2019;4(1):19-30. doi:10.1016/j.oret.2019.05.017.

Clark RAF. Wound repair: overview and general considerations. In: Clark RAF, ed. *The Molecular and Cellular Biology of Wound Repair*. 2nd ed. Plenum; 1996:1-50.

Cohen LH, Noell WK. Relationships between visual function and metabolism. In: Graymore CN, ed. *Biochemistry of the Retina*. Fla Academic Press Inc; 1965:36-50.

Colijn JM, Buitendijk GHS, Prokofyeva E, et al. Prevalence of Age-Related Macular Degeneration in Europe: The Past and the Future. *Ophthalmology*. 2017;124(12):1753-1763. doi:10.1016/j.ophtha.2017.05.035

Cover TM, Thomas JA. *Elements of Information Theory*. John Wiley and Sons; 2006:254.

Dal Bó E. Regulatory capture: a review. *Oxford Rev Econ Policy*. 2006;22(2):203-225. doi:10.1093/oxrep/grj013.

Davis BK, Ting JP. NLRP3 has a sweet tooth. *Nat Immunol*. 2010;11(2):105-106.

Dayalan Naidu S, Kostov RV, Dinkova-Kostova AT. Transcription factors Hsf1 and Nrf2 engage in crosstalk for cytoprotection. *Trends Pharmacol Sci*. 2015;36(1):6-14.

Dayeh MA, Livadiotis G, Aminian F, et al. Effects of Cholesterol in Stress-Related Neuronal Death-A Statistical Analysis Perspective. *Int J Mol Sci*. 2020;21(8):2905. Published 2020 Apr 21. doi:10.3390/ijms21082905

De Cillà S, Vezzola D, Farruggio S, et al. The subthreshold micropulse laser treatment of the retina restores the oxidant/antioxidant balance and counteracts programmed forms of cell death in the mice eyes. *Acta Ophthalmol*. 2019;97(4):e559-e567. doi:10.1111/aos.13995.

de Pedro-Cuesta J, Rábano A, Martínez-Martín P, Ruiz-Tovar M, Alcalde-Cabero E, Almazán-Isla J, et al. Comparative Incidence of Conformational, Neurodegenerative Disorders. *PLoS One*. 2015;10(9):e0137342.

Dennett D. Darwin's *Dangerous Idea* and the *Meanings of Life*. Simon and Shuster; 1995.

Diabetic Retinopathy Clinical Research Network. Randomized trial evaluating ranibizumab plus prompt or deferred laser or triamcinolone plus prompt laser for diabetic macular edema. *Ophthalmology*. 2010;117(6):1064-1077.e35. doi:10.1016/j.ophtha.2010.02.031.

Diabetic Retinopathy Study Research Group. Photocoagulation treatment of proliferative diabetic retinopathy: the second report of Diabetic Retinopathy Study (DRS) findings. *Ophthalmology*. 1978;85:82-106. doi:10.1016/S0161-6420(78)35693-1.

Dorin G. Subthreshold and micropulse diode laser photocoagulation. *Semin Ophthalmol*. 2003;18:147-153. doi:10.1076/soph.18.3.147.29812.

Doyle SL, Campbell M, Ozaki E, Salomon RG, Mori A, Kenna PF, et al. NLRP3 has a protective role in age-related macular degeneration through the induction of IL-18 by drusen components. *Nat Med*. 2012;18(5):791-798.

Dudega V, Vickers SM, Saluja AK. The role of heat shock proteins in gastrointestinal disease. *Gut*. 2009;58(7):1000-1009. doi:10.1136/gut.2007.140194.

Early photocoagulation for diabetic retinopathy. ETDRS report number 9. Early Treatment Diabetic Retinopathy Study Research Group. *Ophthalmol*. 1991;98(5 Suppl):766-785.

Early Treatment Diabetic Retinopathy Study Research Group. Photocoagulation for diabetic macular edema. Early treatment diabetic retinopathy study report number 1. *Arch Ophthalmol*. 1985;103:1796-1806. doi:10.1001/archopht.1985.01050120030015.

Edelstein L. The Hippocratic Oath: Text, Translation and Interpretation. John Hopkins Press; 1943;56.

Edington M, Connolly J, Chong NV. Pharmacokinetics of intravitreal anti-VEGF drugs in vitrectomized versus non-vitrectomized eyes. *Expert Opin Drug Metab Toxicol*. 2017;13(12):1217-1224. doi:10.1080/17425255.2017.1404987

Eng VA, Leng T. Subthreshold laser therapy for macular edema due to branch retinal vein occlusion: a focused review. *Br J Ophthalmol*. 2020;104(9):1184-1189. doi:10.1136/bjophthalmol-2019-315192.

Enomoto Y, Bharti A, Khaleque AA, Song B, Liu C, Apostolopoulos V, et al. Enhanced immunogenicity of heat shock protein 70 peptide complexes from dendritic cell-tumor fusion cells. *J Immunol*. 2006;177(9):5946-5955.

Enríquez AB, Baumal CR, Crane AM, et al. Early experience with Brolucizumab treatment of neovascular age-related macular degeneration. *JAMA Ophthalmol*. 2021;139(4):441-448. doi:10.1001/jamaophthalmol.2020.7085.

Eshtiaghi A, Issa M, Popovic MM, Muni RH, Kertes PJ. Geographic atrophy incidence and progression after intravitreal injections of anti-vascular endothelial growth factor agents for age-related macular degeneration: a meta-analysis. *Retina*. 2021;41(12):2424-2435. doi:10.1097/IAE.0000000000003207.

Facciponte JG, MacDonald IJ, Wang XY, Kim H, Manjili MH, Subjeck JR. Heat shock proteins and scavenger receptors: role in adaptive immune responses. *Immunologic Investig*. 2005;34(3):325-342.

Feigl B, Cao D, Morris CP, Zele AJ. Persons with age-related maculopathy risk genotypes and clinically normal eyes have reduced mesopic vision. *Invest Ophthalmol Vis Sci*. 2011;52(2):1145-1150. doi:10.1167/iovs.10-5967.

Figueira J, Khan J, Nunes S, et al. Prospective randomised controlled trial comparing sub-threshold micropulse diode laser photocoagulation and conventional green laser for clinically significant diabetic macular oedema. *Br J Ophthalmol*. 2009;93:1341-1344. doi:10.1136/bjo.2008.146712.

Flaxel C, Bradle J, Acott T, Samples JR. Retinal pigment epithelium produces matrix metalloproteinases after laser treatment. *Retina*. 2007;27:629-634. doi:10.1097/01.iae.0000249561.02567.fd.

Flaxman SR, Bourne RRA, Resnikoff S, et al; Vision Loss Expert Group of the Global Burden of Disease Study. Global causes of blindness and distance vision impairment 1990-2020: a systematic review and meta-analysis. *Lancet Glob Health*. 2017;5(12):e1221-e1234. doi:10.1016/S2214-109X(17)30393-5.

Fong DS, Aiello L, Gardner TW, et al; American Diabetes Association. Diabetic retinopathy. *Diabetes Care*. 2003;26(suppl 1):S99-S102. doi:10.2337/diacare.26.2007.s99.

Fong DS, Strauber SF, Aiello LP, et al. Comparison of the modified early treatment diabetic retinopathy study and mild macular grid laser photocoagulation strategies for diabetic macular edema. *Arch Ophthalmol*. 2007;125(4):469-480. doi:10.1001/archopht.125.4.469.

Franceschi C, Bonafe M, Valensin S, et al. An evolutionary perspective on immunosenescence. *Ann N Y Acad Sci*. 2000;908:244-254. doi:10.1111/j.1749-6632.2000.tb06651.x.

Franceschi C, Campisi J. Chronic inflammation (inflammaging) and its potential contribution to age-associated diseases. *J Gerontol A Biol Sci Med Sci*. 2014;69 Suppl 1:S4-S9.

Friberg TR, Venkatesh S. Alteration of pulse configuration affects the pain response during diode laser photocoagulation. *Lasers Surg Med*. 1995;16(4):380-383. doi:10.1002/lsm.1900160409.

Friedlander R, Jarosch E, Urban J, Volkwein C, Sommer T. A regulatory link between ER-associated protein degradation and the unfolded-protein response. *Nat Cell Biol*. 2000;2(7):379-384. doi:10.1038/35017001.

Frizziero L, Calciati A, Midena G, et al. Subthreshold micropulse laser modulates retinal neuroinflammatory biomarkers in diabetic macular edema. *J Clin Med*. 2021;10(14):3134. doi:10.3390/jcm10143134.

Frizziero L, Calciati A, Torresin T, et al. Diabetic macular edema treated with 577-nm subthreshold micropulse laser: a real-life, long-term study. *J Pers Med*. 2021;11(5):405. doi:10.3390/jpm11050405.

Fukuda S, Nagano M, Yamashita T, et al. Functional endothelial progenitor cells selectively recruit neurovascular protective monocyte-derived F4/80(+) /Ly6c(+) macrophages in a mouse model of retinal degeneration. *Stem Cells*. 2013;31(10):2149-2161. doi:10.1002/stem.1469

Fulop T, Larbi A, Dupuis G, Le Page A, Frost EH, Cohen AA, et al. Immunosenescence and Inflamm-Aging As Two Sides of the Same Coin: Friends or Foes? *Front Immunol*. 2017;8:1960.

Gabai VL, Mabuchi K, Mosser DD, Sherman MY. Hsp72 and stress kinase c-jun N-terminal kinase regulate the bid-dependent pathway in tumor necrosis factor-induced apoptosis. *Mol Cell Biol*. 2002;22(10):3415-3424.

Gao X, Xing, D. Molecular mechanisms of cell proliferation induced by low power laser irradiation. *J Biomed Sci*. 2009;16:4. doi:10.1186/1423-0127-16-4.

Gawęcki M, Jaszczuk-Maciejewska A, Jurska-Jaśko A, Grzybowski A. Functional and morphological outcome in patients with chronic central serous chorioretinopathy treated by subthreshold micropulse laser. *Graefes Arch Clin Exp Ophthalmol*. 2017;255(12):2299-2306. doi:10.1007/s00417-017-3783-x.

Gawęcki M, Jaszczuk-Maciejewska A, Jurska-Jaśko A, Kneba M, Grzybowski A. Impairment of visual acuity and retinal morphology following resolved chronic central serous chorioretinopathy. *BMC Ophthalmol*. 2019;19(1):160. doi:10.1186/s12886-019-1171-5.

Gawęcki M, Jaszczuk-Maciejewska A, Jusrka-Jaśko A, Kneba M, Grzybowski A. Transfoveal micropulse laser treatment of central serous chorioretinopathy within six months of disease onset. *J Clin Med*. 2019;8:1398. doi:10.3390/jcm8091398.

GBD 2019 Blindness and Vision Impairment Collaborators; Vision Loss Expert Group of the Global Burden of Disease Study. Causes of blindness and vision impairment in 2020 and trends over 30 years, and prevalence of avoidable blindness in relation to VISION 2020: the Right to Sight: an analysis for the Global Burden of Disease Study [published correction appears in Lancet Glob Health. 2021 Apr;9(4):e408]. *Lancet Glob Health*. 2021;9(2):e144-e160. doi:10.1016/S2214-109X(20)30489-7

Gitter KA, ed. *Laser Photocoagulation of Retinal Disease*. Pacific Medical Press; 1989.

Glassman AR, Baker CW, Beaulieu WT, et al; DRCR Retina Network. Assessment of the DRCR retina network approach to management with initial observation for eyes with center-involved diabetic macular edema and good visual acuity: a secondary analysis of a randomized clinical trial. *JAMA Ophthalmol*. 2020;138(4):341-349. doi:10.1001/jamaophthalmol.2019.6035.

Glassman AR, Wells JA 3RD, Josic K, et al; for the Diabetic Retinopathy Clinical Research Network. Five-year outcomes after initial aflibercept, bevacizumab, or ranibizumab treatment for diabetic macular edema (Protocol T Extension Study). *Ophthalmol*. 2020;127(9):1201-1210. doi:10.1001/jamaophthalmol.2019.6035.

Goldberg MF, Jampol LM. Knowledge of diabetic retinopathy before and 18 years after the Airlie House Symposium on Treatment of Diabetic Retinopathy. *Ophthalmol*. 1987 Jul;94(7):741-6. doi:10.1016/s0161-6420(87)33524-9. PMID: 2889177.

Gong J, Zhu B, Murshid A, Adachi H, Song B, Lee A, et al. T cell activation by heat shock protein 70 vaccine requires TLR signaling and scavenger receptor expressed by endothelial cells-1. *J Immunol*. 2009;183(5):3092-3098.

Gotoh T, Terada K, Oyadomari S, Mori M. hsp70-DnaJ chaperone pair prevents nitric oxide- and CHOP-induced apoptosis by inhibiting translocation of Bax to mitochondria. *Cell Death Differ*. 2004;11(4):390-402.

Greenhouse JB. Commentary: cornfield, epidemiology and causality. *Int J Epidemiol*. 2009;38(5):1199-1201. doi:10.1093/ije/dyp299. Epub 2009 Sep 22.

Gross JG, Glassman AR, Jampol LM, et al. Writing committee for the Diabetic Research Clinical Network. Panretinal Photocoagulation vs Intravitreous Ranibizumab for Proliferative Diabetic Retinopathy: a randomized clinical trial [published correction appears in *JAMA*. 2016 Mar 1;315(9):944] [published correction appears in *JAMA*. 2019 Mar 12;321(10):1008]. *JAMA*. 2015;314(20):2137-2146. doi:10.1001/jama.2015.15217.

Guo C, Subjeck JR, Wang XY. Creation of Recombinant Chaperone Vaccine Using Large Heat Shock Protein for Antigen-Targeted Cancer Immunotherapy. *Methods Mol Biol (Clifton, NJ)*. 2018;1709:345-357.

Gurbuxani S, Schmitt E, Cande C, Parcellier A, Hammann A, Daugas E, et al. Heat shock protein 70 binding inhibits the nuclear import of apoptosis-inducing factor. *Oncogene*. 2003;22(43):6669-6678.

Gutstein W, Sinclair SH, Presti P, North RV. Interactive thresholding of central acuity under contrast and luminance conditions mimicking real world environments: 1, evaluation against LogMAR charts. *J Comput Sci Syst Biol*. 2015;8:225-232. doi:10.4172/jcsb.1000193.

Guymer RH, Wu Z, Hodgson LAB, et al. Laser intervention in early stages of age-related macular degeneration study group. Subthreshold nanosecond laser intervention for age-related macular degeneration: the LEAD randomized controlled clinical trial. *Ophthalmology*. 2018;126(6):829-838. doi:10.1016/j.ophtha.2018.09.015.

Halawa OA, Lin JB, Miller JW, Vavvas DG. A review of completed and ongoing complement inhibitor trials for geographic atrophy secondary to age-related macular degeneration. *J Clin Med*. 2021;10(12):2580. doi:10.3390/jcm10122580.

Hall J, Matos S, Gold S, Severino LS. The paradox of sustainable innovation: the 'Eroom' effect (Moore's law backwards). *J Clean Prod*. 2018;172:3487-3497. doi:10.1016/j.jclepro.2017.07.162.

Hamada M, Ohkoshi K, Inagaki K, Ebihara N, Murakami A. Subthreshold Photocoagulation Using Endpoint Management in the PASCAL® System for Diffuse Diabetic Macular Edema. *J Ophthalmol*. 2018;7465794. Published 2018 Jan 31. doi:10.1155/2018/7465794

Han S, Chen J, Hua J, Hu X, Jian S, Zheng G, et al. MITF protects against oxidative damage-induced retinal degeneration by regulating the NRF2 pathway in the retinal pigment epithelium. *Redox Biol*. 2020;34:101537.

Hattenbach LO, Beck KF, Pfeilschifter J, Koch F, Ohrloff C, Schake W. Pigment epithelium-derived factor is up regulated in photocoagulated human retinal pigment epithelial cells. *Ophthalmic Res*. 2005;37:341-346. doi:10.1159/000088263.

Hawkes N. Cancer survival data emphasise importance of early diagnosis. *BMJ*. 2019;364:l408. doi:10.1136/bmj.l408.

Hayreh SS. Photocoagulation for retinal vein occlusion. *Prog Ret Eye Res*. 2021;85:100964. doi:10.1016/j.preteyeres.2021.100964.

Hayreh SS. Photocoagulation for retinal vein occlusion. *Prog Retin Eye Res*. 2021;85:100964. doi:10.1016/j.preteyeres.2021.100964

Hennig P, Garstkiewicz M, Grossi S, Di Filippo M, French LE, Beer HD. The Crosstalk between Nrf2 and Inflammasomes. *Int J Mol Sci*. 2018;19(2).6.186

Hetz C, Zhang K, Kaufman RJ. Mechanisms, regulation and functions of the unfolded protein response. *Nat Rev Mol Cell Biol*. 2020;21(8):421-438. doi:10.1038/s41580-020-0250-z

Hiller MM, Finger A, Schweiger M, Wolf DH. ER degradation of a misfolded luminal protein by the cytosolic ubiquitin-proteasome pathway. *Science*. 1996;273(5282):1725-1728. doi:10.1126/science.273.5282.1725

Hirji SH, Hood DC, Leibmann JM, Blumberg DM. Association of patterns of glaucomatous macular damage with contrast sensitivity and facial recognition in patients with glaucoma. *JAMA Ophthalmol*. 2021;139(1):27-32. doi:10.1001/jamaophthalmol.2020.4749.

Holmström KM, Baird L, Zhang Y, Hargreaves I, Chalasani A, Land JM, et al. Nrf2 impacts cellular bioenergetics by controlling substrate availability for mitochondrial respiration. *Biol Open*. 2013;2(8):761-770.

Holz FG, Sadda SR, Busbee B, et al; Chroma and Spectri Study Investigators. Efficacy and safety of Lampalizumab for geographic atrophy due to age-related macular degeneration: chroma and spectri phase 3 randomized clinical trials. *JAMA Ophthalmol*. 2018;136(6):666-677. doi:10.1001/jamaophthalmol.2018.1544.

Howell GR, Soto I, Libby RT, John SW. Intrinsic axonal degeneration pathways are critical for glaucomatous damage. *Exp Neurol*. 2013;246:54-61. doi:10.1016/j.expneurol.2012.01.014. Epub 2012 Jan 18. PMID: 22285251; PMCID: PMC3831512.

Hull DL, Tessner PD, Diamond AM. Planck's Principle. *Science*. 1978;202(4369):717-723. doi:10.1126/science.202.4369.717.

Inagaki K, Shuo T, Katakura K, Ebihara N, Murakami A, Ohkoshi K. Sublethal photothermal stimulation with a micropulse laser induces heat shock protein expression in ARPE-19 cells. *J Ophthalmol*. 2015;2015:729792. doi:10.1155/2015/729792.

Iwami H, Pruessner J, Shariaki K, Brinkmann R, Miura Y. Protective effect of a laser-induced sub-lethal temperature rise on RPE cells from oxidative stress. *Exp Eye Res*. 2014;124:37-47. doi:10.1016/j.exer.2014.04.014.

Jackson GR, Scott IU, Kim IK, Quillen DA, Iannaccone A, Edwards JG. Diagnostic sensitivity and specificity of dark adaptometry for detection of age-related macular degeneration. *Invest Ophthalmol Vis Sci*. 2014;55(3):1427-1431. doi:10.1167/iovs.13-13745.

Jampol LM, Bressler NM, Glassman AR. Revolution to a new standard treatment of diabetic macular edema. *JAMA*. 2014;311(22):2269-2270. doi:10.1001/jama.2014.2536.

Jaynes ET. *Probability Theory: The Logic of Science*. Cambridge University Press; 2003:592-593.

Jhang JJ, Yen GC. The role of Nrf2 in NLRP3 inflammasome activation. *Cell Mol Immunol*. 2017;14(12):1011-1012.

Jhingan M, Goud A, Peguda HK, Khodani M, Luttrull JK, Chhablani J. Subthreshold microsecond laser for proliferative diabetic retinopathy: a randomized pilot study. *Clin Ophthalmol*. 2018;12:141-145. doi:10.2147/OPTH.S143206.

Johnson TV, Polo AD, Sahel JA, Schuman JS. Neuroprotection, Neuroenhancement, and Neuroregeneration of the Retina and Optic Nerve. *Ophthalmol Sci*. 2022;2(3):100216. Published 2022 Sep 5. doi:10.1016/j.xops.2022.100216

Jonasson F, Arnarsson A, Eiríksdottir G, et al. Prevalence of age-related macular degeneration in old persons: Age, Gene/environment Susceptibility Reykjavik Study. *Ophthalmology*. 2011;118(5):825-830. doi:10.1016/j.ophtha.2010.08.044

Jorge EC, Jorge EN, Botelho M, Farat JG, Virgili G, El Dib R. Monotherapy laser photocoagulation for diabetic macular oedema. *Cochrane Database Syst Rev*. 2018;10(10):CD010859. doi:10.1002/14651858.CD010859.pub2.

Joussen AM, Poulaki V, Le ML, et al. A central role for inflammation in the pathogenesis of diabetic retinopathy. *FASEB J*. 2004;18(12):1450-1452. doi:10.1096/fj.03-1476fje

Jupiter DC. Propensity score matching: retrospective randomization? *J Foot Ankle Surg*. 2017;56(2):417-420. doi:10.1053/j.jfas.2017.01.013.

Karlawish J, Grill JD. The approval of Aduhelm risks eroding public trust in Alzheimer research and the FDA. *Nat Rev Neurol*. 2021;17(9):523-524. doi:10.1038/s41582-021-00540-6.

Karouta C, Kucharski R, Hardy K, et al. Transcriptome-based insights into gene networks controlling myopia prevention. *FASEB J*. 2021;35(9):e21846. doi:10.1096/fj.202100350RR.

Karu T. Photobiology of low-power laser effects. *Health Phys*. 1989;56(5):691-704. doi:10.1097/00004032-198905000-00015

Karu TI, Kolyakov SF. Exact action spectra for cellular responses relevant to phototherapy. *Photomed Laser Surg*. 2005;23:355-361. doi:10.1089/pho.2005.23.355.

Katsumata M. Influence of enzyme activators and inhibitors, present in an enzyme preparation, on the relations between reaction rate and enzyme concentration. *J Theor Biol*. 1969;24(3):294-306. doi:10.1016/s0022-5193(69)80054-8

Katz G, Levkovitch-Verbin H, Treister G, Belkin M, Ilany J, Polat U. Mesopic foveal contrast sensitivity is impaired in diabetic patients without retinopathy. *Graefes Arch Clin Exp Ophthalmol*. 2010;248(12):1699-1703. doi:10.1007/s00417-010-1413-y.

Kauppinen A, Niskanen H, Suuronen T, Kinnunen K, Salminen A, Kaarniranta K. Oxidative stress activates NLRP3 inflammasomes in ARPE-19 cells—implications for age-related macular degeneration (AMD). *Immunol Letters.* 2012;147(1-2):29-33.

Kellert SH. In the Wake of Chaos: Unpredictable Order in Dynamical Systems. University of Chicago Press; 1993.

Kensler TW, Wakabayashi N, Biswal S. Cell survival responses to environmental stresses via the Keap1-Nrf2-ARE pathway. *Annu Rev Pharmacol Toxicol.* 2007;47:89-116.

Kent D, Sheridan C. Choroidal neovascularization: a wound healing perspective. *Mol Vis.* 2003;9:747-755.

Kent D. The pathogenesis of age-related macular degeneration is not inflammatory mediated but is instead due to immunosenescence-related failure of tissue repair. *Med Hypotheses.* 2021;146:110392. doi:10.1016/j.mehy.2020.110392.

Kent D. The stereotypical molecular cascade in neovascular age-related macular degeneration: the role of dynamic reciprocity. *Eye (Lond).* 2015;29(11):1416-1426. doi:10.1038/eye.2015.140

Kern K, Mertineit CL, Brinkmann R, Miura Y. Expression of heat shock protein 70 and cell death kinetics after different thermal impacts on cultured retinal pigment epithelial cells. *Exp Eye Res.* 2018;170:117-126. doi:10.1016/j.exer.2018.02.013.

Keunen JEE, Battaglia-Parodi M, Vujosevic S, Luttrull JK. International retinal laser society guidelines for subthreshold laser treatment. *Transl Vis Sci Technol.* 2020;9(9):15. doi:10.1167/tvst.9.9.15.

Khetarpal S, Kaw U, Dover JS, Arndt KA. Laser advances in the treatment of burn and traumatic scars. *Semin Cutan Med Surg.* 2017;36(4):185-191. doi:10.12788/j.sder.2017.030.

Kiffin R, Christian C, Knecht E, Cuervo AM. Activation of chaperone-mediated autophagy during oxidative stress. *Mol Biol Cell.* 2004;15(11):4829-4840. doi:10.1091/mbc.e04-06-0477

Kim JE, Glassman AR, Josic K, et al; DRCR Retina Network. A randomized trial of Photobiomodulation Therapy for center-involved diabetic macular edema with good visual acuity (Protocol AE). *Ophthalmol Retina.* 2022;6(4):298-307. doi:10.1016/j.oret.2021.10.003.

Klein R, Klein BE, Tomany SC, Meuer SM, Huang GH. Ten-year incidence and progression of age-related maculopathy: The Beaver Dam eye study. *Ophthalmology.* 2002;109(10):1767-1779. doi:10.1016/s0161-6420(02)01146-6

Kohner EM, Hamilton AM, Joplin GF, Fraser TR. Florid diabetic retinopathy and its response to treatment by photocoagulation or pituitary ablation. *Diabetes.* 1976 Feb;25(2):104-110. doi:10.2337/diab.25.2.104. PMID: 1248671

Kolomyer AM, Zarbin MA. Trophic factors in the pathogenesis and therapy for retinal degenerative diseases. *Surv Ophthalmol.* 2014;59:135-165. doi:10.1016/j.survophthal.2013.09.004.

Komarova EY, Afanasyeva EA, Bulatova MM, Cheetham ME, Margulis BA, Guzhova IV. Downstream caspases are novel targets for the antiapoptotic activity of the molecular chaperone hsp70. Cell Stress Chaperones. 2004;9(3):265-275.

Komatsu M, Kurokawa H, Waguri S, Taguchi K, Kobayashi A, Ichimura Y, et al. The selective autophagy substrate p62 activates the stress responsive transcription factor Nrf2 through inactivation of Keap1. *Nat Cell Biol.* 2010;12(3):213-223.

Kozak I, Luttrull JK. Modern retinal laser therapy. *Saudi J Ophthalmol.* 2015;29(2):137-146. doi:10.1016/j.sjopt.2014.09.001.

Kregel K. Invited review: heat shock proteins: modifying factors in physiological stress responses and acquired thermotolerance. *J Appl Physiol.* 2002;92(5):2177-2186. doi:10.1152/japplphysiol.01267.2001.

L'Esperance FA Jr. Clinical comparison of xenon-arc and laser photocoagulation of retinal lesions. *Arch Ophthalmol.* 1966;75(1):61-67. doi:10.1001/archopht.1966.00970050063012.

L'Esperance FA Jr. Diabetic retinopathy. *Med Clin North Am.* 1978;62(4):767-785. doi:10.1016/S0025-7125(16)31772-2.

Lahav K, Levkovitch-Verbin H, Belkin M, Glovinsky Y, Polat U. Reduced mesopic and photopic foveal contrast sensitivity in glaucoma. *Arch Ophthalmol.* 2011;129(1):16-22. doi:10.1001/archophthalmol.2010.332.

Lai K, Zhao H, Zhou L, et al. Subthreshold Pan-Retinal Photocoagulation Using Endpoint Management Algorithm for Severe Nonproliferative Diabetic Retinopathy: A Paired Controlled Pilot Prospective Study. *Ophthalmic Res.* 2021;64(4):648-655. doi:10.1159/000512296

Lai TT, Ho TC, Yang CM. Spontaneous resolution of foveal detachment in traction maculopathy in high myopia unrelated to posterior vitreous detachment. *BMC Ophthalmol.* 2016;16:18. Published 2016 Feb 11. doi:10.1186/s12886-016-0195-3

Lains I, Punklik SJ, Ye AN, et al. Baseline predictors associated with 3-year changes in dark adaptation in age-related macular degeneration. *Retina.* 2021;41(10):2098-2105. doi:10.1097/IAE.0000000000003152.

Lancaster GI, Febbraio MA. Exosome-dependent trafficking of HSP70: a novel secretory pathway for cellular stress proteins. *J Biol Chem.* 2005;280(24):23349-23355.

Landa G. Micropulse laser for persistent subretinal fluid in a patient previously treated for rhegmatogenous retinal detachment. *Med Hypothesis Discov Innov Ophthalmol.* 2018;7(4):190-194.

Lanzetta P, Dorin G, Pirracchio A, Bandello F. Theoretical bases of non-ophthalmoscopically visible endpoint photocoagulation. *Semin Ophthalmol.* 2001;16(1):8-11. doi:10.1076/soph.16.1.8.4216

Lanzetta P, Furlan F, Morgante L, Veritti D, Bandello F. Nonvisible subthreshold micropulse diode laser (810 nm) treatment of central serous chorioretinopathy. A pilot study. *Eur J Ophthalmol*. 2008;18:934-940. doi:10.1177/112067210801800613.

Laursen ML, Moeller F, Sander B, Sjoelie AK. Subthreshold diode micropulse laser treatment in diabetic macular edema. *Br J Ophthalmol*. 2004;88:1173-1179. doi:10.1136/bjo.2003.040949.

Lavinsky D, Cardillo JA, Melo LA Jr, Dare AR, Farah ME, Belfort R. Randomized clinical trial evaluating mETDRS versus normal or high-density micropulse photocoagulation for diabetic macular edema. *Invest Ophthalmol Vis Sci*. 2011;52:4314-4323. doi:10.1167/iovs.10-6828.

Lavinsky D, Wang J, Huie P, et al. Nondamaging retinal laser therapy: rationale and applications to the macula. *Invest Ophthalmol Vis Sci*. 2016;57(6):2488-2500. doi:10.1167/iovs.15-18981.

L'Esperance FA Jr. The treatment of ophthalmic vascular disease by argon laser photocoagulation. *Trans Am Acad Ophthalmol Otolaryngol*. 1969;73(6):1077-1096.

Levin LA, Crowe ME, Quigley HA; Lasker/IRRF initiative on astrocytes and glaucomatous neurodegeneration participants. Neuroprotection for glaucoma: requirements for clinical translation. *Exp Eye Res*. 2017;157:34-37. doi:10.1016/j.exer.2016.12.005.

Levine S, Malone E, Lekiachvili A, Briss P. Health care industry insights: why the use of preventive services is still low. *Prev Chronic Dis*. 2019;16:180625. doi:10.5888/pcd16.180625.

Li W, Li Y, Guan S, Fan J, Cheng CF, Bright AM, et al. Extracellular heat shock protein-90alpha: linking hypoxia to skin cell motility and wound healing. *Embo J*. 2007;26(5):1221-1233.

Lin A, Giuliano CJ, Palladino A, et al. Off-target toxicity is a common mechanism of cancer drugs undergoing clinical trials. *Sci Transl Med*. 2019:11(509):eaaw8412. doi:10.1126/scitranslmed.aaw8412.

Lu RC, Tan MS, Wang H, Xie AM, Yu JT, Tan L. Heat shock protein 70 in Alzheimer' disease. *Biomed Res Int*. 2014;2014:435203. doi:10.1155/2014/435203.

Lukacs, E. "A Characterization of the Normal Distribution". *Ann Math Stat*. 1942: 13(1): 91–93. doi:10.1214/AOMS/1177731647. ISSN 0003-4851.

Lundh A, Lexchin J, Mintzes B, Schroll JB, Bero L. Industry sponsorship and research outcome. *Cochrane Database Syst Rev*. 2017;2(2):MR000033. doi:10.1002/14651858.MR000033.pub3.

Luttrull JK, Tzekov R, Bhavan SV. Positive trends in retinal nerve fiber layer and ganglion cell complex thickness in open angle glaucoma Bhavan SV. Positive trends in retinal nerve fiber layer and ganglion cell complex thickness in open angle glaucoma and age-related macular degeneration following SDM laser vision protection therapy for neuroprotection. *Evidence of Neuroregeneration*. 2023.

Luttrull JK, Chang DB, Margolis BWL, Dorin G, Luttrull DK. Laser re-sensitization of medically unresponsive neovascular age-related macular degeneration: efficacy and implications. *Retina*. 2015;35(6):1184-1194. doi:10.1097/IAE.0000000000000458.

Luttrull JK, Dorin G. Subthreshold diode micropulse photocoagulation as invisible retinal phototherapy for diabetic macular edema. A review. *Curr Diabetes Rev*. 2012;8:274-284. doi:10.2174/157339912800840523.

Luttrull JK, Gray G. Real world data comparison of standard care vs SDM laser vision protection therapy for prevention of neovascular AMD. *Clin Ophthalmol*. 2022;16:1555-1568. doi:10.2147/OPTH.S366150.

Luttrull JK, Kent D. Laser therapy to prevent choroidal neovascularization. In: Chhablanni J, ed. *Choroidal Neovascularization*. Springer Verlag; 2020:401–423. doi:10.1007/978-981-15-2213-0_30.

Luttrull JK, Kent D. Modern retinal laser for neuroprotection in open-angle glaucoma. In: Samples JR, Ahmed IIK, eds. *New Concepts in Glaucoma Surgery*, Vol. 1. Kugler Publications; September 2019:255-274.

Luttrull JK, Margolis BWL. Functionally guided retinal protective therapy as prophylaxis for age-related and inherited retinal degenerations. A pilot study. *Invest Ophthalmol Vis Sci*. 2016;57(1):265-275. doi:10.1167/iovs.15-18163.

Luttrull JK, Musch D, Spink CJ. Subthreshold diode micropulse photocoagulation for proliferative diabetic retinopathy. *Letter (Reply) Eye*. Advance online publication Jan 2009; doi:10.1038/eye.2008.418.

Luttrull JK, Musch MC, Mainster MA. Subthreshold diode micropulse photocoagulation for the treatment of clinically significant diabetic macular edema. *Br J Ophthalmol*. 2005;89(1):74-80. doi:10.1136/bjo.2004.051540.

Luttrull JK, Samples JR, Kent D, Lum BJ. Panmacular subthreshold diode micropulse laser (SDM) as neuroprotective therapy in primary open-angle glaucoma. In: Samples JR, Knepper PA, eds. *Glaucoma Research 2018-2020*. Kugler Publications; 2018:281-294.

Luttrull JK, Sinclair SD. Safety of transfoveal subthreshold diode micropulse laser for intra-foveal diabetic macular edema in eyes with good visual acuity. *Retina*. 2014;34(10):2010-2020. doi:10.1097/IAE.0000000000000177.

Luttrull JK, Sinclair SH, Elmann S, Chang DB, Kent D. Slowed progression of age-related geographic atrophy following subthreshold laser. *Clin Ophthalmol*. 2020;14:2983-2993. doi:10.2147/OPTH.S268322.

Luttrull JK, Sinclair SH, Elmann S, Glaser BM. Low incidence of choroidal neovascularization following subthreshold diode micropulse laser (SDM) for high-risk AMD. *PLoS ONE*. 2018;13(8):e0202097. doi:journal.pone.0202097.

Luttrull JK, Spink CJ, Musch DA. Subthreshold diode micropulse panretinal photocoagulation for proliferative diabetic retinopathy. *Eye*. 2008;22(5):607-612. doi:10.1038/sj.eye.6702725.

Luttrull JK, Spink CJ. Prolonged choroidal hypofluorescence following verteporfin photodynamic therapy combined with intravitreal triamcinolone acetonide injection. *Retina*. 2007; 27(6):688-692. doi:10.1097/IAE.0b013e318030e999.

Luttrull JK, Spink CJ. Serial optical coherence tomography of subthreshold diode laser micropulse photocoagulation for diabetic macular edema. Ophthalmic Surg Lasers Imaging. 2006;37:370-377. doi:10.3928/15428877-20060901-03.

Luttrull JK, Sramek C, Palanker D, Spink CJ, Musch DC. Long-term safety, high-resolution imaging, and tissue temperature modeling of subvisible diode micropulse photocoagulation for retinovascular macular edema. *Retina*. 2012;32(2):375-386. doi:10.1097/IAE.0b013e3182206f6c.

Luttrull JK. Comment on: van Rijssen TJ, van Dijk EHC, Scholz P, et al. PLACE trial report no. 3 (Letter). *Am J Ophthalmol*. 2020;212:186-187.

Luttrull JK. Epiretinal membrane and traction retinal detachment complicating laser-induced chorioretinal venous anastomosis. *Am J Ophthalmol*. 1997;123:698-699. doi:10.1016/S0002-9394(14)71088-8.

Luttrull JK. Improved retinal and visual function following subthreshold diode micropulse laser (SDM) for retinitis pigmentosa. *Eye (London)*. 2018;32(6):1099-1110. doi:10.1038/s41433-018-0017-3.

Luttrull JK. Laser is the first-choice treatment for diabetic retinopathy. Amsterdam Retina Debate. Annual meeting of the European Society of Retina Specialists (Euretina); September 8, 2017, Barcelona, Spain.

Luttrull JK. Low-intensity / high-density subthreshold diode micropulse laser (SDM) for central serous chorioretinopathy. *Retina*. 2016;36(9):1658-1663. doi:10.1097/IAE.0000000000001005.

Luttrull JK. Subthreshold diode micropulse laser (SDM) for persistent macular thickening and limited visual acuity after epiretinal membrane peeling. *Clin Ophthalmol*. 2020:14;1177-1188. doi:10.2147/OPTH.S251429.

Lynn SA, Keeling E, Munday R, Gabha G, Griffiths H, Lotery AJ, et al. The complexities underlying age-related macular degeneration: could amyloid beta play an important role? *Neural Regener Res*. 2017;12(4):538-548.

Mainster MA. Decreasing retinal photocoagulation damage: principles and techniques. *Semin Ophthalmol*. 1999;14:200-209. doi:10.3109/08820539909069538.

Majeski AE, Dice JF. Mechanisms of chaperone-mediated autophagy. *Int J Biochem Cell Biol*. 2004;36(12):2435-2444. doi:10.1016/j.biocel.2004.02.013

Malik KJ, Sampat KM, Mansouri A, Mansouri A, Steiner JN, Glaser BM. Low-intensity/high density subthreshold micropulse diode laser for chronic central serous chorioretinopathy. *Retina*. 2015;35:532-536. doi:10.1097/IAE.0000000000000285.

Mambula SS, Calderwood SK. Heat shock protein 70 is secreted from tumor cells by a nonclassical pathway involving lysosomal endosomes. *J Immunol*. 2006;177(11):7849-7857.

Mansouri A, Sampat KM, Malik KJ, Steiner JN, Gaser BM. Efficacy of subthreshold micropulse laser in the treatment of diabetic macular edema is influenced by pre-treatment central foveal thickness. *Eye (Lond)*. 2014;28(12):1418-1424. doi:10.1038/eye.2014.264.

Marmor MF. Structure and function of the retinal pigment epithelium. *Int Ophthalmol Clin*. 1975;15(1):115-130. doi:10.1097/00004397-197501510-00010

Martin NA, Tepper JE, Giri VN, et al. Adopting consensus terms for testing in precision medicine. *JCO Precis Oncol*. 2021;5:PO.21.00027. doi:10.1200/PO.21.00027.

Martine P, Chevriaux A, Derangere V, Apetoh L, Garrido C, Ghiringhelli F, et al. HSP70 is a negative regulator of NLRP3 inflammasome activation. *Cell Death & Disease*. 2019;10(4):256.

Maturi RK, Glassman AR, Josic K, et al; DRCR Retina Network. Effect of intravitreous anti-vascular endothelial growth factor vs sham treatment for prevention of vision-threatening complications of diabetic retinopathy: the protocol W randomized clinical trial. *JAMA Ophthalmol*. 2021;139(7):701-712. doi:10.1001/jamaophthalmol.2021.0606.

Mazzoni F, Müller C, DeAssis J, Lew D, Leevy WM, Finnemann SC. Non-invasive *in vivo* fluorescence imaging of apoptotic retinal photoreceptors. *Sci Rep*. 2019;9:1590. doi:10.1038/s41598-018-38363-z.

Medzhitov R. Origin and physiological roles of inflammation. *Nature*. 2008;454(7203):428-35. doi:10.1038/nature07201.

Mehrtash M, Bakker JP, Ayas N. Predictors of continuous positive airway pressure adherence in patients with obstructive sleep apnea. *Lung*. 2019;197(2):115-121. doi:10.1007/s00408-018-00193-1.

Melo EP, Konno T, Farace I, et al. Stress-induced protein disaggregation in the endoplasmic reticulum catalysed by BiP. *Nat Commun*. 2022;13(1):2501. doi:10.1038/s41467-022-30238-2.

Mendell JR, Al-Zaidy SA, Rodino-Klapac LR, et al. Current clinical applications of in vivo gene therapy with AAVs. *Mol Ther*. 2021;29(2):464-488. doi:10.1016/j.ymthe.2020.12.007.

Meusser B, Hirsch C, Jarosch E, Sommer T. ERAD: the long road to destruction. *Nat Cell Biol*. 2005;7(8):766-772. doi:10.1038/ncb0805-766.

Midena E, Bini S, Martini F, et al. Changes of aqueous humor Muller cells' biomarkers in human patients affected by diabetic macular edema after subthreshold micropulse laser treatment. *Retina*. 2020;40(1):126-134. doi:10.1097/IAE.0000000000002356.

Midena E, Micera A, Frizziero L, Pilotto E, Esposito G, Bini S. Sub-threshold micropulse laser treatment reduces inflammatory biomarkers in aqueous humour of diabetic patients with macular edema. *Sci Rep.* 2019;9(1):10034. doi:10.1038/s41598-019-46515-y.

Miki A, Medeiros FA, Weinreb RN, et al. Rates of retinal nerve fiber layer thinning in glaucoma suspect eyes. *Ophthalmology.* 2014;121(7):1350-1358. doi:10.1016/j.ophtha.2014.01.017.

Minowa Y, Ohkoshi K, Ozawa Y. Subthreshold Laser Treatment for Serous Retinal Detachment Associated with Tilted Disc Syndrome. *Case Rep Ophthalmol.* 2021;12(3):978-986. Published 2021 Dec 28. doi:10.1159/000520570

Mohammadzadeh V, Su E, Rabiolo A, et al. Ganglion cell complex: the optimal measure for detection of structural progression in the macula. *Am J Ophthalmol.* 2022;237:71-82. doi:10.1016/j.ajo.2021.12.009.

Moisseiev E, Smit-McBride Z, Oltjen S, et al. Intravitreal administration of human bone marrow CD34+ stem cells in a murine model of retinal degeneration. *Invest Ophthalmol Vis Sci.* 2016;57(10):4125-4135. doi:10.1167/iovs.16-19252.

Moore SM, Chao DL. Application of subthreshold laser therapy in retinal diseases: a review. *Expert Rev Ophthalmol.* 2018;13:311-320.

Moorman CM, Hamilton AM. Clinical applications of the micropulse diode laser. *Eye (Lond).* 1999;13(Pt 2):145-150. doi:10.1038/eye.1999.41.

Mordant DJ, Al-Abboud I, Muyo G, et al. Spectral imaging of the retina. *Eye (Lond).* 2011;25(3):309-320. doi:10.1038/eye.2010.222.

Morgan CM, Schatz H. Atrophic creep of the retinal pigment epithelium after focal macular photocoagulation. *Ophthalmology.* 1989;96:96-103. doi:10.1016/S0161-6420(89)32924-1.

Mori K. Tripartite management of unfolded proteins in the endoplasmic reticulum. *Cell.* 2000;101(5):451-454.

Morimoto RI. Cell-nonautonomous regulation of proteostasis in aging and disease. *Cold Spring Harb Perspect Biol.* 2020;12(4):a034074. doi:10.1101/cshperspect.a034074.

Morris ZS, Wooding S, Grant J. The answer is 17 years, what is the question: understanding time lags in translational research. *J R Soc Med.* 2011;104(12):510-520. doi:10.1258/jrsm.2011.110180.

Moynihan R. Key opinion leaders: independent experts or drug representatives in disguise? BMJ. 2008 Jun 21;336(7658):1402-1403. doi:10.1136/bmj.39575.675787.651. PMID: 18566074; PMCID: PMC2432185.

Munk MR, Fernandes J, Mets M, Patel JD, Johnson ML, Jampol LM. Reversible nyctalopia and retinopathy in a patient with metastatic cancer treated with anti-heat-shock protein 90 therapy. *JAMA Ophthalmol.* 2014;132(7):899-901. doi:10.1001/jamaophthalmol.2014.409.

Murshid A, Theriault J, Gong J, Calderwood SK. Investigating receptors for extracellular heat shock proteins. *Methods in Molecular Biology.* Clifton, NJ. 2011;787:289-302.

Nape I, Singh K, Klug A, et al. Revealing the invariance of vectorial structured light in complex media. Nat Photon. 2022;16(7):538-546. doi:10.1038/s41566-022-01023-w.

Neely KA, Quillen DA, Schachat AP, Gardner TW, Blankenship GW. Diabetic retinopathy. *Med Clin North Am.* 1998;82(4):847-876. doi:10.1016/s0025-7125(05)70027-4.

Nguyen QD, Brown DM, Marcus DM, et al; RISE and RIDE Research Group. Ranibizumab for diabetic macular edema: results from 2 phase III randomized trials: RISE and RIDE. *Ophthalmology.* 2012;119(4):789-801. doi:10.1016/j.ophtha.2011.12.039.

Nordgaard CL, Berg KM, Kapphahn RJ, et al. Proteomics of the retinal pigment epithelium reveals altered protein expression at progressive stages of age-related macular degeneration. *Invest Ophthalmol Vis Sci.* 2006;47(3):815-822. doi:10.1167/iovs.05-0976.

Ohno-Matsui K, Ikuno Y, Lai TYY, Gemmy Cheung CM. Diagnosis and treatment guideline for myopic choroidal neovascularization due to pathologic myopia. *Prog Retin Eye Res.* 2018;63:92-106. doi:10.1016/j.preteyeres.2017.10.005.

Okeagu CU, Agrón E, Vitale S, Domalpally A, Chew EY, Keenan TDL; Age-Related Eye Disease Study 2 Research Group. Principal cause of poor visual acuity after neovascular age-related macular degeneration: age-related eye disease study 2 report number 23. *Ophthalmol Retina.* 2021;5(1):23-31. doi:10.1016/j.oret.2020.09.025.

O'Koren EG, Yu C, Klingeborn M, Wong AYW, Prigge CL, Mathew R, et al. Microglial Function Is Distinct in Different Anatomical Locations during Retinal Homeostasis and Degeneration. *Immunity.* 2019;50(3):723-37.e7.

Otani A, Dorrell MI, Kinder K, et al. Rescue of retinal degeneration by intravitreally injected adult bone marrow-derived lineage-negative hematopoietic stem cells. *J Clin Invest.* 2004;114:765-774. doi:10.1172/JCI200421686.

Othman IS, Eissa SA, Kotb MS, Sadek SH. Subthreshold diode-laser micropulse photocoagulation as a primary and secondary line of treatment in management of diabetic macular edema. *Clin Ophthalmol.* 2014;8:653-659. Published 2014 Mar 31. doi:10.2147/OPTH.S59669

Oxford English Dictionary, 2nd ed. Clarendon Press; March 30, 1989.

Pandey P, Saleh A, Nakazawa A, Kumar S, Srinivasula SM, Kumar V, et al. Negative regulation of cytochrome c-mediated oligomerization of Apaf-1 and activation of procaspase-9 by heat shock protein 90. *Embo J.* 2000;19(16):4310-4322.

Pandey SK, Milverton EJ, Maloof AJ. A tribute to Charles David Kelman, MD: ophthalmologist, inventor and pioneer of phacoemulsification. *Clin Exp Ophthalmol.* 2004;32(5):529-533. doi:10.1111/j.1442-9071.2004.00887.x.

Park HS, Cho SG, Kim CK, Hwang HS, Noh KT, Kim MS, et al. Heat shock protein hsp72 is a negative regulator of apoptosis signal-regulating kinase 1. *Mol Cell Biol.* 2002;22(22):7721-7730.

Park SS, Moisseiev E, Bauer G, et al. Advances in bone marrow stem cell therapy for retinal dysfunction. *Prog Retin Eye Res.* 2017;56:148-165. doi:10.1016/j.preteyeres.2016.10.002..

Parodi MB, Iacono P, Ravalico G. Intravitreal triamcinolone acetonide combined with subthreshold grid laser treatment for macular oedema in branch retinal vein occlusion: a pilot study. *Br J Ophthalmol.* 2008;92:1046-1050. doi:10.1136/bjo.2007.128025.

Parodi MB, Spasse S, Iacono P, Di Stephano G, Canziani T, Ravalico G. Subthreshold grid laser treatment of macular edema secondary to branch retinal vein occlusion with micropulse infrared (810 nano meter) diode laser. *Ophthalmology.* 2006;113(12):2237-2242. doi:10.1016/j.ophtha.2006.05.056.

Patz A, Maumenee AE, Ryan SJ. Argon laser photocoagulation. Advantages and limitations. *Trans Am Acad Ophthalmol Otolaryngol.* 1971;75(3):569-579.

Piippo N, Korhonen E, Hytti M, Skottman H, Kinnunen K, Josifovska N, et al. Hsp90 inhibition as a means to inhibit activation of the NLRP3 inflammasome. *Sci Rep.* 2018;8(1):6720.

Pillar S, Moisseiev E, Sokolovska J., Grzybowski A. Recent developments in diabetic retinal neurodegeneration: a literature review. *J Diabetes Res.* 2020;2020:5728674. doi:10.1155/2020/5728674.

Plafker SM. Oxidative stress and the ubiquitin proteolytic system in age-related macular degeneration. *Adv Exp Med Biol.* 2010;664: 447-456.

Polyzos SA, Mantzoros CS. Diabetes mellitus: 100 years since the discovery of insulin. *Metabolism.* 2021 May;118:154737. doi:10.1016/j.metabol.2021.154737. Epub 2021 Feb 18. PMID: 33610498.

Prestera T, Talalay P, Alam J, Ahn YI, Lee PJ, Choi AM. Parallel induction of heme oxygenase-1 and chemoprotective phase 2 enzymes by electrophiles and antioxidants: regulation by upstream antioxidant-responsive elements (ARE). *Mol Med.* 1995; 1(7):827-837.

Puell MC, Barrio AR, Palomo-Alvarez C, Gómez-Sanz FJ, Clement-Corral A, Pérez-Carrasco MJ. Impaired mesopic visual acuity in eyes with early age-related macular degeneration. *Invest Ophthalmol Vis Sci.* 2012;53(11):7310-7314. doi:10.1167/iovs.11-8649.

Quin Y, Huttlin EL, Winsnes CF, et al. A multi-scale map of cell structure fusing protein images and interactions. 2021;600(7889):536-542. doi:10.1038/s41586-021-04115-9.

Ramaiah MJ, Tangutur AD, Manyam RR. Epigenetic modulation and understanding of HDAC inhibitors in cancer therapy. *Life Sci.* 2021;277:119504. doi:10.1016/j.lfs.2021.119504

Ravin JG. Gullstrand, Einstein, and the Nobel Prize. *Arch Ophthalmol.* 1999;117(5):670-672. doi:10.1001/archopht.117.5.670.

Reza FM. An Introduction to Information Theory. Dover Publications, Inc.; 1994 [1961].

Richter K, Haslbeck M, Buchner J. The heat shock response: life on the verge of death. *Mol Cell.* 2010;40(2):253-266. doi:10.1016/j.molcel.2010.10.006.

Riggs LA. Electroretinography. *Vision Res.* 1986;26:1443-1459. doi:10.1016/0042-6989(86)90167-7.

Roh JS, Sohn DH. Damage-associated molecular patterns in inflammatory diseases. *Immune Netw.* 2018;18(4):e27. doi:10.4110/in.2018.18.e27.

Roider J, Brinkmann R, Wirbelauer C, Laqua H, Birngruber R. Subthreshold (retinal pigment epithelium) photocoagulation in macular diseases: a pilot study. *Br J Ophthalmol.* 2000;84:40-47. doi:10.1136/bjo.84.1.40.

Roider J, Liew SH, Klatt C, et al. Selective retina therapy (SRT) for clinically significant diabetic macular edema. *Graefes Arch Clin Exp Ophthalmol.* 2010;248(9):1263-1272. doi:10.1007/s00417-010-1356-3

Roisman L, Magalhães FP, Lavinsky D, et al. Micropulse diode laser treatment for chronic central serous chorioretinopathy: a randomized pilot trial. *Ophthalmic Surg Lasers Imaging Retina.* 2013;44:465-470. doi:10.3928/23258160-20130909-08.

Romero-Aroca P, Baget-Bernaldiz M, Pareja-Rios A, Lopez-Galvez M, Navarro-Gil R, Verges R. Diabetic Macular Edema Pathophysiology: Vasogenic versus Inflammatory. *J Diabetes Res.* 2016;2016:2156273. doi:10.1155/2016/2156273

Rosenbaum PR, Rubin DB. The central role of the propensity score in observational studies for causal effects. *Biometrika.* 1983;70(1):41-55. doi:10.1093/biomet/70.1.41.

Rosenfeld PJ, Feuer WJ. Warning: do not treat intermediate AMD with laser therapy. *Ophthalmology.* 2019;126(6):834-840. doi:10.1016/j.ophtha.2018.12.016.

Rybinski M, Szymanska Z, Lasota S, Gambin A. Modeling the efficacy of hyperthermia treatment. *J R Soc Interface.* 2013;10:20130527. doi:10.1098/rsif.2013.0527.

Sachdeva MM, Cano M, Handa JT. Nrf2 signaling is impaired in the aging RPE given an oxidative insult. *Exp Eye Res.* 2014;119:111-114.

Saleh A, Srinivasula SM, Balkir L, Robbins PD, Alnemri ES. Negative regulation of the Apaf-1 apoptosome by Hsp70. *Nat Cell Biol.* 2000;2(8):476-483.

Salimi L, Rahbarghazi R, Jafarian V, et al. Heat shock protein 70 modulates neural progenitor cells dynamics in human neuroblastoma SH-SY5Y cells exposed to high glucose content. *J Cell Biochem.* 2018;119(8):6482-6491. doi:10.1002/jcb.26679

San Gil R, Ooi L, Yerbury JJ, Ecroyd H. The heat shock response in neurons and astroglia and its role in neurodegenerative diseases.

Mol Neurodegener. 2017;12(1):65. doi:10.1186/s13024-017-0208-6.

Schatz H, Madeira D, McDonald HR, Johnson RN. Progressive enlargement of laser scars following grid laser photocoagulation for diffuse diabetic macular edema. *Arch Ophthalmol*. 1991;109(11):1549-1551. doi:10.1001/archopht.1991.01080110085041.

Scholz P, Altay L, Fauser S. A review of subthreshold micropulse laser for treatment of macular disorders. *Adv Ther*. 2017;34(7):1528-1555. doi:10.1007/s12325-017-0559-y.

Schott G, Pachi H, Limbach U, Gundert-Remy U, Lieb K, Ludwig W. The financing of drug trials by pharmaceutical companies and its consequences. *Dtsch Arztebl Int*. 2010;107(17):295-301. Published online. 2010;107(17):295-301. doi:10.3238/arztebl.2010.0295.

Schröder M, Kaufman RJ. The mammalian unfolded protein response. *Annu Rev Biochem*. 2005;74:739-789. doi:10.1146/annurev.biochem.73.011303.074134.

Schwartz M, Shechter R. Systemic inflammatory cells fight off neurodegenerative disease. *Nat Rev Neurol*. 2010;6(7):405-410.

Selvarani R, Mohammed S, Richardson A. Effect of rapamycin on aging and age-related diseases-past and future. *Geroscience*. 2021;43(3):1135-1158. doi:10.1007/s11357-020-00274-1

Shah J, Nguyen V, Hunt A, et al. Characterization of poor visual outcomes of diabetic macular edema: the fight retinal blindness! Project. *Ophthalmol Retina*. 2022;6(7):540-547. doi:10.1016/j.oret.2022.03.007.

Shen L, Liu F, Grossetta Nardini H, Del Priore LV. Natural History of Geographic Atrophy in Untreated Eyes with Nonexudative Age-Related Macular Degeneration: A Systematic Review and Meta-analysis. *Ophthalmol Retina*. 2018;2(9):914-921. doi:10.1016/j.oret.2018.01.019

Shimura M, Yasuda K, Nakazawa T, Tamai M. Visual dysfunction after panretinal photocoagulation in patients with severe diabetic retinopathy and good vision. *Am J Ophthalmol*. 2005;140(1):8-15. doi:10.1016/j.ajo.2005.02.029

Shpilka T, Haynes CM. The mitochondrial UPR: mechanisms, physiological functions and implications in ageing. *Nat Rev Mol Cell Biol*. 2018;19(2):109-120. doi:10.1038/nrm.2017.110.

Sinclair SH, Luttrull JK. Diabetes Mellitus Associated Progressive Neurovascular Retinal Injury: Recommendations for Imaging and Functional Testing and Potential Role for Early Intervention with Modern Retinal Laser Therapy. *J Ophth Rev Rep*. July 2022; 3(3):1-17.

Sinclair SH, Schwartz SS. Diabetic retinopathy-an underdiagnosed and undertreated inflammatory, neuro-vascular complication of diabetes. *Front Endocrinol (Lausanne)*. 2019;10:843. doi:10.3389/fendo.2019.00843.

Singer AJ, Clark RA. Cutaneous wound healing. *N Engl J Med*. 1999;341(10):738-746. doi:10.1056/NEJM199909023411006.

Sivaprasad S, Dorin G. Subthreshold diode laser micropulse photocoagulation for the treatment of diabetic macular edema. *Expert Rev Med Devices*. 2012;9(2):189-197. doi:10.1586/erd.12.1.

Sivaprasad S, Sandhu R, Tandon A, Sayed-Ahmed K, McHugh DA. Subthreshold micropulse diode laser photocoagulation for clinically significant diabetic macular oedema: a a three-year follow up. *Clin Exp Ophthalmol*. 2007;35:640-644. doi:10.1111/j.1442-9071.2007.01566.x.

Smith HL, Mallucci GR. The unfolded protein response: mechanisms and therapy of neurodegeneration. *Brain*. 2016;139(Pt 8):2113-2121. doi:10.1093/brain/aww101

Snodderly DM, Sandstrom MM, Leung IYF, Neuringer M. Retinal pigment epithelial distribution in central retina of rhesus monkeys. *Invest Ophthalmol Vis Sci*. 2002;43:2815-2818.

Solomon SD, Lindsley K, Vedula SS, Ksystolik MG, Hawkins BS. Anti-vascular endothelial growth factor for neovascular age-related macular degeneration. *Cochrane Database Syst Rev*. 2019;4(3):CD005139. doi:10.1002/14651858.CD005139.pub4.

Spaide RF, Gemmy Cheung CM, Matsumoto H, et al. Venous overload choroidopathy: a hypothetical framework for central serous chorioretinopathy and allied disorders. *Prog Retin Eye Res*. 2022;86:100973. doi:10.1016/j.preteyeres.2021.100973.

Sramek C, Mackanos M, Spitler R, et al. Non-damaging retinal phototherapy: dynamic range of heat shock protein expression. *Invest Ophthalmol Vis Sci*. 2011;52:1780-1787. doi:10.1167/iovs.10-5917.

Srivastava K, Narang R, Bhatia J, Saluga D. Expression of heat shock protein 70 gene and its correlation with essential hypertension. *PLoS One*. 2016;11(3):e0151060. doi:10.1371/journal.pone.0151060.

Stankiewicz AR, Lachapelle G, Foo CP, Radicioni SM, Mosser DD. Hsp70 inhibits heat-induced apoptosis upstream of mitochondria by preventing Bax translocation. *J Biol Chem*. 2005;280(46):38729-38739.

Stella SL Jr, Geathers JS, Weber SR., et al. Neurodegeneration, neuroprotection and regeneration in the zebrafish retina. *Cells*. 2021;10(3):633. doi:10.3390/cells10030633.

Stetler RA, Gan Y, Zhang W, et al. Heat shock proteins: cellular and molecular mechanisms in the central nervous system. *Prog Neurobiol*. 2010;92(2):184-211. doi:10.1016/j.pneurobio.2010.05.002.

Stringham JM, Garcia PV, Smith PA, et al. Macular pigment and visual performance in low-light conditions. *Invest Ophthalmol Vis Sci*. 2015;56(4):2459-2468. doi:10.1167/iovs.14-15716.

Strowig T, Henao-Mejia J, Elinav E, Flavell R. Inflammasomes in health and disease. Nature. 2012;481(7381):278-286.

Suzuki T, Motohashi H, Yamamoto M. Toward clinical application of the Keap1-Nrf2 pathway. *Trends Pharmacol Sci*. 2013;34(6):340-346.

Szymanska Z, Zylicz M. Mathematical modeling of heat shock protein synthesis in response to temperature change. *J Theo Bio*. 2009;259:562-569. doi:10.1016/j.jtbi.2009.03.021.

Taleb NN. Antifragile: Things That Gain from Disorder. Random House; 2012:430.

Tarallo V, Hirano Y, Gelfand BD, Dridi S, Kerur N, Kim Y, et al. DICER1 loss and Alu RNA induce age-related macular degeneration via the NLRP3 inflammasome and MyD88. Cell. 2012;149(4):847-859.

Tatsumi T, Takatsuna Y, Oshitari T, et al. Randomized clinical trial comparing intravitreal aflibercept combined with subthreshold laser to intravitreal aflibercept monotherapy for diabetic macular edema. *Sci Rep*. 2022;12(1):10672. doi:10.1038/s41598-022-14444-y.

Terashima H, Hasebe H, Okamoto F, Matsuoka N, Sato Y, Fukuchi T. Combination therapy of intravitreal ranibizumab and subthreshold micropulse photocoagulation for macular edema secondary to branch retinal vein occlusion: 6 month results. *Retina*. 2019;39(7):1377-1384. doi:10.1097/IAE.0000000000002165.

Terrab L, Wipf P. Hsp70 and the unfolded protein response as a challenging drug target and an inspiration for probe molecule development. *ACS Med Chem Lett*. 2020;11(3):232-236. doi:10.1021/acsmedchemlett.9b00583.

Toth CA, Tai V, Pistilli M, et al; Comparison of Age-related Macular Degeneration Treatments Trials Research Group. Distribution of OCT features within areas of macular atrophy or scar after 2 years of Anti-VEGF treatment for neovascular AMD in CATT. *Ophthalmol Retina*. 2019;3(4):316-325. doi:10.1016/j.oret.2018.11.011. Epub 2018 Dec 3.

Townsend C, Hamilton AM, Cheng H. Photocoagulation in diabetic retinopathy: III. Complications. *Int Ophthalmol Clin*. 1978 Winter;18(4):121-131. PMID: 721380.

Travers KJ, Patil CK, Wodicka L, Lockhart DJ, Weissman JS, Walter P. Functional and genomic analyses reveal an essential coordination between the unfolded protein response and ER-associated degradation. *Cell*. 2000;101(3):249-258. doi:10.1016/s0092-8674(00)80835-1

Tschopp J, Schroder K. NLRP3 inflammasome activation: the convergence of multiple signalling pathways on ROS production? *Nat Rev Immunol*. 2010;10(3):210-215. doi:10.1038/nri2725.

Tsen F, Bhatia A, O'Brien K, Cheng CF, Chen M, Hay N, et al. Extracellular heat shock protein 90 signals through subdomain II and the NPVY motif of LRP-1 receptor to Akt1 and Akt2: a circuit essential for promoting skin cell migration in vitro and wound healing in vivo. *Mol Cell Biol*. 2013;33(24):4947-4959.

Tseng WA, Thein T, Kinnunen K, Lashkari K, Gregory MS, D'Amore PA, et al. NLRP3 inflammasome activation in retinal pigment epithelial cells by lysosomal destabilization: implications for age-related macular degeneration. *Invest Ophthalmol Vis Sci*. 2013;54(1):110-120.

Uji A, Nittala MG, Hariri A, Velaga SB, Sadda SR. Directional kinetics analysis of the progression of geographic atrophy. *Graefes Arch Clin Exp Ophthalmol*. 2019;257(8):1679-1685. doi:10.1007/s00417-019-04368-1

Van Rijssen TJ, van Dijk EHC, Scholz P, et al. Focal and diffuse chronic central serous chorioretinopathy treated with half-dose photodynamic therapy or subthreshold micropulse laser: PLACE Trial Report No. 3. *Am J Ophthalmol*. 2019;205:1-10. doi:10.1016/j.ajo.2019.03.025.

Van Rijssen TJ, Van Dijk EHC, Scholz P, et al. Reply to: Comment on Place Trial No. 3. *Am J Ophthalmol*. 2020;212:187-188. doi:10.1016/j.ajo.2019.11.022.

Varkey B. Principles of clinical ethics and their application to practice. *Med Princ Pract* 2021;30:17-28. doi:10.1159/000509119.

Ventura LM, Feuer WJ, Porciatti V. Progressive loss of retinal ganglion cell function is hindered with IOP-lowering treatment in early glaucoma. *Invest Ophthalmol Vis Sci* 2012;53(2):659-663.

Ventura LM, Porciatti V. Pattern electroretinogram in glaucoma. *Curr Opin Ophthalmol*. 2006;17(2):196-202. doi:10.1097/01.icu.0000193082.44938.3c

Verdina T, Ferrari C, Valerio E, et al. Subthreshold micropulse yellow laser for the management of refractory cystoid macular edema consequent to complicated cataract surgery. *Eur J Ophthalmol*. 2021;31:NP93-NP98. doi:10.1177/1120672120928008.

Vitale M, Bakunts A, Orsi A, et al. Inadequate BiP availability defines endoplasmic reticulum stress. *eLife*. 2019;8:e41168. doi:10.7554/eLife.41168.

Von Clausewitz, C. Howard, Michael; Paret, Peter (eds.). *On War* [*Vom Krieg*] (Indexed ed.). New Jersey: Princeton University Press; 1984 (1832). p. 87. ISBN 978-0-691-01854-6.

Vujosevic S, Bottega E, Casciano M, Pilotto E, Convento E, Midena E. Microperimetry and fundus autofluorescence in diabetic macular edema: subthreshold micropulse diode laser versus modified early treatment diabetic retinopathy study laser photocoagulation. *Retina*. 2010;30(6):908-916. doi:10.1097/IAE.0b013e3181c96986.

Vujosevic S, Frizziero L, Martini F, et al. Single retinal layer changes after subthreshold micropulse yellow laser in diabetic macular edema. *Ophthalmic Surg Lasers Imaging Retina*. 2018;49(11):e218-e225. doi:10.3928/23258160-20181101-22.

Vujosevic S, Gatti V, Muraca A, et al. Optical coherence tomography angiography changes after subthreshold micropulse yellow laser in diabetic macular edema. *Retina*. 2020;40(2):312-321. doi:10.1097/IAE.0000000000002383.

Vujosevic S, Martini F, Convento E, et al. Subthreshold laser therapy for diabetic macular edema: metabolic and safety issues. *Curr Med Chem*. 2013;20:3267-3271. doi:10.2174/09298673113209990030.

Vujosevic S, Martini F, Longhin E, Convento E, Cavarzeran F, Midena E. Subthreshold micropulse yellow laser versus subthreshold micropulse infrared laser in center-involving diabetic macular edema: morphologic and functional safety. *Retina*. 2015;35:1594-1603. doi:10.1097/IAE.0000000000000521.

Vujosevic S, Toma C, Villani E, et al. Subthreshold micropulse laser in diabetic macular edema: 1-year improvement in OCT/OCT-angiography biomarkers. *Transl Vis Sci Technol*. 2020;9(10):31. doi:10.1167/tvst.9.10.31.

Wakabayashi Y, Usui Y, Okunuki Y, et al. Intraocular VEGF level as a risk factor for postoperative complications after vitrectomy for proliferative diabetic retinopathy. *Invest Ophthalmol Vis Sci*. 2012;53(10):6403-6410. Published 2012 Sep 21. doi:10.1167/iovs.12-10367

Walther DM, Kasturi P, Zheng M, et al. Widespread proteome remodeling and aggregation in aging C. elegans. *Cell*. 2015;161(4):919-932. doi:10.1016/j.cell.2015.03.032.

Wang F, Liu Y, Du C, Gao R. Current Strategies for Real-Time Enzyme Activation. *Biomolecules*. 2022;12(5):599. Published 2022 Apr 19. doi:10.3390/biom12050599

Wang L, Cano M, Handa JT. p62 provides dual cytoprotection against oxidative stress in the retinal pigment epithelium. *Biochimica et Biophysica Acta*. 2014;1843(7):1248-1258.

Wang-Michelitsch J, Michelitsch, T. Aging as a process of accumulation of misrepairs. 2015. arXiv:1503.07163.

Wei X, Cho KS, Thee EF, Jager MJ, Chen DF. Neuroinflammation and microglia in glaucoma: time for a paradigm shift. *J Neurosci Res*. 2019;97(1):70-76. doi:10.1002/jnr.24256.

Wen JC, Reina-Torres E, Sherwood JM, et al. Intravitreal anti-VEGF injections reduce aqueous outflow facility in patients with neovascular age-related macular degeneration. *Invest Ophthalmol Vis Sci*. 2017;58(3):1893-1898. doi:10.1167/iovs.16-20786.

Wood JP, Shibeeb O, Plunkett M, Casson RJ, Chidlow G. Retinal damage profiles and neuronal effects of laser treatment: comparison of a conventional photocoagulator and a novel 3-nanosecond pulse laser. *Invest Ophthalmol Vis Sci*. 2013;54(3):2305-2318. Published 2013 Mar 28. doi:10.1167/iovs.12-11203

Wu MY, Yiang GT, Lai TT, Li CJ. The oxidative stress and mitochondrial dysfunction during the pathogenesis of diabetic retinopathy. *Oxid Med Cell Longev*. 2018;2018:3420187. doi:10.1155/2018/3420187.

Xu H, Chen M, Forrester JV. Para-inflammation in the aging retina. *Prog Retin Eye Res*. 2009;28(5):348-368. doi:10.1016/j.preteyeres.2009.06.001.

Xu Q, Metzler B, Jahangiri M, Mandal K. Molecular chaperones and heat shock proteins in atherosclerosis. *Am J Physiol Heart Circ Physiol*. 2012;302(3):H506-H514. doi:10.1152/ajpheart.00646.2011.

Xu Z, Wei Y, Gong J, Cho H, Park JK, Sung ER, et al. NRF2 plays a protective role in diabetic retinopathy in mice. *Diabetologia*. 2014;57(1):204-213.

Yan LJ, Christians ES, Liu L, Xiao X, Sohal RS, Benjamin IJ. Mouse heat shock transcription factor 1 deficiency alters cardiac redox homeostasis and increases mitochondrial oxidative damage. *Embo J*. 2002;21(19):5164-5172.

Zhang L, Lu Q, Chang C. Epigenetics in Health and Disease. *Adv Exp Med Biol*. 2020;1253:3-55. doi:10.1007/978-981-15-3449-2_1

Zhou R, Yazdi AS, Menu P, Tschopp J. A role for mitochondria in NLRP3 inflammasome activation. *Nat.* 2011;469(7329):221-225.

Zweng HC, Little HL, Peabody RR. Argon laser photocoagulation of diabetic retinopathy. *Arch Ophthalmol*. 1971 Oct;86(4):395-400. doi:10.1001/archopht.1971.01000010397006. PMID: 5110132.